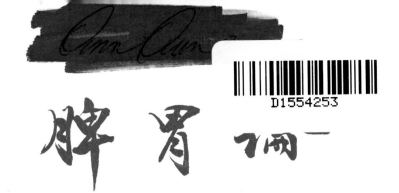

脾 胃 7兩一

LI DONG-YUAN'S
Treatise On The Spleen & Stomach

A TRANSLATION OF THE PI WEI LUN

NEW EDITION

Translated & Annotated
by Bob Flaws

BLUE POPPY PRESS

Published by:

BLUE POPPY PRESS
A Division of Blue Poppy Enterprises, Inc.
5441 Western Avenue #2
BOULDER, CO 80301

SECOND EDITION OCTOBER 2004

ISBN 0-936185-41-4
Library of Congress #92-75135

Printed at Johnson Printing, Boulder, Colorado

COMP Designation: Denotative translation

Printed on recycled paper products with soy-based ink.

10 9 8 7 6 5 4 3 2

Table of Contents

BOOK THREE

Translator's Preface

This book is a translation of and commentary on Li Gao's *Pi Wei Lun (Treatise on the Spleen & Stomach)*. Li Gao, a.k.a. Li Dong-yuan and Li Ming-zhi, was arguably the greatest of the four great masters of the Jin-Yuan dynasties (1115-1386 CE). The other three of these four great masters of this time were Liu He-jian, a.k.a., Liu Wan-su, Zhang Cong-zheng, a.k.a. Zhang Zi-he, and Zhu Zhen-heng, a.k.a. Zhu Dan-xi. Li Dong-yuan was the founder of the school of supplementing earth, and the *Pi Wei Lun* is regarded as Li's final book and greatest masterpiece.

The Jin-Yuan dynasties are considered the renaissance of Chinese medicine. Most of the seminal theories of Chinese medicine were set down in the Han dynasty (206 BCE-220 CE) in such classics as the *Nei Jing (Inner Classic), Nan Jing (Classic of Difficulties)*, and *Shang Han Lun/Jin Gui Yao Lue (Treatise on Damage [Due to] Cold/Essentials from the Golden Cabinet)*. For the next thousand years, there was little radical development in these theories. However, during the Song dynasty (960-1279 CE), the development of Neoconfucianism allowed Chinese thinkers the freedom to posit entirely new ideas, and the four great schools of the Jin-Yuan that followed grew directly out of this philosophical revolution. Although many Chinese medical histories present the four great schools of the Jin-Yuan as four separate theoretical approaches to the practice of Chinese medicine, in fact, three out of four were a clear progression or evolution from one to the next. In this case, Liu Wan-su's school of cool and cold (medicines) emphasized the role of heat evils in disease. Li Dong-yuan then further refined this observation with his development of the theory of yin fire which explains where these heat evils frequently come from when engendered internally. And finally, Zhu Dan-xi further refined Li's praxis by routinely adding moist, yin-enriching medicinals to Li's commonly sweet, acrid, and warm formulas. Therefore, we can now speak of Li-Zhu medicine, meaning the theories and practices of Li Dong-yuan and Zhu Dan-xi as a single school of or approach to the practice of Chinese medicine.

Recently, many Chinese doctors in Asia and abroad have realized that the theories and prescriptive methodology of Li-Zhu medicine are some of the most

effective and appropriate for treating the knotty, difficult-to-treat diseases which
have become the stock in trade of contemporary Chinese medicine. As I hope
to show in this book, the theories and treatments of Li Dong-yuan and Zhu Dan-
xi are especially appropriate for chronic diseases with multi-pattern presentations, such as allergies, endocrine disorders, chronic viral disorders, immune
deficiencies, autoimmune diseases, and cancers. However, till now, these theories have not been generally well known, and Blue Poppy Press's first translation
of this work appeared without commentary, making it difficult for most readers to extract the clinical gist of what Li was trying to say. Therefore, I have retrans-
lated this important Chinese medical text and added commentaries and case
histories in order to make its wisdom more accessible to modern readers. There
is no way I would have attempted this new edition of the *Pi Wei Lun* were it not
for the pioneering translation of Yang Shou-zhong and Li Jian-yong, Blue Poppy's
first translators of this important text. Thus I am grateful and indebted for their
ground-breaking work.

Li Gao (1180-1251 CE) was one of the most eminent Chinese medical scholars
of his time. He was born in Zhending (present day Baoding in Hebei province)
into a very wealthy family which owned thousands of acres of land and enjoyed
the company of the highest officials and most distinguished scholars of their day.
From his childhood, Li received an excellent education in the Confucian classics, and, rolling in wealth, he did not need to learn a profession to earn his living. At that time, the practice of medicine, though a respectable profession, was
inferior to official position in the Confucian bureaucracy, and most intellectu-
als preferred to spend their lives climbing the bureaucratic ladder. However, one
year while Li was still young, his mother fell ill. One after another doctor was
sent for, but none was able to even diagnose Li's mother let alone help her even
a little. When Li's mother eventually died, Li blamed himself for a lack of filial
piety. As his mother's son, he reproached himself that should have known enough
medicine to take care of her himself. Therefore, similar to Zhang Zhong-jing in
the Han dynasty, Li determined to learn medicine. Money being no object, Li
did not hesitate to pay a small fortune in silver in order to study directly under
Zhang Yuan-su, one of the greatest doctors and teachers of medicine of his time.

At the outbreak of war against the Mongols, Li moved to Henan where he lived
among a number of highranking officials. Being from a rich family, Li did not
practice medicine as a livelihood. Instead, Li practiced medicine as an expression of Confucian benevolence. Over the years, Li became a distinguished practitioner in nearly all the specialties of Chinese medicine, including internal
medicine, acupuncture, pathology, pharmacology, gynecology, and pediatrics.
In fact, Li so distinguished himself above and beyond simply being a disciple of

Zhang that Wang Hang-gu, also an outstanding student of Zhang's and a famous medical scholar in his own right, formally acknowledged Li as his master. Within Chinese culture, such an acknowledgment by a classmate who might otherwise claim equal status has profound implications. Wang said:

> I have been studying medicine for scores of years... but I am eager to have an excellent teacher for a guide... This desire has been occupying my mind day and night, but I have yet thought of no suitable candidate except for Elder-born Li.

According to one of Li's biographies, there was a famine in the area in which he was living from 1201-1208 CE and the people were also suffering from various epidemics. Other doctors in the area relied on either the sweating or precipitation (*i.e.*, purgation) methods for any and every patient, and, therefore, many of these died. Among the local doctors, it is said that only Li Dong-yuan traced the disease causes and mechanisms, reviewed the signs and symptoms, conducted physical examinations, and then prescribed appropriate medicinals.

In terms of the evolution of Chinese medicine, it was Li Dong-yuan who emphasized internal damage as opposed to external contraction as the main cause of chronic, enduring diseases and raised the spleen and stomach to pivotal and preeminent importance among the five viscera and six bowels. It was also Li Dong-yuan who developed the theory of yin fire and then designed a host of brilliant Chinese medicinal formulas to address so many of the clinical manifestations of this species of internally engendered heat. Li left behind a number of important works in the literature of Chinese medicine. These include the *Nei Wai Shang Bian Huo Lun (Treatise on Solving Confusion in Discriminating Internal & External Damages)*; the *Lan Shi Mi Cang (Secret Collection of the Orchid Chamber)*; the *Yi Xue Fa Ming (The Study of Medicine Made Clear)*; the *Yong Yao Fa Xiang (Methods & Approaches to Using Medicinals)*; and the *Pi Wei Lun*. Of these, the *Pi Wei Lun* is Li's undisputed masterpiece and was probably the last work he wrote before he died at 71 years of age.

This translation is based on three editions of the *Pi Wei Lun* currently available in the People's Republic of China. The *Gu Qin Yi Tong Zheng Mai Quan Shu (The Complete Book of All Collected Ancient & Modern Medicine & Orthodox Pulse [Lore])* is a photolithograph of a Ming dynasty book published by the People's Health & Hygiene Press in 1957 which includes several Jin-Yuan texts. In 1976, the People's Health & Hygiene Press published an annotated version of the *Pi Wei Lun* with commentaries developed by the Hunan Chinese Medical Research Institute. In 1995, another edition of the *Pi Wei Lun* was included in Ye Chuan and Jian Yi's *Jin Yuan Si Da Yi Xue Jia Ming Zhu Ji Cheng (A Compilation of Famous Texts from the Masters of the Four Great Schools of Medicine of the Jin-Yuan)* published by the Chinese National Chinese Medicine & Medicinals Publishing House in Beijing. This English version is a collation based on these three editions. Following ancient Chinese tradition, all commentaries and foot-notes added to the original text are printed in ink, while the original text is printed in black. Chapter numbers have been added for the sake of convenient reference. In addition, the table of contents reflects the title of the chapters as they appear in this English text, not as they appear in the source text. Materials within the text in parentheses were made by some previous editor(s). Materials in brackets have been inserted by the present translator to make the meaning more intelligible and readily understandable in English while yet preserving some of the flavor of the original for serious scholars.

The English language Chinese medical terminology used in this book is based on Nigel Wiseman and Feng Ye's *A Practical Chinese Medical Dictionary* published by Paradigm Publications (Brookline, MA, 1998). Divergences from this standard are footnoted the first time they appear. Formulas are identified by their Chinese names in Pinyin romanization followed by my own English language translation in parentheses. Similarly, ingredients in these formulas are identified first in Chinese in Pinyin romanization followed by Latinate pharmacological nomenclature in parentheses. The main sources for the identifications of these medicinals in preparing this work were Bensky and Gamble's *Chinese Herbal Medicine: Materia Medica* (Eastland Press, Seattle, 1993), Hong-yen Hsu's *Oriental Materia Medica: A Concise Guide* (Oriental Healing Arts Institute, Long Beach, CA, 1986), Stuart and Read's *Chinese Materia Medica* (Southern Materials Center, Inc., Taipei, 1979), and Jiangsu New Medical Academy's *Zhong Yao Da Ci Dian (Dictionary of Chinese Medicinals*, Shanghai Science & Technology Press, Shanghai, 1991). All Chinese medicinal identifications have been translated into their standard modern Chinese names. Thus *Shao Yao* has become *Bai Shao, Ju Pi* has become *Chen Pi, Suo Sha Ren* has simply become *Sha Ren*, etc. Acupuncture points are identified first in Chinese in Pinyin romanization followed by standard channel-numeric notation in parentheses. And finally, the 10 heavenly stems and 12 earthly branches are identified in Chinese in Pinyin romanization first followed by an alpha-numeric code in parentheses. Hence (S1) refers to the first heavenly stem, while (B12) refers to the 12th earthly branch. These changes have been made in an attempt to make the text as easily approachable to modern readers as possible.

Bob Flaws
Summer, 2004

脾胃論

Book One

1

Treatise on the Transmutation of Vacuity & Repletion of the Spleen & Stomach

This opening chapter sets the theoretical stage for Li's more clinically oriented chapters to follow. Those who are interested in the evolution of Chinese medical thought concerning the role of the spleen-stomach and internal engenderment (as opposed to external contraction) will find it interesting. However, for those interested only in clinical practice, it does not contain much of importance. All Li's relatively novel (at the time) insights and interpretations in this chapter have long since become a standard part of professional Chinese medicine.

The *Wu Zang Bie Lun (A Divergent Treatise on the Five Viscera)* states:

> The stomach, large intestine, small intestine, triple burner, and urinary bladder, these five are engendered by the qi of heaven and, their qi resembling heaven, they drain but do not store. Receiving the turbid qi from the five viscera, they are named bowels of conveyance and transformation. They do not keep [things] long but transport and drain.
>
> What are known as the five viscera store essence qi without draining it, and, therefore, they can be full but not replete. [While] the six bowels convey and transform substances rather than store, and, therefore, they can be replete but not full. The reason is that, when water and grains enter through the mouth, the stomach is full and the intestines are empty. As food goes down, the intestines become full and the stomach becomes empty. This is what is meant by [the six bowels being] replete but not full, whereas [the five viscera are] full but not replete.[1]

The *Yin Yang Ying Xiang Da Lun (Great Treatise on the Mutual Correspondence of Yin & Yang)* states:

> The valley qi flows to the spleen. Valley here refers to the interstices between the muscles. The six channels are rivers. The stomach and intestines are the sea, while the nine orifices are [the places where] water pours its qi.[2]

The nine orifices are governed by the five viscera, but the five viscera are free and uninhibited only when they are supplied with stomach qi. The *Tong Ping Xu Shi Lun (Comprehensive Treatise on the Investigation of Vacuity & Repletion)* states: "Headache, ringing in the ears, and inhibition of the nine orifices are generated by the spleen and stomach."[3] If stomach qi becomes vacuous, the ears, mouth, and nose may all contract disease.

The *Jing Mai Bie Lun (A Divergent Treatise on the Channels & Vessels)* states:

> Food qi, entering the stomach, spreads essence to the liver and diffuses qi into the sinews. Entering the stomach, food qi, the turbid of which gathers at the heart, diffuses essence into the vessels. With vessel qi flowing in the channels, channel qi gathers in the lungs which face the hundred of vessels and transport essence to the skin and hair. The minute vessels, having taken in essence, move the qi to the bowels. When bowel essence and spirit brightness are maintained in the four viscera, qi tends toward balance. To examine this balance, the qi mouth or opening [pulse] is the gauge which decides life and death.[4]

> Having entered the stomach, fluids float the essence qi and transport it up to the spleen. The spleen qi spreads the essence which comes up home to the lungs and frees the flow of the water passageways, transporting [water essence] down to the urinary bladder. Water essence spreads in the four directions and the five channels run side by side in agreement with the four seasons, the five viscera, and yin and yang measurements. Thus normalcy is kept.[5]

It is also stated that yin is produced from the five flavors. However, the five flavors may also damage the five palaces of yin [*i.e.* the five viscera]. As to the five flavors, [one] must be abstemious to avoid surfeit even if the mouth has a taste and a desire for them, for surfeit will damage the correct or righteous [qi].

> With the five flavors kept balanced carefully, the bones are straight and the sinews are flexible, qi and blood flow [freely], and the interstices are compact. Thus the bone qi is vigorous. Carefully following these instructions, [one] will enjoy a long life decreed by heaven.[6]

The *Ping Ren Qi Xiang Lun (The Treatise on Qi Images [of the Pulse] in Healthy People)* states:

> The root of a person is water and grains. Therefore, one dies when one

runs out of water and grains and so will one when stomach qi is absent from the pulse.[7]

This so-called absence of stomach qi does not mean a liver [pulse] which is not bowstring[8] or a kidney [pulse] which is not stone[like]. Stones are heavy and thus tend to fall or sink. Therefore, a deep pulse is figuratively referred to as stone-like. The presence of stomach qi is indicated by a moderate pulse image. In this case, a moderate pulse means a pulse which is neither too fine and weak or too large, forceful, and/or bowstring. According to five phase theory, there is a distinctive pulse image that is prevalent in and corresponds to each of the seasons. According to this theory, in winter the pulse should naturally be deep like a stone, while in summer it should be surging. However, no matter what its seasonal image, the pulse should also be moderate, thus expressing the presence of stomach qi and a modicum of good health.

A perusal and study of the [above] several quotes show that original qi is always abundant as long as it is enriched and nourished by spleen and stomach qi when they are free from any damage. If the stomach qi is weak and food intake is doubled, then not only will spleen and stomach qi be damaged, but original qi cannot be replenished. As a result, various diseases will arise.

Brilliant like the sun and stars though the import of the *Nei Jing (Inner Classic, i.e.,* the *Su Wen* or *Simple Questions)* is, for fear that it should be beyond the reach of later generations, this same teaching is reiterated in the *Ling Shu Jing (The Spiritual Pivot Classic)*. This classic states:

> After water and grains have entered through the mouth, their flavors which are five in number pour respectively into their own seas, whereas fluids and humors take respectively their own courses.[9]

> The stomach is the sea of water and grains with its transporting points at *Qi Chong* (St 30) above and [*Zu*] *San Li* (St 36) below.

> The sea of water and grain causes abdominal fullness if it is superabundant or [constant] hunger with rejection of food taken in if it is insufficient.[10]

> Humans receive qi from grain. The place which grains pour into is the stomach. The stomach is the sea of water and grain, qi and blood. [The place] where seas spread their cloud qi is under heaven. [The place] into which the stomach discharges qi and blood are the channel canals. What are called the channel canals are the major connecting vessels of the five viscera and the six bowels.[11]

Again it says:

> After the five grains enter the stomach, their wastes, fluids and humors, and the ancestral qi separate into three canals. The ancestral qi gathers in the chest, coming out through the throat so that it penetrates the heart and lungs and operates respiration. The constructive qi distills fluids and humors, pouring them into the vessels and transforming them into blood so that [blood] can nurture the extremities of the limbs and pour into the five viscera and six bowels in the interior in step with the moments of time [in the day]. The defensive qi makes 100 circuits of the body in one day and night. Thus, one moment of time in this cycle is approximately one quarter of an hour as measured by water dripping in the clepsydra or ancient water clock.
>
> The defensive qi comes out swiftly as an impetuous qi. It runs without end in the four extremities and through the spaces between flesh and skin.[12]

It adds:

> The middle burner also originates in the stomach behind the upper burner. After receiving qi, it separates wastes, steams the fluids and humors, and transforms them into purified essence. It pours [this purified essence] up into the lungs and then transforms it into blood as supplies for the living body. [As such, blood] is more valuable than anything else.[13]

It is very compassionate of the sage to take all the trouble of making these repetitions over and again. This shows his boundless kindness toward later generations.

The first part of this chapter is essentially an argument for the special importance of the spleen-stomach in the engenderment and transformation of source or original qi. Till now within Chinese medicine, no important medical texts had privileged any of the five viscera or six bowels. Within five phase theory, all the viscera and bowels are coequal in importance. Now, Li is saying that, among the five viscera and six bowels, the spleen-stomach hold a special place and importance as the fount of source qi. Readers should note that, in this text and from hereon out, source or original qi means the latter heaven source qi emanating from the spleen and stomach, not the original or source qi stored and governed by the kidneys.

It follows that dietary irregularity and lack of moderation in [eating] cold and hot [foods] will damage the spleen and stomach. Joy, anger, worry, and fear may damage the original qi and heart fire will consequently be abetted. Fire and the original qi are mutually irreconcilable. If fire triumphs, it will overwhelm the earth phase. This causes disease.

Also up until the *Pi Wei Lun*, the emphasis on disease causes and mechanisms had been on the six environmental excesses. Now Li is saying that, because immoderate eating and unregulated emotions may adversely effect the spleen-stomach, these internal or neither internal nor external causes should also be seen as being coequally or even pre-eminently important.

The *Tiao Jing Pian (On Balancing the Channels)* states, "Disease arising in yin is generated from eating, drinking, and living environment, yin and yang, joy and anger." In this context, yin and yang refer to sexual intercourse. It further explains:

Yin vacuity leads to internal heat. [It is manifested by] fatigue, decrepit and diminished form qi, meager grain qi, upper burner obstruction, and blockage of the lower duct. Stomach qi becomes hot and this hot qi steams the chest giving rise to [a sensation] of internal heat.[14]

Previously, Liu Wan-su had elevated fire-heat among the six environmental excesses to pre-eminence among disease evils. Here, Li is showing how heat evils may be engendered internally. In essence, Li is accpeting Liu's emphasis on heat evils but further evolving that point of view by delineating their internal engenderment as opposed to external contraction.

Once the spleen and stomach are damaged, the concomitant five turmoils will arise. The five turmoils refer to disorders of the heart, the lungs, stomach and intestines, the limbs, and the head. [The signs at the] outset are intense generalized fever, headache, visual dizziness, heavy limbs, debilitated limbs, fatigue, and somnolence. Damaged by heat, the original qi loses its function and, as a result, the limbs are cumbersome and fatigued.

In the classics, the sage concludes that the stomach qi is the root of humanity. The sage composed these essays to bring out the meaning, throwing light [on the problem] by means of juxtaposition. He has explained all this on numerous occasions. But bad physicians read but do not understand him and make wanton use [of attacking therapy]. Much as they want to save people, they do harm to them.

As with many Chinese doctors of varying ages, Li was not comfortable simply asserting new medical teachings. Instead, he is arguing that he is merely bringing out the true meaning of previous classics that other Chinese doctors have misinterpreted or failed to take to their logical conclusions.

Thus [I will] quote explanations from the classics about disease arising from the spleen and stomach and the necessity of replenishing the original qi to nurture life item by item.

The *Sheng Qi Tong Tian Lun (Treatise on the Communication of Life Qi with Heaven)* states:

> When the qi of the azure [*i.e.*, the sky and the weather it contains] is clear and clean, orientation and reflection [within the human body] operate [well]. When [the qi of the azure] is followed, yang qi is secure and thieving evils, even though they may have entered the body, can do no harm. This means adaptation to the laws of the seasons. Therefore, sages concentrate their essence spirit on acclimatizing to the heavenly qi so that they enjoy access to spirit brightness. [If one] fails to follow [the heavenly qi], the nine orifices will become obstructed from the interior, [yang or hot qi] congestion will occur in the muscles in the exterior, and the defensive qi will be dispersed and become disintegrated. This is called self-damaging. It is frittering away of one's qi.

> With vexation and taxation, yang qi becomes tense, [making] essence expire. If this lingers and accumulates till summer, it will cause people boiling reversal with blindness and ear obstruction, [a violent problem] like an overflooding lake with broken dams. Boiling reversal refers to fright reversal with irascibility caused by yin being burned by internal heat. Ear obstruction means deafness.

Therefore, the qi of heaven values clarity and yang qi is averse to vexation and taxation. This is the first cause of disease starting from the spleen and stomach. This suggests that both the six external qi and emotional factors may lead to disease of the spleen and stomach.

The *Wu Chang Zheng Da Lun (Great Treatise on the Government of the Five Constants)* states:

> When yin essence mounts, people enjoy longevity. When yang essence descends, people die prematurely.[15]

Mounting of yin essence means that grain qi ascends owing to harmony of the spleen and stomach. Since spring and summer exercise government, people enjoy longevity. Spring and summer exercise of government refers to prevalence of the kind of weather usually seen in spring and summer when every living thing springs up, grows, and thrives. A normal abundance of yang qi is thus implied by analogy. Descending of yang essence means that grain qi flows down owing to disharmony of the spleen and stomach. Since astringing and storage exercise government, people suffer shortened lives. "Astringing and storage" refers to prevalence of a kind of weather usually seen in fall and winter when living things stop growing, become withered, and are harvested. This is also referred to as malfunction of the yang qi within the body. This is the second cause of disease starting from the spleen and stomach. This paragraph further emphasizes the vital significance of the harmony of the spleen and stomach or digestion.

The *Liu Jie Zang Xiang Lun (Treatise on the Mutual [Reflections] of the Six Periods of the Year and the Viscera)* explains:

> The spleen, stomach, large intestine, small intestine, triple burner, and urinary bladder are the root of the granaries, the abode of the constructive [qi]. They are all called organs able to transform wastes and change flavors and [are responsible for] entrance and egress. Their efflorescence is [reflected in] the four whites around the lips. The four whites refer to the comparatively white-colored areas adjacent to the lips. What they replenish is the muscles. Their flavor is sweet and their color is yellow. They are consummate yin and have access to the qi of the earth [*i.e.*, stomach qi]. All 11 viscera depend on the gallbladder for decision.[16]

The gallbladder is the upbearing qi of shao yang or spring. When spring qi upbears, the ten thousand transformations are ensured. On that account, when the gallbladder spring qi upbears, the other viscera follow suit. If the gallbladder qi fails to upbear, swill diarrhea, intestinal afflux [*i.e.*, dysentery], and various other illnesses will arise. This is the third cause of disease starting from the spleen and stomach.

I.e., failure to upbear. In actuality, the gallbladder per se is not very important, but the upbearing of the clear is. Later Chinese doctors have come to emphasize the spleen's upbearing of the yang. This is but a step in that eventual evolution.

The classic states:

> Heaven feeds humanity with five qi, while the earth feeds humanity with five flavors. The five qi are the fishy, burning, aromatic, urine-like, and

putrid smells. The five flavors are acrid, bitter, sweet, salty, and sour. The five qi enter through the nose and are stored in the heart and the lungs, making [vision of] the five colors bright and clear and the voice resonant. The five flavors enter through the mouth and are stored in the stomach and intestines. It is to nourish the five qi that the flavors are stored. Here the five qi refer to the qi of the five viscera. When harmonious, qi engenders. [Thus] fluids and humors are developed together and spirit engenders itself.[17]

What is called qi here is that which "the upper burner opens and effuses and [which is] distilled from the flavors of the five grains to fume the skin, replenish the body, and moisten the hair as mist and irrigate as dew."[18] If qi is in chaos, how can people live on? This is the fourth cause of disease starting from the spleen and stomach.

There are definitely more than these four. In discussing the evil qi of heaven and earth, the classics say that once people are affected by them, the five viscera and the six bowels are damaged. [However,] they can only suffer from external evils when both form and qi are [already] vacuous. Without vacuity evil present, thieving evils [from outside] alone can do no harm to people. Thus it is evident that disease starts from the spleen and stomach. Since the sage has reiterated his views [on this] on so many occasions and goes into such detail [about it], comprehension of this must be grasped.

Li is unambiguous in his assertion above that, for external evils to enter the body, the righteous qi must already be vacuous and that the spleen-stomach is the root of the engenderment and transformation of the righteous qi. As we will see later, this belief has profound implications in contemporary clinical practice. However, as one example of how this theory has affected contemporary Chinese medicine I would draw readers' attention to an article published in issue #3, 2004 of the *Shang Hai Zhong Yi Yao Za Zhi (Shanghai Journal of Chinese Medicine & Medicinals)* titled, "Lifting the Essentials of Xie Guang-ru's Experience in the Treatment of Cancer Based on *The Treatise of the Spleen & Stomach.*" This article appeared on pages 18-20 of that journal. In it, Zhang Ting describes how Xie Guang-ru, a professor of oncology at Tianjin Medical University with over 30 years experience in the integrated Chinese-Western medical treatment of cancer, believes that cancer is due to either former heaven natural endowment insufficiency, later heaven loss of regulation, or unregulated eating and drinking which damage and cause detriment to the spleen and stomach. Thus the spleen is not able to move and transform water dampness. Instead, water dampness accumulates and gathers, thus causing loss of normalcy in the movement and circulation of qi and blood. Over time, this gives rise to the production of concretions

and conglomerations. In addition, spleen qi vacuity leading to defensive qi vacuity allows for easy contraction of external evils, while fallen and depressed central qi plus damp evils easily give rise to damp heat. Either brewing of damp heat
evils or contraction of external evils can give rise to cancer toxins. Therefore, in
the treatment of all kinds of cancer, Prof. Xie believes it is vitally important to
fortify the spleen and upbear the clear as well as attacking evils in the form of
dampness, phlegm, blood stasis, heat, and toxins. According to Zhang Ting,
Prof. Xie is unequivocal in positing that original qi insufficiency, downward falling
of clear yang, and upward attack of yin fire are the main mechanisms of cancer.
This theory dovetails very nicely with contemporary Western theories about the
role of digestive enzymes in the prevention of cancer first put forward by biolo-
gist John Beard and Dr. Max Wolf and later championed by Drs. William D. Kelley
and Nick Gonzalez.

Go by the law of yin and yang, act in conformity with the art of numbers, keep
a moderate diet, keep regular hours of life, and do not tax oneself wantonly
[through sexual indulgence]. The art of numbers refers to the study and application of yin-yang, the five phases, 10 stems, and 12 branches. Then form and
spirit both will be in harmony and heaven's [decreed] life span will be lived out.
Demise will never come before the hundredth birthday is celebrated.[19]

From this point of view, how can diet and daily life activities be considered
negligible?

Again, Li is trying to reposition diet and lifestyle as disease causing agents within
Chinese medicine. For 1000 years, the emphasis has been on external contraction. Li is arguing for a shift in emphasis to internal engenderment, at least for
chronic, enduring diseases.

Endnotes

[1] *Nei Jing Su Wen*, Ch. 11
[2] *Su Wen*, Ch. 5
[3] *Su Wen*, Ch. 28
[4] *Su Wen*, Ch. 21
[5] *Su Wen*, Ch. 3
[6] *Ibid.*
[7] *Su Wen*, Ch. 18
[8] Wiseman translates *xian* as "stringlike." I prefer bowstring, since stringlike does not convey the sense of tautness described by this pulse image.
[9] *Ling Shu*, Vol. 6, Ch. 36
[10] *Ling Shu*, Vol. 6, Ch. 33
[11] *Ling Shu*, Vol. 9, Ch. 60

[12] *Ling Shu,* Vol. 10, Ch. 71
[13] *Ling Shu,* Vol. 4, Ch. 18
[14] *Su Wen,* Ch. 62
[15] *Su Wen,* Ch. 70
[16] *Su Wen,* Ch. 9
[17] *Ibid.*
[18] *Ling Shu,* Vol. 6, Ch. 30
[19] *Su Wen,* Ch. 1

2

Diagram of Upbearing & Downbearing, Floating & Sinking, Supplementing & Draining of the Visceral Qi in Different Seasons

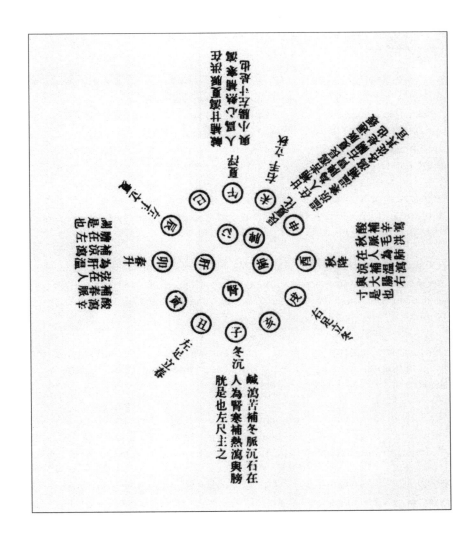

This chapter primarily consists of a diagram showing the five viscera and their relationship to the 12 terrestrial branches and the four seasons (see previous page). Interest in the stems and branches and their application to Chinese herbal medicine is one of the hallmarks of Jin-Yuan dynasty medicine. Until this time, these theories were not widely used in Chinese medicine outside the practice of specifically acupuncture-moxibustion. Introducing this diagram at this point in this book puts Li clearly within the line of tradition exemplified by Liu Wan-su. Otherwise, this diagram has little practical utility. It is my opinion that five phase, 10 stem, and 12 branch theory are some of the most theoretical and least clinically useful parts of Chinese medicine.

(A) Sour drains and acrid supplements; spring pulse: bowstring; liver in humans; warm [medicinals] supplement and cool drain; together with the gallbladder [the liver is reflected] at the left bar.

The *cun kou* or inch mouth pulse at the styloid process on the wrists is divided into three sections. The *cun* or inch section is distal to the styloid process; the *chi* or cubit section is proximal to the styloid process; and the *guan* or barrier section is located in between these two or directly over the styloid process. This short passage describes, among other things, the rules for choosing medicinals in the different seasons. The following sections should be read in the same way.

(B) Salty supplements and sweet drains; summer pulse: surging; the heart in humans; hot [medicinals] supplement and cold drain; together with the small intestine [the heart is reflected] at the left inch.

(C) Sweet supplements and bitter drains; long summer pulse: slow and moderate; the spleen and stomach in humans; [these two are reflected] at the right bar; cool, cold, and warm [medicinals] as well as supplementation and drainage [should be prescribed] in accordance with [natural] inclinations.

(D) Sour supplements and acrid drains; autumn pulse: hairy and surging; the lungs in humans; cool [medicinals] supplement and warm drain; together with the large intestine [the lungs are reflected] at the right inch.

(E) Salty drains and bitter supplements; winter pulse: deep and stone-like; the kidneys in humans; cold [medicinals] supplement and hot drain; together with the large intestine and urinary bladder [the kidneys are reflected] at both cubits.

Within the above correspondences, the reader should note that Li is using the pulse position correspondences of the Nan Jing (Classic of Difficulties) and Mai

Jing (Pulse Classic). Today within standard professional Chinese medicine, we use the pulse position correspondences set forward by such Ming dynasty sources as Li Shi-zhen and Zhang Jie-bin.

The five phases mutually generate in an endless cycle of wood, fire, earth, metal, and water. [Of these,] only earth has no season of its own, being effulgent in the last eighteen days of each of the four seasons in order to generate the other four viscera. The four seasons are *chen, xu, chou,* and *wei* [or B5, B11, B2, and B8 respectively]. The formal body of man corresponds to the nine fields. The nine fields refer to the eight quarters of the compass with the center, *i.e.,* the east, west, south, north, southeast, northeast, southwest, northwest, and center. Another interpretation is the nine prefectures of the ancient Chinese empire. The left foot rules the beginning of spring, the *chou* phase; the left hand rules the beginning of summer, the *chen* phase; the right hand rules the beginning of autumn, the *wei* phase; the right foot rules the beginning of winter, the *xu* phase. The root qi of *wu* dampness is moderate, while its ancillary qi are warm, cool, cold, and hot. Earth is associated with two heavenly stems, *wu* and *ji.* Dampness belongs to earth, or, in other words, dampness and earth correspond, occupying *wu* and *ji* respectively. Humans' stomachs correspond to this. The root flavor of *ji*[1] earth is salty, while its ancillary flavors are acrid, sweet, sour, and bitter. Humans' spleens correspond to this. The spleen and stomach together transform [*i.e.,* contract or manifest] disease in the seasons [*wu* and *ji*]. Such disease can be treated in no formulaic way but [only] in accordance with its inclinations. As diseases of the liver and lungs lie between water and fire, their favorable and unfavorable transmutations vary with each other and are uncertain, possibly warm and possibly cool. Water corresponds with the kidneys which lie in the lower part of the body, while fire corresponds with the heart which lies in the upper. Thus, this sentence suggests that the liver and lungs are located in between. Moreover, because the lungs/metal are the mother of the kidneys/water, while the liver/wood is the mother of the heart/fire, diseases involving the lungs and liver will typically spread to the heart and kidneys. [Treatment] should aim at the cause.

Upbearing and downbearing, floating and sinking are the four movements of the qi. What they mean is ascension, descension, exteriorization, and interiorization respectively. These four movements of the qi are intimately associated with the qi mechanism. Upbearing and downbearing have to do with the upbearing of the clear and the downbearing of the turbid, and the spleen-stomach is the pivot of this division or separation. Floating and sinking describe the movement of the defensive qi to and from the exterior in correspondence with the daily diurnal cycle. It was Li who emphasized the importance of the upbearing of the qi mechanism within Chinese medicine. Li made disinhibition of the qi mechanism through upbearing clear yang an integral part of all of his most famous formulas. It is also important to point out that the upbearing of the clear and downbearing of the turbid are interdependent. Only if the clear is upborne can the turbid be downborne and vice versa. Therefore, by upbearing the clear, Li is automatically helping to assure the proper downbearing of the turbid.

Endnote

[1] The original has *si*. This must be a misprint for *ji*, B6.

3

Treatise on the Waxing & Waning[1] of the Spleen & Stomach

If original qi is exuberant within the stomach, [the stomach] is capable of large food intake without damage, nor does it feel hungry well past mealtime. If the spleen and stomach are both effulgent, food intake may be large and one gets fat. If they are both vacuous, [one] is unable to eat and gets thin or gets fat in spite of low food intake but is unable to lift the limbs in spite of being fat. Fatness in China is a neutral word, denoting sometimes a healthy state, sometimes an unhealthy condition. This is because the spleen is replete and evil qi [*i.e.*, phlegm dampness] is exuberant. There are also cases of thinness despite large food intake. [In this case,] fire hidden in the qi phase in the stomach results in large food intake, while spleen vacuity leads to withered flesh. This is known as food languor. Food languor refers to lethargy and drowsiness, especially following meals, despite large food intake. Shu-he[2] has said, "Large food intake is not incompatible with weak muscles." He is referring to the case discussed [above].

If the original qi in the spleen-stomach is exuberant, the spleen and stomach are able to disperse and transform or digest food properly as well as engender and transform qi and blood properly. Therefore, the stomach is not damaged by large food intake, nor is the person immediately too hungry, a symptom of qi vacuity, if one is late for one's meal. If, on the other hand, the spleen and stomach become vacuous and weak, this may result in either emaciation or weight gain. In the latter case, there is both spleen qi vacuity and phlegm damp exuberance. Li also points out that a hot stomach always results in a larger than normal appetite with rapid hungering and that stomach heat may coexist with spleen vacuity. In fact, this latter scenario is quite common among Westerners.

Dietary irregularity causes stomach disease, and stomach disease is responsible for shortness of breath, scanty essence spirit, engenderment of intense heat, and occasionally a visible fire going up to glow in no other place but the face. The *Huang Di Zhen Jing (Yellow Emperor's Acupuncture Classic)* states, "Hot face is a disease of the foot yang ming."[3] Once the stomach is diseased, the spleen has nowhere from which to receive its supplies. The spleen is dead yin, governing no definite period, and, therefore, it too can become diseased [in any of the seasons]. As a viscus, the spleen is justifiably regarded as yin, but there are two different interpretations for the term dead yin. Some say the spleen is called dead yin because it does not govern any one of the four seasons. Another interpretation is that the spleen is dead yin when being overwhelmed by its restraining phase, *i.e.*, liver wood.

If the formal body is overtaxed, the spleen will contract disease, giving rise to fatigue, somnolence, debilitated limbs, and diarrhea. Once the spleen is diseased, the stomach alone cannot move fluids and humors and consequently also becomes diseased.

This underscores the deleterious effect of taxation fatigue on the spleen.

Generally speaking, if the spleen and stomach are vacuous and weak, yang qi is unable to engender or grow. In other words, spring and summer fail to govern and the qi of the five viscera fail to engender. Spring and summer are seasons when every living thing begins to or is prospering. Yang qi functions like these two seasons and the things which flourish in these two seasons. Therefore, normal physiological function is compared to spring and summer or that which they govern. When the spleen is diseased, [yang qi] flows down to overwhelm the kidneys. That is, earth restrains water and, as a result, there occurs weak and flaccid bones. This is called bone wilting. It causes the bones to become empty and vacuous of marrow and the legs unable to walk on the ground. This is superimposition of yin qi, a pattern of exuberant yin and vacuous yang. Superimposition means that two yin organs, the spleen and kidneys, are both affected. The fundamental principle shows that sweating effects recuperation, whereas precipitation leads to death. If acrid and sweet medicinals are employed to enrich the stomach, this will result in upbearing and floating and the qi of generation and growth will be made effulgent. [In this case,] diaphoresis is not used to promote perspiration so much as to assist yang.

Here Li is talking about failure of the spleen to upbear clear yang. Instead, the yang qi falls downward to become depressed in the lower burner. As for sweating being the correct treatment principle in this case, Li recognizes that acrid, windy-natured, exterior-resolving medicinals can also be used to rectify the qi and resolve depression. Because they are upbearing and out-thrusting or effusing in nature, they upbear the clear yang and out-thrust depression. This is an extremely important fact in clinical practice, and Li frequently uses exterior-resolving and/or wind-treating medicinals in exactly this way, for instance *Chai Hu* (Radix Bupleuri), *Sheng Ma* (Rhizoma Cimicifugae), and *Ge Gen* (Radix Puerariae).

When the stomach is diseased, the pulse is moderate [or relaxed]. The *huan mai* can either be normal or pathological. If normal, the word *huan* may be translated as moderate. But if pathological it is better translated as relaxed or retarded since it is slightly slow. When the spleen is diseased, the pulse is slow and, in addition, the patient has throbbing qi around their navel which is felt firm and painful when pressure is applied. Throbbing qi around the navel means a sensation of throbbing or pulsing around the navel.

If fire overwhelms the earth phase, the pulse is surging and moderate [or relaxed] besides there being signs of generalized fever and discomfort in the heart. This is because yang qi is too decrepit and weak to engender and emit. To treat this, one should not use medication methods designed for [diseases of] the five viscera. [Rather,] medicinals should be meted out in compliance with the methods of upbearing and downbearing, floating and sinking, supplementing and draining instructed in the *Zang Qi Fa Shi Lun* (*Treatise on Visceral Qi Following the Seasons*).

A relaxed pulse, fatigue, somnolence, and debilitated limbs with possible diarrhea demonstrate overwhelming dampness. [In that case,] use *Ping Wei San* (Level the Stomach Powder).[4] In case of a bowstring pulse, qi weakness, spontaneous perspiration, and heat in the limbs with possible diarrhea or dry, withered skin and hair and the head hair falling out, use *Huang Qi Jian Zhong Tang* (Astragalus Fortify the Center Decoction).[5] In case of a vacuous pulse and weak blood, add to this one or two ingredients chosen from *Si Wu Tang* (Four Materials Decoction)[6] as indicated by the apparent signs. In case of vacuous and weak true qi, shortness of breath, and weak pulse, prescribe *Si Jun Zi Tang* (Four Gentleman Decoction).[7] In case of thirst or urinary blockage or inhibition, whether the urine be reddish or yellowish, profuse or scanty, choose one or two ingredients from *Wu Ling San* (Five [Ingredients] Poria Powder)[8] except for *Gui Zhi* (Ramulus Cinnamomi Cassiae) and add these to the principal formula, [*i.e., Bu Pi Wei Xie Yin Huo Sheng Yang Tang*, Supplement the Spleen & Stomach, Drain Yin Fire, and Upbear Yang Decoction]. The above five formulas should be applied with variation in accordance with the signs shown in addition to the principal pattern, [*i.e.*, the pattern that indicates the principal formula].

In this passage, Li is essentially saying that, when treating the spleen and stomach, one can add other ingredients to accomplish a variety of other treatment principles as required by the patient's signs and symptoms.

If there is exterior vacuity with spontaneous perspiration, add *Huang Qi* (Radix Astragali Membrancei) in spring and summer but *Gui Zhi* (Ramulus Cinnamomi Cassiae) in autumn and winter. In case of acute abdominal spasm or bowstring pulse, add *Fang Feng* (Radix Ledebouriellae Divaricatae). In case of extremely acute spasm, [also] add *Gan Cao* (Radix Glycyrrhizae Uralensis). In case of abdominal constriction or shortness of breath, also add this. In case of abdominal fullness with no qi rolling, do not add it. Qi rolling means flatulence and qi not rolling means qi stuffiness and fullness in the abdomen. In case of disharmony of the qi in the spleen and stomach, do not, despite qi not rolling, exclude it and, to break qi stagnation, add *Hou Po* (Cortex Magnoliae Officinalis) which cannot be used in large quantities, one-fifth of the amount of *Gan Cao* (Radix Glycyrrhizae Uralensis) being appropriate. Oppression and heaviness in the abdomen is not abdominal distention but dispersion or noncollection [of the spleen qi]. This calls for adding *Bai Shao* (Radix Albus Paeoniae Lactiflorae) to effect collection. In case of short, rapid, or insufficient lung qi, add *Ren Shen* (Radix Panacis Ginseng) and *Bai Shao*. In relation to the middle burner, the use of *Bai Shao* can upbear yang in the spleen to deter evils in the liver and gall-bladder from attacking. [If there is] abdominal constriction, spasm, and tension, then one must remove *Bai Shao*. [These symptoms] make the use of any kind of sour, astringing medicinals impossible. [In case of] abdominal pain, add *Gan Cao* and *Bai Shao*. The crop, which produces sweetness, is *ji* (S6). Crop usually refers to the spleen and stomach, but here it refers to *Gan Cao* or other sweet-flavored ingredients. The curved and straight, which produces sourness, is *jia* (S1). Curved and straight usually refer to wood or trees, but here it means *Bai Shao* or other sour ingredients. [Using] *jia* and *ji* to transform earth is a wonderful method invented by Zhong-jing.[9] *Jia* (S1), the first celestial stem, wood, represents the gallbladder as well as sourness, and *ji* (S6), earth, the spleen as well as sweetness. *Bai Shao* is sour (*jia*), while *Gan Cao* is sweet (*ji*). The combined use of *Gan Cao* (*ji*) and *Bai Shao* (*jia*) is designed to palliate the spleen by *ji* and inhibit the gallbladder by *jia* to cure abdominal pain. This condition involves spleen earth but is due to gallbladder wood. [In case of] fever in addition to abdominal pain, add *Huang Qin* (Radix Scutellariae Baicalensis). [In case of] aversion to cold or a cold sensation in the abdomen, add *Gui Zhi* (Ramulus Cinnamomi Cassiae). [In case of] fatigue, somnolence, the existence of dampness, and inability to eat due to stomach vacuity, heavy drowsiness, or diarrhea, add *Cang Zhu* (Rhizoma Atractylodis). [In case of] spontaneous perspiration, add *Bai Zhu* (Rhizoma Atractylodis Macrocephalae). [In case of] inhibited urination, add white *Fu Ling* (Sclerotium Poriae Cocos). Also add this [in case of] thirst. In case of weak qi, add *Fu Ling* and *Ren Shen*. In case of exuberant qi, add *Chi Fu Ling* (red Sclerotium Poriae Cocos) and *Sha Ren* (Fructus Amomi). In case of inability to convey recovered qi and the existence of heat, add *Huang Lian* (Rhizoma Coptidis Chinensis) in small quantities. Recovered qi may refer to relief of abdominal distention and fullness. Failure to convey qi implies discomfort in the abdomen with flatulence. Also add this in case of vexation and restlessness of the heart.

In case of scanty urination, add *Zhu Ling* (Sclerotium Polypori Umbellati) and *Ze Xie* (Rhizoma Alismatis Orientalis) but do not add these [in case of] profuse perspiration and exhaustion of fluids in the upper [burner], for it is desirable for fluids themselves to return to the stomach. [In case of] urinary blockage with no thirst, add stir-fried *Huang Bai* (Cortex Phellodendri) and *Zhi Mu* (Rhizoma Anemarrhenae Aspheloidis). In case of inhibited urination, add stir-fried *Hua Shi* (Talcum). In case of inhibited urination and dribbling voiding, add *Ze Xie*. In addition, *Wu Ling San* (Five [Ingredients] Poria Powder) treats thirst with inhibited urination. [However, if there is] no aversion to cold, the use of *Gui Zhi* (Ramulus Cinnamomi Cassiae) is prohibited. Confused vision and hearing with absence of thirst and uninhibited urination is a blood stasis pattern. [Therefore,] use stir-fried *Huang Bai* and *Zhi Mu* to clear the kidneys of dry heat. [In case of] inhibited orifice with strangury, add *Ze Xie* and stir-fried *Hua Shi* (Talcum). To treat solely inhibited orifice, it is equally appropriate to add *Mu Tong* (Caulis Akebiae) to *Liu Yi San* (Six to One Powder).[10] In case of heat in the heart, prescribe Qian's formula, *Dao Chi San* (Abduct the Red Powder).

In case of fullness in the center or simply abdominal distention, add *Hou Po* (Cortex Magnoliae Officinalis). In case of impeded qi, add *Chen Pi* (Pericarpium Citri Reticulatae). In case of qi stagnation, add *Qing Pi* (Pericarpium Citri Reticulatae Viride) and *Chen Pi* (Pericarpium Citri Reticulatae), [the ratio of the amounts being] one to three [respectively]. In case of uninhibited urination with shortness of breath, remove *Fu Ling* and add *Huang Qi* (Radix Astragali Membranacei) to supplement the qi to *Si Jun Zi Tang* (Four Gentlemen Decoction). In case of qi not rolling in the abdomen, add a half amount of *Gan Cao*. Abdominal stabbing pain or pricking pain all over the body, abdominal urgency, an uncomfortable [feeling] in the abdomen, or going to defecate without being able to relieve oneself are all ascribed to blood vacuity. Either blood vacuity giving rise to abdominal urgency or qi and blood vacuity and weakness with pain in the eye [calls for] adding whole *Dang Gui* (Radix Angelicae Sinensis). In case of headache, add *Chuan Xiong* (Radix Ligustici Wallichii). In case of tormenting headache, a headache of the shao yin, add *Xi Xin* (Herba Asari Cum Radice). In case of hair falling out and pain below the umbilicus, add *Shu Di* (cooked Radix Rehmanniae Glutinosae).

To treat spleen and stomach vacuity weakness, I used to limit myself to the [above] five formulas with some variation. *I.e.*, *Ping Wei San* (Level the Stomach Powder), *Huang Qi Jian Zhong Tang* (Astragalus Fortify the Center Decoction), *Si Wu Tang* (Four Materials Decoction), *Si Jun Zi Tang* (Four Gentlemen Decoction), and *Wu Ling San* (Five [Ingredients] Poria Powder). If there were one or two signs of patterns of the five viscera, I never failed to achieve [the desired] effect by adding certain medicinals to these formulas in accordance with those signs. However, I did not succeed in effecting a complete cure. Some patients turned up again for one or another reason or possibly because their conception, governing, and penetrating vessels were struck by evils. [In the last analysis, however,] the cause was always spleen and stomach vacuity weakness. Limiting myself to certain formulas to treat disease was a violation of the norms stipulated in the *Su Wen (Simple Questions)* even though the method followed was the formula variation method in accordance with signs. This refers to the principles and methods explained in Chapter 22 of the *Su Wen*.

Because of this, [I] carried out a probing inquiry into the theories expounded by the *Su Wen (Simple Questions)*, *Nan Jing (Classic of Difficulties)*, and *Huang Di Zhen Jing (Yellow Emperor's Acupuncture Classic)*. The origin of spleen and stomach insufficiency is insufficiency of yang qi and surplus of yin qi. To treat this, formula composition in accordance with signs must be made in light of the methods of upbearing and downbearing, floating and sinking in relation to insufficient original qi. For these methods, one should see the diagram at the beginning of Chapter 2. It shows that different medication methods should be followed in different seasons. The reason is that insufficiency of the spleen and stomach is different from that of other viscera in that [the spleen and stomach] are not a fixed entity. Unlike the other four viscera, the spleen prevails during the 18 days between each season instead of governing one definite season. Thus it is closely related to all the other viscera. In treating the liver, heart, lungs, and kidneys, whether they are vacuous or replete, whether by supplementation or drainage, what is vital is that the medicinals should always boost the spleen and stomach.

In terms of visceral vacuity, the heart and lungs both get their qi from the spleen. All medicinals which supplement the heart and lungs do so via supplementation of the spleen. In contemporary Chinese medicine, no pattern of liver qi vacuity is currently recognized (at least not as standard). What some Chinese doctors argue is a liver qi vacuity is actually a liver-spleen disharmony with marked symptoms of qi vacuity. In this case, the qi vacuity is remedied via supplementation of the spleen qi. Because former and latter heavens are mutually rooted and mutually engendering, spleen qi vacuity may eventually result in kidney qi vacuity. If this continues on long enough, then there will be a spleen-kidney yang vacuity or a qi and yin vacuity, meaning a spleen qi-kidney yin vacuity. In any of these three cases, one must supplement the spleen as well as the kidneys in order to achieve the correct therapeutic effect. In actual fact, although textbooks talk about simple kidney yin or yang vacuity patterns, there is rarely kidney yin or yang vacuity without concomitant spleen qi vacuity as Li correctly saw.

The classic explains, "[Because] whatever fails to arrive when it ought leads to deficiency, the restrained will move frenetically, the engendered will suffer from disease, and the restraining will overwhelm." What fails to arrive when it ought refers to the delayed comer which is a vacuity evil. That which fails to arrive refers to the delayed arrival of the seasons. Note that the paragraphs following, except when explained otherwise, are all based on the premise that winter comes later than usual or, in other words, that kidney water is insufficient. According to five phase theory, if, for example, we experience a cold spring, which implies a liver wood deficiency, its restrained phase, spleen earth, will become frenetic. Its engendered phase, heart fire, will contract disease, and its restraining phase, lung metal, will become overwhelming. All this refers to five transports and six qi theory which was one of the theories emphasized by doctors in the Jin-Yuan. This theory has to do with climatology as described by yin-yang, the five phases, six qi, and the 10 heavenly stems and 12 earthly branches.

[Suppose winter comes later than it should. In that case,] the heart and small intestine will overwhelm the spleen and stomach. The spleen and stomach pulses will manifest as large, floating, and bowstring, and the disease [will manifest] as vexation, agitation, oppression, and stuffiness or heat in the limbs, or a bitter taste in the mouth, and dry tongue and throat. This is damage done by dietary irregularity and overtaxation which results in spleen and stomach vacuity weakness, a disease involving the blood. Mainly [this results in] stopping fluids from flowing into the mouth. Hence the mouth and throat become dry. The patient feels thirsty, but, if the physician treats them with *Wu Ling San* (Five [Ingredients] Poria Powder), thirst and agitation will be made worse in spite of the intention to quench them. This is because [these water-seeping ingredients make] fluids now suffer double exhaustion. This may even cause crisis and death. The classic instructs, "In case of vacuity, supplement the mother." It is necessary to supplement the root, [*i.e.,*] the spleen and stomach while treating the heart and small intestine with the sweet, warm medicinals as the ruler, bitter, cold medicinals as the envoy, and sour ingredients as the ministers and assistants. The heart is bitter about slackening and, by promptly using sour, it can be astringed. Effulgent heart fire subjects lung metal to evils, and metal vacuity should be supplemented by sour. Secondly, sweet and warm and sweet and cold agents should be used to drain hyperactive and superabundant heart fire through [supplementing] the spleen and stomach. This is the way to treat the root.

Frenetic movement of the restrained refers to effulgent heart fire. The child is capable of making the mother replete. The mother [in this case] is liver wood. When liver wood becomes effulgent, it takes advantage of the raging fire and becomes audacious, moving frenetically. It follows that the spleen and stomach become the first victims. Generalized heaviness and migratory pain may arise.

This is because, with dampness and heat locked in contention, wind heat is depressed and confined, having to attach to the tangible, bodily form. [Thus] irascibility may arise. This is because wind heat has sunken into the earth [*i.e.*, the lower burner]. Eye disease with growth of internal obstruction may [also] arise. This is because the liver wraps [*i.e.*, controls] the blood, the stomach governs the blood, and the heart governs the vessels which are the abode of the blood. This sentence implies that the spleen, stomach, heart, and the below-mentioned liver are all involved in the condition under discussion. One should note, however, that the liver is the center of interest in this paragraph. Since, as some people say, the heart governs the blood, or, as others say, the liver governs blood and opens into the eyes, there may arise confused vision, confused hearing, hallucinations, dreams of the dead, and aching distention of the limbs with spasms. All this indicates that liver wood is too exuberant not to be an evil. There may arise wilting or impediment, inversion or cold stroke, malign sores or kidney atony, or heat above but cold below. These evils, though [each] different [one from the other], all indicate wind heat which stops growth and wood fire which is confined in the tangible bodily form.

Contraction of disease of the engendered refers to the subjection of the lungs by the evils of earth, fire, and wood. This means that when spleen/earth/mother is vacuous, the lungs/metal/child are affected. If the lungs' restraining function is affected, frenetic liver wood, which should otherwise be restrained, turns to conquer them with heart fire or that which restrains the lungs joining in. Since clearing and depurative qi is damaged, chest fullness, diminished qi, and shortness of breath arise. This is because the lungs govern all kinds of qi, and the qi of the five viscera all have become insufficient. Hence the yang tract stops working. The yang tract refers to the qi of the heart and lungs in the upper burner. Coughing and cold and heat may also arise, since damp heat overwhelms the interior.

Overwhelming the restraining refers to water taking advantage of frenetic wood to rebel against earth. It follows that the kidneys [*i.e.*, kidney yin/kidney water] become perspiration after entering the heart, tears after entering the liver, drool after entering the spleen, and phlegm, coughing, sticky nasal mucous, sneezing, and watery nasal discharge after entering the lungs. Another explanation says that [by dint of] the lower origin [*i.e.*, kidney yang], earth becomes exuberant enough to conquer water so that the three vessels, the governing, conception, and penetrating, also become exuberant [with effulgent fire]. The kidneys constitute both true yin and true yang. When kidney yang or rather kidney fire becomes effulgent, its child, earth, becomes effulgent too. As a result, kidney water is overwhelmed. This fire burns water to a boil and overwhelms the spleen and lungs. Thus phlegm, drool, and spittle come out of the mouth. If these descend, they issue as genital sweating, cold in the external kidneys [or testicles], inability of the legs to carry the body, and dull pain in the soles of the feet. Or, if by the strength of wood, water may ascend to issue in dry eyes, gum in the eyes, and cold tears. All this is due to lung metal being too vacuous to hold any-one in awe. This implies that liver wood is frenetic since its restraining phase metal is vacuous.

Insufficiency of the spleen and stomach invariably leads to blood disease. In this case, yang qi is insufficient and yin qi is superabundant, and, therefore, the nine orifices become blocked. All yang qi has its root in yin blood. When yin blood is subjected to fire evils, yin becomes exuberant [with fire] and exuberant yin ascends to overwhelm the yang phase. If the yang tract fails to work, no engendering and soaring qi is left. It is yang qi which penetrates the orifices. It is yin qi which attaches to the bodily form. [Only] if yin qi attaches to the upper and yang qi rises to heaven, do both then execute their respective duties. The last three sentences are a further explanation of blocked nine orifices. It is important that when yang qi, which is an engendering and soaring qi, is short, yin qi cannot be upborne by it. Consequently, the orifices, which are the openings of the bodi-ly form, are affected.

In contemporary Chinese medicine, we say that the spleen governs the engen-derment and transformation of blood. Therefore, if the spleen qi becomes vac-uous and weak, the spleen will typically not engender new blood sufficiently. In addition, because the qi moves the blood, spleen qi vacuity may lead to blood stasis. Because the spleen qi governs the movement and transformation of water fluids in the body, if the spleen qi is too vacuous and weak to govern this func-tion, fluids may collect and transform into dampness. If dampness lingers and endures, it may congeal into phlegm. In that case, phlegm dampness with or without blood stasis may block any of the nine orifices. If heat enters the blood aspect or division, it may cause the blood to move frenetically. Often this results in upward counterflow with epistaxis, hematemesis, and hemoptysis.

Now, in composing formulas, acrid, sweet, and warm medicinals should not be used alone. This was one of the failings of the extremely popular formulas in the Song dynasty *Tai Ping Hui Min He Ji Ju Fang (Imperial Grace Collected Formulas & Harmonizing Prescriptions of the Tai Ping [Era])* which Li was trying to remedy. Nor should sweet, bitter, and intensely cold medicinals be used alone. This was the failing of Liu Wan-su's heat-clearing formulas.

From the time of Zhang Zhong-jing up till Liu Wan-su, many Chinese doctors used acrid, sweet, warm medicinals excessively or even exclusively. In contrast,

Liu Wan-su recommended using formulas that are bitter and cold. However, some of Liu's formulas are excessively bitter and cold. Here, Li is advocating a more complex and, at the same time, more harmonious and balanced prescriptive practice.

With the wine-processed twins as envoys, the bitter, sweet, cold medicinals are conducted to the top of the head and then ushered into the kidneys and liver below. The wine-processed twins refers to *Huang Qin* (Radix Scutellariae Baicalensis) and *Huang Lian* (Rhizoma Coptidis Chinensis). This is what is called upbearing and downbearing, floating and sinking. [It requires the alternating use] of an even to odd numbered [formula] and from an odd to even numbered [formula]. (Odd numbers are yang and even numbers are yin. [Later editor]) To drain yin fire, various wind agents are used to upbear and perfuse yang qi. Windy medicinals include, for example, *Sheng Ma* (Rhizoma Cimicifugae), *Chai Hu* (Radix Bupleuri), and *Fang Feng* (Radix Ledebouriellae Divaricatae), all of which are acrid, upbearing, and effusing. In other words, they are like wind in nature. Additionally, they all course wind and effuse it from the exterior. If one does not understand this upbearing, effusing nature these medicinals, there is much about the practice of Chinese herbal medicine which will remain opaque. These are employed to enrich the function of the liver and gallbladder so that yang qi will be engendered and emerge in the yin phase above. Finally, use acrid, sweet, warm medicinals to reinforce the upbearing agents in order that these agents may be perfuse and disperse in the yang phase and be conducted into the nine orifices. The classic states:

> Food, having entered the stomach, spreads essence to the liver and diffuses qi into the sinews. Having entered the stomach, food, the turbid of which gathers in the heart, diffuses essence into the vessels. With vessel qi flowing in the channels, channel qi gathers in the lungs. The lungs, facing the hundreds of vessels, transport essence to the skin and hair. [And] the minute vessels, having taken in essence, move qi to the bowels.

This is the first mention of the term "yin fire" in the *Pi Wei Lun*. While I will discuss yin fire in greater depth below, please note that Li is advocating the use of acrid, windy-natured, upbearing, and effusing medicinals as a way to clear yin fire. He then goes on to say that these windy medicinals should be combined with acrid, sweet, warm medicinals to enhance their overall effect.

In addition, after water and grains enter the stomach, they first travel in the yang tract and the yang qi begins to upbear and float. Floating enables the yang qi to spread and fill the skin and hair. Upbearing [enables it to] replenish the top of the head. Because of this, the nine orifices are rendered open and uninhibited.

If dietary irregularity causes detriment to the stomach qi, [the stomach qi] is no longer able to capture and transform [food]. Then [nothing] will spread to the liver, [nothing] will gather in the heart, and [nothing] will permeate the lungs. [In consequence,] lethargy and drowsiness will arise after eating. When lying down, food settles on one side and the qi is soothed for a while. This shows that the upbearing and effusing qi is no longer able to work. The classic states:

Having entered the stomach, fluids float the essence qi and transport it up to the spleen. The spleen qi spreads essence which gathers in the lungs.

Immediately as fluids enter the stomach, such patients feel them already reach somewhere below the umbilicus with a desire to urinate. Since no essence qi is transported to the spleen or gathers in the lungs, heart fire attacks upward, causing dry mouth and throat. All this is too apparent not to see that it is due to yin qi which is greatly exuberant. What is more, [in the case of] spleen and stomach disease, there is a throbbing qi around the navel which is felt firm and painful when pressure is applied. The presence of this indicates spleen and stomach vacuity, while its absence indicates otherwise. This serves as a sure indicator. It is important to understand that either stomach heat or spleen qi vacuity can cause excessively profuse urination, and excessively profuse urination is even more likely when these two disease mechanisms occur together. Such profuse urination may eventually give rise to signs and symptoms of dryness. Stomach heat may also and often does give rise to heart heat.

Spleen and stomach insufficiency [may] result in fire being unable to engender earth and erroneously attack and repel [the spleen-stomach instead. In this case,] whatever fails to arrive when it ought leads to deficiency. Because the spleen and stomach are earth, while earth is damp, this sentence implies that, in long summer, a period governed by the spleen, if dampness fails to prevail, the spleen and stomach become weak. In this case, Li recommends the following formula which is essentially a spleen-fortifying, qi-supplementing formula that only secondarily clears heart fire.

> *Bai Zhu* (Rhizoma Atractylodis Macrocephalae), sovereign
> *Ren Shen* (Radix Panacis Ginseng)
> *Huang Qi* (Radix Astragali Membranacei), ministers
> *Bai Shao* (Radix Albus Paeoniae Lactiflorae)
> *Gan Cao* (Radix Glycyrrhizae Uralensis)
> *Sang Bai Pi* (Cortex Radicis Mori Albi), assistants
> *Huang Lian* (Rhizoma Coptidis Chinensis), envoy

The various windy [natured] medicinals are all able to conquer dampness with wind, and so can the various sweet, warm medicinals.

Heart fire hyperactivity and exuberance overwhelming the spleen and stomach position is also [an example of] something failing to arrive when it ought leading to deficiency. Fire is supposed to engender earth, but, if dampness fails to arrive in due time, the spleen and stomach become weak and heart fire, far from engendering earth, will overwhelm it. In this case, Li recommends primarily clearing heat and draining fire with bitter, cool and cold medicinals as in the following formula.

Huang Lian (Rhizoma Coptidis Chinensis), sovereign
Huang Bai (Cortex Phellodendri)
Sheng Di (uncooked Radix Rehmanniae Glutinosae), ministers
Bai Shao (Radix Albus Paeoniae Lactiflorae)
Shi Gao (Gypsum Fibrosum)
Zhi Mu (Rhizoma Anemarrhenae Aspheloidis)
Huang Qin (Radix Scutellariae Baicalensis)
Gan Cao (Radix Glycyrrhizae Uralensis), assistants

Frenetic movement of liver wood [gives rise to] chest and rib-side pain, a bitter [taste in the] mouth, a dry tongue, alternating cold and heat, retching, irascibility, aching and distention of the limbs, dribbling urination, difficult defecation, and spasms and sudden abdominal pain. All this is [a result of] the overwhelming of the restraining. Liver wood is supposed to restrain spleen earth, but if liver wood moves frenetically, the restraining phase is said to overwhelm that which it ordinarily only restrains. This is what we now commonly refer to as a liver-spleen disharmony with depressive heat.

Chai Hu (Radix Bupleuri), sovereign
Fang Feng (Radix Ledebouriellae Divaricatae)
Bai Shao (Radix Albus Paeoniae Lactiflorae)
Rou Gui (Cortex Cinnamomi Cassiae), ministers
Qiang Huo (Radix Et Rhizoma Notopterygii)
Du Huo (Radix Angelicae Pubescentis)
Ze Xie (Rhizoma Alismatis Orientalis)
Huang Bai (Cortex Phellodendri), assistants
Sheng Ma (Rhizoma Cimicifugae), envoy
Zhu Ling (Sclerotium Polypori Umbellati)
Gao Ben (Radix Et Rhizoma Ligustici Sinensis)
Chuan Xiong (Radix Ligustici Wallichii)
Xi Xin (Herba Asari Cum Radice)
Man Jing Zi (Fructus Viticis)
Bai Zhi (Radix Angelicae Dahuricae)
Shi Gao (Gypsum Fibrosum)

Zhi Mu (Rhizoma Anemarrhenae Aspheloidis)
Hua Shi (Talcum)

Although not one of Li's most famous formulas, readers should recognize how Li is using certain ingredients for more than one purpose. For instance, *Fang Feng, Qiang Huo,* and *Du Huo* are all meant to treat the aching and distention in the limbs at the same time as aiding *Chai Hu* and *Sheng Ma* to upbear the clear. In addition, Li eliminates depressive heat via 1) acridly upbearing and out-thrusting, 2) bitter and coldly draining and clearing, and 3) seeping water and disinhibiting urination, thus guiding yang evils into the yin tract. In addition, because upbearing and downbearing are mutually interdependent, seeping downward promotes the upbearing of the clear at the same time that upbearing of the clear promotes downward seepage.

Lung metal suffering from evils is due to spleen and stomach vacuity weakness being too great to engender the lungs. This is a disease contracted by the engendered. Hence coughing, shortness of breath, ascent of qi, inability of the skin and hair to resist cold, scant, exhausted essence spirit, melancholy, and depression arise. All this is a result of insufficient yang qi with superabundant yin qi and of superabundant substance with insufficient function. Some interpret this as bodily form is superabundant while essence spirit is insufficient.

In the 20th century, Zhang Xi-chun also recognized the importance of the spleen qi to the heart and lung qi. His formula *Sheng Xian Tang* (Upbear the Sunken Decoction) for a great qi vacuity, meaning an upper burner qi vacuity, is directly derived from Li Dong-yuan's theory and praxis.

Ren Shen (Radix Panacis Ginseng), sovereign
Huang Qi (Radix Astragali Membranacei)
Chen Pi (Pericarpium Citri Reticulatae), ministers
Bai Zhu (Rhizoma Atractylodis Macrocephalae)
Bai Shao (Radix Albus Paeoniae Lactiflorae)
Gui Zhi (Ramulus Cinnamomi Cassiae)
Sang Bai Pi (Cortex Radicis Mori Albi)
Gan Cao (Radix Glycyrrhizae Uralensis), any kind of sour agent can do [*sic*]
Mu Xiang (Radix Auklandiae Lappae)
Bin Lan (Semen Arecae Catechu)
Wu Wei Zi (Fructus Schisandrae Chinensis), the above three assistants
    remove intruding qi

Jie Geng (Radix Platycodi Grandiflori), conductor
Qing Pi (Pericarpium Citri Reticulatae Viride), to break stagnant qi

Although this formula is not one of Li's famous ones, it is an interesting one for the treatment of depression and/or chronic fatigue immune deficiency syndrome (CFIDS) where there is a liver-spleen disharmony resulting in a lung qi vacuity and some deep-lying heat in the lungs. In addition, due to the inclusion of *Mu Xiang* and *Bin Lan*, the patient may also be suffering from irritable bowel syndrome (IBS) with intestinal dysbiosis.

Kidney water rebelling against earth is a frenetic movement of the restrained. It produces drool, clear snivel, copious spittle, profuse urination, and aversion to cold. If there is retaliation between earth and fire and the two vessels [*i.e.*, the penetrating and conception vessels] are affected by evils, there will be inability of the legs to carry the body, the soles of the feet will be too painful to touch the ground, [and there will be] fatigued and weakened bones, somnolence, cold in the testicles, dull abdominal pain, confused hearing, confused vision, and pain all along the low back, spine, upper back, and scapula. Kidney water is supposed to restrain heart fire and be restrained in turn by spleen earth. If earth is insufficient and liver wood becomes pathogenic, heart fire, the mother of spleen earth, will run rampant, overwhelming earth. This is called a kind of retaliation.

Gan Jiang (dry Rhizoma Zingiberis Officinalis), sovereign
Bai Zhu (Rhizoma Atractylodis Macrocephalae)
Chuan Wu (Radix Aconiti Carmichaeli), ministers
Cang Zhu (Rhizoma Atractylodis)
Fu Zi (Radix Lateralis Praeparatus Aconiti Carmichaeli), blast-fried, a small amount
Rou Gui (Cortex Cinnamomi Cassiae), debarked, a small amount
Fu Ling (Sclerotium Poriae Cocos)
Zhu Ling (Sclerotium Polypori Umbellati), assistants
Ze Xie (Rhizoma Alismatis Orientalis), envoy

Today, we would probably describe this scenario as a spleen-kidney yang vacuity with marked cold and possible flooding of water.

After water and grain enter the stomach, yang qi moves upward. Fluids and humors plus qi enter the heart and penetrate the lungs to fill and replete [*i.e.*, replenish] the skin and hair and to scatter [or disperse] in the hundreds of vessels. The spleen is endowed with qi from the stomach to irrigate the four sides [*i.e.*, the four limbs] and to construct and nourish the qi and blood. [If] food and drink cause detriment to the stomach and taxation fatigue damages the spleen, spleen and stomach vacuity lead to fire evils overwhelming them and the engenderment of great heat. [In that case,] one should first [address] the heart aspect [or division in order to] supplement the origin of the spleen. This sentence implies draining the heart to supplement the spleen. Since earth is engendered by fire, simultaneously draining any fire within the spleen [and/or] stomach combats this. [In other words,] first one [should] treat the tip [or branch], and afterwards one should treat the root.

This is the first place in the *Pi Wei Lun* that Li states a vacuous spleen-stomach may result in some kind of heat evils and heat evils, especially associated with the heart, can damage the spleen and stomach. He will develop this idea further on. It is an important part of yin fire theory.

[If] dampness and heat mutually unite, yang qi becomes [more] vacuous day [by day]. Yang qi vacuity leads to inability of ascension and upbearing. Instead, the qi of the spleen and stomach pour downward to the liver and kidneys. This is fall and winter and no spring and summer. Spring governs upbearing and summer governs floating. Within humans, these correspond to the liver and heart, and their weakness leads to yin qi exuberance. Therefore, the yang qi does not gain the channels and constructive. The classic says:

> Yang is rooted in yin. [Therefore,] draining [any] fire within yin by upbearing and effusing with thin flavors and windy medicinals in order to extend yang qi leads to yin qi not being diseased and yang qi living [or growing].

The *Zhuan (Transmission)* states, "By honoring the end within the beginning, putting in order leads to no fault." Truly it is said.

The *Si Qi Tiao Shen Da Lun (Great Treatise on the Four Qi & the Regulation of the Spirit)* says:

> [If] heaven [is too] bright, then [neither] the sun nor moon are bright. [Thus] evils may lodge in the cavities and orifices and yang qi may become blocked and obstructed. [If] the earth emits brightness, then the clouds and mist lack essence. Correspondingly above the white dew does not descend.

In humans, this is like stomach vacuity resulting in fire assailing it. [If] the spleen is damaged by taxation fatigue, taxation leads to the consumption of qi as well as to heart fire blazing and stirring. [Then] the blood vessels may boil and cook, leading to blood disease as well as yang qi not being punished. Yin fire may also flame upward by itself arising from the cavities and orifices and resulting in singing all around the body. [In that case,] contrarily using hot medicinals in order to dry the spleen and stomach leads to one mistake on top of another.

The stomach is the pivot of the spleen, [while] the spleen is the softness of the stomach, and these are spoken of as exterior and interior. [If] food and drink are not regulated, this leads to the stomach first becoming diseased. [However,] the spleen, having no place from which [to receive] its endowment, it later becomes diseased. Taxation and fatigue first lead to spleen disease. [However, due to subsequent] inability of the stomach to move the qi, it later becomes diseased. Although there may be differences in the engenderment of disease first or later, contraction of evils by the one [eventually] leads to disease of the other.

The stomach is the sea of the 12 channels, and the 12 channels are endowed by it with their blood and qi [in order] to enrich and nourish the body. If the yang ming is involved in a disease, together with, say, the jue yin or some other channel, reasoned consideration is demanded when prescribing medication. [In weighing,] the weight should be made [correctly] at the steelyard. When [weighing things] by the *liang*, the weight should operate within the range of the *liang*. When [weighing things] by the *jin*, the weight should operate within the range of the *jin*. This allusion is given to clarify that spleen and stomach disease cannot be looked at by a fixed standard or treated by one and the same method. People should be made aware that the hundreds of diseases are all generated as a result of decrepit spleen and stomach. A miscalculation by the *li* or *hao* may incur instant disaster. One *hao* equals 1/10 *li* equals 1/1000 *qian*. Suppose a formula is composed in the season of long summer. This season is thought to be a time when the host or ruling qi is declining, while the guest qi is effulgent. Host or ruling qi refers to the prevailing weather in a certain season. The host qi for each season is the same every year. For instance, the host qi of winter is cold and the host qi of summer is hot. Guest qi refers to specific weather changes within a season, including wind, fire, great heat, dryness, and cold. Guest qi may vary in a given season from year to year. Both host and guest qi are calculated by *wu yun liu qi* or five transport, six qi theory. The formula given below [as an example], which is named *Bu Pi Wei Xie Yin Huo Sheng Yang Tang* (Supplement the Spleen & Stomach, Drain Yin Fire, & Upbear Yang Decoction), should be expanded by certain seasonal ingredients as instructed.

Bu Pi Wei Xie Yin Huo Sheng Yang Tang (Supplement the Spleen & Stomach, Drain Yin Fire & Upbear Yang Decoction)

Chai Hu (Radix Bupleuri), 1.5 *liang*, sovereign

mix-fried *Gan Cao* (Radix Glycyrrhizae Uralensis)
Huang Qi (Radix Astragali Membranacei), ministers
Cang Zhu (Rhizoma Atractylodis), soaked with rice water, stripped
    of the black skin, sliced, sun-dried, grated into dust, stir-fried
Qiang Huo (Radix Et Rhizoma Notopterygii), 1 *liang* each
Sheng Ma (Rhizoma Cimicifugae), 8 *qian*
Ren Shen (Radix Panacis Ginseng), ministers
Huang Qin (Radix Scutellariae Baicalensis), 7 *qian* each
Huang Lian (Rhizoma Coptidis Chinensis), stripped of hair, wine-
    processed, stir-fried, at once minister and assistant, 5 *qian*
Shi Gao (Gypsum Fibrosum), a small amount; use a tiny amount
    in long summer; may be removed after that time; particular
    amount at one's discretion

While this formula is not one which is commonly used today, it is the only one of Li's formulas in the *Pi Wei Lun* to contain the words "yin fire" in its name, and, in terms of its overall composition, it is emblematic of Li's style of prescription. Typical Li-Zhu formulas consist of three basic groups of medicinals. These are 1) spleen-fortifying, qi-supplementing medicinals, 2) qi-rectifying medicinals, and 3) heat-clearing medicinals. In the above formula, *Huang Qi, Ren Shen,* mix-fried *Gan Cao,* and *Cang Zhu* all fortify the spleen and supplement or boost the qi. *Chai Hu, Qiang Huo,* and *Sheng Ma* rectify the qi and upbear the clear, thus dis-inhibiting the qi mechanism. *Huang Qin, Huang Lian,* and *Shi Gao* clear heat and drain fire from the heart and stomach. As we will see below, Most Li-Zhu formulas then go on to add one more category of medicinals, *i.e.,* any other medicinals required to remedy any other simultaneously occurring disease mechanisms or to treat any main symptoms.

Slice all the above, [and take] three *qian* per dose. Boil in two cups of water down to one cupful and take while quite warm after removing the dregs between breakfast and lunch every other day. In the course of administration, it is appropriate to reduce food intake, to have delicious food, and, after taking the medicine, to refrain from talking for 1-2 watches' time [*i.e.,* several hours]. Refrain from wine, sodden wheat foods, and spices for fear that food of great dampness and heat might assist fire evils and bring detriment to the original qi again. Also keep away from cold water as well as cold or cool, bland, percolating substances and fruits for fear that yang qi should fail to engender and become effulgent. It is appropriate to have warm food and less of the tasty and flavorful. Tasty, flavorful foods refer to fatty, greasy foods. Generally speaking, this method and this formula are intended to float and upbear the yang qi. Bland, percolating, and draining flavors, which are all flavors which enrich yin, should be rigidly prohibited. It is true that they are sometimes used [in such cases] as a makeshift measure. For example, in case of effulgent kidney fire and exuberant governing, conception, and penetrating vessels, *Huang Bai* (Cortex Phellodendri) and *Zhi Mu* (Rhizoma Anemarrhenae Aspheloidis) can be used after being washed in wine and stir-fried. As to their quantities, this should depend on the particular disease. However, they cannot be administered for long for fear that yin qi will be assisted to do harm. Reddish urine or inhibited voiding can be [treated] by disinhibitors. Bound stools can be [treated] by moving medicinals. [However,] these, too, serve as nothing more than makeshift measures. When disinhibition is realized, they should be discontinued. On the other hand, if one were to abide by the food prohibitions and all edible things were prohibited, there would be nothing to nourish the stomach qi. [Therefore, in spite of the above commandments,] foods can be chosen with discretion to enrich the stomach.

There are several notable things about Li's post-formula directions. First, he implies that the medicinals alone, without dietary and lifestyle changes, cannot affect a perfect cure. Secondly, in terms of dietary therapy, he is advocating what is now known in Chinese medicine as a "clear, bland" diet. This means a relatively light diet of easily digestible foods which is not too greasy nor too spicy. In Chinese dietary therapy, there is a dichotomy between qi and *wei* or flavor. All foods have varying proportions of these two yang or yin qualities. The more flavor a food has (flavor in this technical Chinese medical sense), the more nutritious it is but also the harder to digest and the more likely to engender spleen-damaging dampness. For instance, sausage and eggs would be high in *wei* or flavor. As such, they are good for nourishing the blood and enriching yin, but, if eaten to excess, can damage the spleen-stomach. The clear bland diet also eschews alcohol or anything else made through fermentation. This includes cheese, vinegar, and breads, what Li refers to as "sodden wheat foods." These foods tend to damage the spleen and engender dampness and heat, and above, Li has pointed out how damp heat may further damage the spleen.

In effect, the clear, bland diet of Chinese medicine is very similar to Western hypoallergenic and anticandidal diets. Interestingly, almost a thousand years ago, Li recognized that one cannot be too restrictive with such diets or one is left with nothing to eat. This is a common complaint of modern patients who are put on such hypoallergenic and/or anticandidal diets. Another interesting point is Li's recognition of how draining and dispersing talking is. As mentioned above, the heart and lung qi come from the spleen, and talking consumes large amounts of heart and lung qi. Therefore, Li recommends that, to get the best effect from taking qi-supplementing medicinals, one should decrease the amount they talk.

Endnotes

[1] Wiseman & Feng give "prevalence" for *sheng*, waxing, and "debility" for *shuai*, waning.

[2] Wang Shu-he (3rd Cent. CE), author of the *Mai Jing (Pulse Classic)*, the first work in history specifically devoted to pulse diagnosis.

[3] *Ling Shu*

[4] The ingredients of this formula are: *Cang Zhu* (Rhizoma Atractylodis), *Chen Pi* (Pericarpium Citri Reticulatae), *Hou Po* (Cortex Magnoliae Officinalis), and *Gan Cao* (Radix Glycyrrhizae Uralensis).

[5] This formula is composed of: *Huang Qi* (Radix Astragali Membranacei), *Bai Shao* (Radix Albus Paeoniae Lactiflorae), *Gui Zhi* (Ramulus Cinnamomi Cassiae), mix-fried *Gan Cao* (Radix Glycyrrhizae Uralensis), *E Jiao* (Gelatinum Corii Asini), *Sheng Jiang* (uncooked Rhizoma Zingiberis Officinalis), *Da Zao* (Fructus Zizyphi Jujubae).

[6] This formula is composed of: *Dang Gui* (Radix Angelicae Sinensis), *Shu Di* (cooked Radix Rehmanniae Glutinosae), *Bai Shao* (Radix Albus Paeoniae Lactiflorae), *Chuan Xiong* (Radix Ligustici Wallichii).

[7] This formula is composed of: *Ren Shen* (Radix Panacis Ginseng), *Bai Zhu* (Rhizoma Atractylodis Macrocephalae), *Fu Ling* (Sclerotium Poriae Cocos), and mix-fried *Gan Cao* (Radix Glycyrrhizae Uralensis).

[8] This formula is composed of: *Fu Ling* (Sclerotium Poriae Cocos), *Zhu Ling* (Sclerotium Polypori Umbellati), *Bai Zhu* (Rhizoma Atractylodis Macrocephalae), *Ze Xie* (Rhizoma Alismatis Orientalis), and *Gui Zhi* (Ramulus Cinnamomi Cassiae).

[9] Zhang Zhong-jing (*circa* 150-219 CE), author of the *Shang Han Lun/Jin Gui Yao Lue (Treatise on Damage [Due to] Cold/Essentials from the Golden Cabinet)*, the pioneer work on Chinese internal medicine.

[10] The ingredients in this formula are: *Hua Shi* (Talcum) and *Gan Cao* (Radix Glycyrrhizae Uralensis) in a ratio of six to one in weight.

4
Treatise on the Lungs in Relation to Spleen-stomach Vacuity

[When] the spleen and stomach are vacuous, [there may arise] fatigue, somno-lence, and lack of reception of the four limbs [of qi and blood]. Fatigue, som-nolence, and lack of strength in the four limbs are three of the most reliable symptoms of spleen qi vacuity. If there is a little abatement of dampness and heat when autumn dryness begins to move [or prevail, there may arise] gener-alized heaviness, painful joints, a bitter [taste in] the mouth, a dry tongue, inabil-ity to taste food, unregulated defecation, frequent urination, no desire to eat, and inability to disperse [or digest] food. In this case, the generalized heaviness is due to damp encumbrance, and the painful joints are due to damp heat imped-iment. The bitter taste in the mouth is due to heat floating upward to steam the liver-gallbladder, while the dry tongue is due to heat floating upward to dam-age and consume fluids in the mouth. The frequent urination is due to an over-heated stomach sending too many fluids downward for excretion along with a vacuous spleen sending too few fluids upward for dispersal around the body by the lungs. Then the inability to taste food and lack of desire to eat further evi-dence the spleen vacuity. [These] may be accompanied by aversion to cold as after a soaking, melancholy, despondency, and a malign and inharmonious facial complexion due to a combination with lung illness. It is extremely important to understand that the lung (and heart) qi essentially comes from the spleen. Therefore, in real life, most patients who exhibit signs and symptoms of lung qi vacuity also exhibit signs and symptoms of spleen qi vacuity. Lung qi vacuity includes the respiratory qi as well as the defensive qi. All this indicates yang qi is not extending [or diffusing. Therefore,] it is necessary to upbear yang and boost the stomach [with the formula] called *Sheng Yang Yi Wei Tang* (Upbear Yang & Boost the Stomach Decoction).

Sheng Yang Yi Wei Tang (Upbear Yang & Boost the Stomach Decoction)

Huang Qi (Radix Astragali Membranacei), 2 *liang*

Ban Xia (Rhizoma Pinelliae Ternatae), washed with boiled water. This
   ingredient should (not [later editor]) be used in case of a rough [or
   choppy] pulse.
Ren Shen (Radix Panacis Ginseng), stemmed
mix-fried Gan Cao (Radix Glycyrrhizae Uralensis), 1 liang for each of the
   above
Bai Shao (Radix Albus Paeoniae Lactiflorae)
Fang Feng (Radix Ledebouriellae Divaricatae). Acrid warm should be
   employed to effectuate drainage due to effulgent autumn.
Qiang Huo (Radix Et Rhizoma Notopterygii)
Du Huo (Radix Angelicae Pubescentis), 5 qian for each of the above
Chen Pi (Pericarpium Citri Reticulatae), 4 qian
Fu Ling (Sclerotium Poriae Cocos). Do not use in case of uninhibited urine
   with no thirst.
Ze Xie (Rhizoma Alismatis Orientalis). Do not use without strangury.
Chai Hu (Radix Bupleuri)
Bai Zhu (Rhizoma Atractylodis Macrocephalae), 3 qian for each of the above
Huang Lian (Rhizoma Coptidis Chinensis), 2 qian

The reason Li says not to use Fu Ling and Ze Xie without the presence of strangury is that this formula seeks to upbear the qi from the spleen to the lungs. If
one disinhibits urination, one guides the yang qi downward into the yin tract,
i.e., the urinary tract in the lower burner. However, the main thrust of this formula seeks to lead the clear yang upward into the yang tract, the heart and
lungs. If there is strangury, such disihibition of urination is warranted. Since
upbearing and downbearing are interdependent, if turbidity is not properly
downborne, the clear cannot be properly upborne. Otherwise, disinhibition is
potentially counterproductive.

Why should the lungs be supplemented with Ren Shen, Bai Zhu, Bai Shao, and
the like when autumn is effulgent? The reason is that, since the spleen and stomach are vacuous, the lungs are what are afflicted by disease most severely of all.
Know that opportune supplementation works easily. Readers should note that
lung qi supplementing medicinals are essentially spleen-fortifying medicinals.
While, theoretically, it is possible to supplement the lungs without supplementing the spleen, in internal medicine, there is simply no other way.

This formula is still very useful today, and not just in the fall. It can be used whenever there is a liver-spleen disharmony with some element of depressive heat in
the heart and stomach complicated by wind damp impediment. It is also pro-
totypical of what I consider a Li-Zhu formula. Within it, Huang Qi, Ren Shen, Bai

Zhu, and mix-fried *Gan Cao* all fortify the spleen and supplement the qi. *Fang Feng, Ban Xia, Qiang Huo, Du Huo, Chai Hu*, and *Chen Pi* all rectify the qi and upbear the qi, thus resolving depression and disinhibiting the qi mechanism. *Huang Lian* clears heat from the heart, liver-gallbladder, and stomach. If spleen vacuity has resulted in dampness, with such symptoms as thirst and frequent and/or difficult urination, then *Fu Ling* and *Ze Xie* seep dampness and disinhibit urination. Thus these two ingredients fall under the category of doing whatever else is necessary as indicated by the presenting patterns. *Bai Shao* is a grace note to this formula. As the reader will see, Li regularly adds at least one blood-supplementing medicinal to many of his formulas. This helps nourish the liver so that the liver is empowered to control its function of coursing and discharge. Technically, the combination of liver-coursing, qi-rectifiers, and blood-supplements is called "harmonizing the liver." In addition, adding one or more blood-supplements also makes supplementing the qi more effective and efficient.

Slice all the above [and take] three *qian* per dose, boiled with 5 slices of ginger (*jiang*) and 2 cored dates (*zao*) in 3 cups of water down to 2 cupfuls. Take while warm between breakfast and lunch after removing the dregs. [Food] prohibitions are the same as above. This dosage should be gradually increased up to 5 *qian*. If, after administering this formula, the disease deteriorates following urination, disinhibition of urine is shown to be improper. [In that case,] *Fu Ling* and *Ze Xie* should be reduced a little. If there is a liking for food, do not eat to one's heart's content on the first or second day for fear that the stomach might be damaged again since the strength of the medicinals is not yet big enough for stomach qi to convey, upbear, and effuse. It is proper to have a little tasty, flavorful [food] or to have delicious food to assist the strength of the medicinals. Again, tasty, flavorful food means fatty, greasy food. This will boost the upbearing and floating qi and hence enrich the stomach qi. Be careful not to take bland-flavored food. This will reduce the strength of the medicinals and help the evil qi (evil qi must have been mistakenly used in place of stomach qi [later editor]) downbear and sink.

Bland foods tend to seep dampness and disinhibit urination. Because the yang qi both moves and follows water fluids, this downward movement of fluids also leads the yang qi to move downward at a time when the emphasis should be on its upbearing and floating or ascending.

The formal body can be worked [*i.e.*, exercised] some in order to help the stomach and medicinals convey, upbear, and emit. Physical exercise moves the qi and, therefore, helps disinhibit the qi mechanism. Thus a moderate amount of physical exercise helps the spleen-stomach recuperate. [But] be careful not to tax the body too much and thus incur new damage. However, too much exercise results in overconsumption of the qi and blood. Since the spleen is the root of qi and blood engenderment and transformation, such overconsumption or taxation damages the spleen. It is much better if the spleen and stomach obtain quiet and stillness [or rest]. When the stomach qi is commonly a little stronger, a small amount of fruit can be eaten to assist the strength of grains and medicinals. The classic states, "The five grains are [the main] nourishment, while the five fruits assist them."[1]

Chinese have long believed that cereals are the foundation of the human diet. However, this belief may be a cultural artifact based on genetic predisposition. In other words, it may not be a universal truth. Other human gene pools may not metabolize cereals the same way as the Chinese. Therefore, one needs to be careful not to take everything Li says at face value.

REPRESENTATIVE CASE HISTORIES:

From "New Uses of *Sheng Yang Yi Wei Tang* (Upbear Yang & Boost the Stomach Decoction)" by Chen Hai-zhao *et al.*, *Xin Zhong Yi (New Chinese Medicine)*, #1, 2004, p. 69-70

CASE 1: Chronic fatigue syndrome

The patient was a 44 year-old male who was first examined on Jan. 5, 2002. For the last year, the man had been under a lot of stress and had become excessively fatigued. Gradually, he had lost strength throughout his body. His four limbs were sore and painful. He had difficulty relaxing. There was heat in the centers of his palms and soles. His memory had gotten worse. He was dizzy and had headaches. In addition, his appetite was poor, he had difficulty sleeping and profuse dreams, and his stools were sometimes loose. The man's tongue was pale with white, slimy fur, and his pulse was soggy. Electrocardiogram, liver and kidney function tests, and CT scan all ruled out organic disease. Therefore, the man was diagnosed with chronic fatigue syndrome. The treatment principles were to fortify the spleen and boost the qi, boost the stomach and upbear yang, and the formula employed consisted of *Sheng Yang Yi Wei Tang*: *Huang Qi* (Radix Astragali Membranacei) and *Fu Ling* (Sclerotium Poriae Cocos), 20g each, *Dang Shen* (Radix Codonopsitis Pilosulae), *Ze Xie* (Rhizoma Alismatis Orientalis), and stir-fried *Bai Zhu* (Rhizoma Atractylodis Macrocephalae), 30g each, *Chen Pi* (Pericarpium Citri Reticulatae) and *Bai Shao* (Radix Albus Paeoniae Lactiflorae), 15g each, *Ban Xia* (Rhizoma Pinelliae Ternatae), 12g, *Chai Hu* (Radix Bupleuri), *Qiang Huo* (Radix Et Rhizoma

Notopterygii), *Du Huo* (Radix Angelicae Pubescentis), *Fang Feng* (Radix Ledebouriellae Divaricatae), *Huang Lian* (Rhizoma Coptidis Chinensis), and mix-fried *Gan Cao* (Radix Glycyrrhizae Uralensis), 10g each. One packet of these medicinals was decocted in water and administered per day in two divided doses. After taking 21 packets, the man's lack of strength and encumbered limbs had disappeared and his eating and sleep had returned to normal. The patient was counseled to limit his fatigue and get adequate rest.

CASE 2: Emotional depression

The patient was a 17 year-old male who was initially examined on May 30, 2001. Recently this young man had been under a lot of stress. Therefore, he had become depressed and seldom spoke. He said he felt as if his brain was reacting slowly and that his whole body lacked strength. His memory was poor and his grades had also deteriorated. The patient seemed listless, his appetite was poor, and he reported that he had lost one kilogram of weight over the last month. In addition, his sleep was poor. This meant that going to sleep was difficult and the patient was easily wakened. His tongue was pale with thick, slimy, white fur, and his pulse was deep and fine. After being diagnosed as depressed, his pattern was discriminated as too much worry and thinking damaging the spleen with spleen vacuity and damp encumbrance. Thus the treatment principles were to fortify the spleen and transform dampness, boost the qi and upbear yang. The formula employed was *Sheng Yang Yi Wei Tang* with additions and subtractions: *Huang Qi* (Radix Astragali Membranacei), stir-fried *Bai Zhu* (Rhizoma Atractylodis Macrocephalae), *Ze Xie* (Rhizoma Alismatis Orientalis), and *Dang Shen* (Radix Codonopsitis Pilosulae), 30g each, *Fu Ling* (Sclerotium Poriae Cocos), 20g, *Chen Pi* (Pericarpium Citri Reticulatae), *Ban Xia* (Rhizoma Pinelliae Ternatae), and *Bai Shao* (Radix Albus Paeoniae Lactiflorae), 15g each, *Chai Hu* (Radix Bupleuri), *Sheng Ma* (Rhizoma Cimicifugae), *Qiang Huo* (Radix Et Rhizoma Notopterygii), *Fang Feng* (Radix Ledebouriellae Divaricatae), *Huang Lian* (Rhizoma Coptidis Chinensis), and mix-fried *Gan Cao* (Radix Glycyrrhizae Uralensis), 10g each. One packet of these medicinals was decocted in water and administered per day. After one continuous month of administration, accompanied by less time each day studying, the young man's symptoms all remitted and he was judged cured.

CASE 3: Spontaneous perspiration

The patient was a 35 year-old male who was first seen on Oct. 10, 2001. The man said that, when he exerted himself, he sweated profusely. However, now, even with slight exertion he was sweating more and that he easily caught cold. He had already been given *Yu Ping Feng San* (Jade Windscreen Powder) and other such formulas but without any obvious change for the better. At the time of examination, there was spontaneous perspiration, aversion to wind, chilled extremities, lack of strength, a pale tongue with thin, white fur, and a deep, fine pulse. Therefore, the man was diagnosed with exterior vacuity spontaneous perspiration. The treatment principles were to warm the kidneys and fortify the spleen, boost the qi and secure the exterior, and the formula used was *Sheng Yang Yi Wei Tang* with additions and subtractions: *Huang Qi* (Radix Astragali Membranacei), stir-fried *Bai Zhu* (Rhizoma Atractylodis Macrocephalae), and *Dang Shen* (Radix Codonopsitis Pilosulae), 30g each, *Fu Ling* (Sclerotium Poriae Cocos) and *Ze Xie* (Rhizoma Alismatis Orientalis), 20g each, *Chen Pi* (Pericarpium Citri Reticulatae) and *Bai Shao* (Radix Albus Paeoniae Lactiflorae), 15g each, *Ban Xia* (Rhizoma Pinelliae Ternatae), 12g, *Chai Hu* (Radix Bupleuri), *Qiang Huo* (Radix Et Rhizoma Notopterygii), *Fang Feng* (Radix Ledebouriellae Divaricatae), *Du Huo* (Radix Angelicae Pubescentis), *Rou Gui* (Cortex Cinnamomi Cassiae), *Fu Zi* (Radix Lateralis Praeparatus Aconiti Carmichaeli), and mix-fried *Gan Cao* (Radix Glycyrrhizae Uralensis), 10g each. One packet of these medicinals was decocted in water and administered per day in two divided doses. After taking these medicinals for one month, the sweating and aversion to wind had markedly decreased. After taking the same prescription for another month, all the symptoms had completely disappeared. Therefore, the man was prescribed *Bu Zhong Yi Qi Wan* (Supplement the Center & Boost the Qi Pills) along with *Jin Gui Shen Qi Wan* (*Golden Cabinet Kidney Qi Pills*) for one year. At the end of one year, the man returned for a follow-up examination. During that time, none of his symptoms had recurred and his bodily constitution was much improved overall.

From *Ming Fang Xin Yong (Famous Formulas, New Uses)* by Wang Xin-min & Han Guan-xian, Chinese National Chinese Medicine & Medicinals Press, Beijing, 1998, p. 191-194

CASE 4: Leukorrhea

The patient was a 37 year-old female who had continuous abnormal vaginal discharge which was clear in consistency and slightly malodorous. The patient had already taken hundreds of packets of Chinese medicinals without effect. When she had taken 15 packets of *Wan Dai Tang* (End Vaginal Discharge Decoction), this had actually made her symptoms worse. At the time of examination, there was a white facial complexion, lassitude of the spirit, decreased appetite, loose stools, fatigued limbs, occasionally a feeling of qi falling, a pale tongue with white fur, and a fine, weak pulse. Based on these signs and symptoms, it was determined that the woman suffered from non-upbearing of clear yang with spleen dampness pouring downward. Therefore, she was prescribed the following version of *Sheng Yang Yi Wei Tang*: *Huang Qi* (Radix Astragali Membranacei), 30g, *Qian Shi* (Semen Euryalis Ferocis) and *Hong Shen* (Radix Rubrus Panacis Ginseng), 20g each, *Bai Zhu* (Rhizoma Atractylodis Macrocephalae), *Fu Ling* (Sclerotium Poriae Cocos), and *Ze Xie* (Rhizoma Alismatis Orientalis), 12g each, lime-processed *Ban Xia* (Rhizoma Pinelliae Ternatae), *Chen Pi* (Pericarpium Citri Reticulatae), *Fang Feng* (Radix Ledebouriellae Divaricatae), *Qiang Huo* (Radix Et Rhizoma Notopterygii), *Du Huo* (Radix Angelicae Pubescentis), and *Bai Shao* (Radix Albus Paeoniae Lactiflorae), 10g each, *Chai Hu* (Radix Bupleuri) and mix-fried *Gan Cao* (Radix Glycyrrhizae Uralensis), 6g each, *Huang Lian* (Rhizoma Coptidis Chinensis), 3g, *Da Zao* (Fructus Zizyphi Jujubae), 6 pieces, and *Sheng Jiang* (uncooked Rhizoma Zingiberis Officinalis), 3 slices. Three packets were prescribed, one packet to be decocted in water and administered per day. After taking these medicinals, the patient's leukorrhea was reduced by half and her mood had improved. Therefore, another 10 packets of the above formula were administered plus 15 grams each of *Shan Yao* (Radix Dioscoreae Oppositae) and *Jin Ying Zi* (Fructus Rosae Laevigatae). At this point the woman's leukorrhea was cured. In addition to the above treatment methods, kidney-supplementing medicinals were administered in pill form. On follow-up after three years, there had been no recurrence and the woman's health was normal.

CASE 5: Urticaria

The patient was a 36 year-old male with urticaria and itching which was sometimes better and sometimes worse. The man had been treated with both Chinese and Western medicines for half a year with small results. In fact, his symptoms had increased when he had taken 24 packets of *Xiao Feng San* (Disperse Wind Powder). At the time of examination, there were wheals on one side of his body which were more extreme on his extremities. These wheals varied in size from as small as a bean to as large as the palm of a hand. They were pale red in color and itched severely. In addition, the man complained of abdominal pain, loose stools, and spontaneous perspiration. His tongue was covered in thick, white fur, and his pulse was fine and weak. Therefore, his pattern was categorized as non-upbearing of the spleen and stomach clear yang, disharmony of the constructive and defensive, and wind damp depressed and stagnant in the interstices. The formula prescribed consisted of: *Huang Qi* (Radix Astragali Membranacei), 20g, *Dang Shen* (Radix Codonopsitis Pilosulae), *Bai Zhu* (Rhizoma Atractylodis Macrocephalae), *Fu Ling* (Sclerotium Poriae Cocos), *Fang Feng* (Radix Ledebouriellae Divaricatae), *Qiang Huo* (Radix Et Rhizoma Notopterygii), *Bai Ji Li* (Fructus Tribuli Terrestris), and *Bai Shao* (Radix Albus Paeoniae Lactiflorae), 15g each, *Ban Xia* (Rhizoma Pinelliae Ternatae), *Chen Pi* (Pericarpium Citri Reticulatae), *Ze Xie* (Rhizoma

Alismatis Orientalis), and *Gui Zhi* (Ramulus Cinnamomi Cassiae), 12g each, mix-fried *Gan Cao* (Radix Glycyrrhizae Uralensis), 8g, *Chai Hu* (Radix Bupleuri), 6g, *Da Zao* (Fructus Zizyphi Jujubae), 5 pieces, and *Sheng Jiang* (uncooked Rhizoma Zingiberis Officinalis), 3 slices. After taking five packets of these medicinals, the rash had decreased by 80%. Therefore, 15 grams each of *Ji Xue Teng* (Caulis Milletiae Seu Spatholobi) and *Dan Shen* (Radix Salviae Miltiorrhizae) and 20 grams each of *Yi Yi Ren* (Semen Coicis Lachryma-jobi) and *Bai Bian Dou* (Semen Dolichoris Lablab) were added to the original formula and another 10 packets were prescribed. At the end of this time, the rash was completely eliminated. On follow-up after two years, there had been no recurrence.

CASE 6: Chronic cough

The patient was a 79 year-old male. After catching a cold, the man had developed a continuous cough which previous long-term treatment had failed to cure. The man had frequent recurrent bouts of coughing with profuse phlegm which was easy to expectorate. In addition, there was lassitude of the spirit, spontaneous perspiration, loose stools, qi sagging, white, slimy tongue fur, and a fine, slippery pulse. Whenever the man urinated, he would cough. His four limbs were also encumbered and fatigued. Based on these findings, the patient's pattern was categorized as downward falling of the clear yang, and *Sheng Yang Yi Wei Tang* with additions and subtractions was prescribed: *Huang Qi* (Radix Astragali Membranacei), 30g, *Dang Shen* (Radix Codonopsitis Pilosulae), *Bai Zhu* (Rhizoma Atractylodis Macrocephalae), and *Fu Ling* (Sclerotium Poriae Cocos), 15g each, *Gui Zhi* (Ramulus Cinnamomi Cassiae), *Ban Xia* (Rhizoma Pinelliae Ternatae), *Ze Xie* (Rhizoma Alismatis Orientalis), *Hong Shen* (Radix Rubrus Panacis Ginseng), 12g each, *Qiang Huo* (Radix Et Rhizoma Notopterygii), *Du Huo* (Radix Angelicae Pubescentis), *Fang Feng* (Radix Ledebouriellae Divaricatae), *Bai Shao* (Radix Albus Paeoniae Lactiflorae), and *Wu Mei* (Fructus Pruni Mume), 10g each, mix-fried *Gan Cao* (Radix Glycyrrhizae Uralensis), 8g, *Chai Hu* (Radix Bupleuri) and *Wu Wei Zi* (Fructus Schisandrae Chinensis), 6g each, *Yi Yi Ren* (Semen Coicis Lachryma- jobi), 20g, *Da Zao* (Fructus Zizyphi Jujubae), 6 pieces, and *Sheng Jiang* (uncooked Rhizoma Zingiberis Officinalis), 5 slices. After taking four packets of these medicinals, the man's cough was reduced by half, his slimy tongue further had gradually improved, and his sleep and eating were good. Therefore, 12 grams each of *Zi Wan* (Radix Asteris Tatarici) and *Bai Bu* (Radix Stemonae) were added to the above formula. After taking eight packets of this, the patient was cured. The previous formula plus *Ji Nei Jin* (Endothelium Corneum Gigeriae Galli) was made into pills which the man took three times per day. On follow-up after one year, the man was healthy and fit and there had been no recurrence of the cough.

Case 7: Purpuric nephritis

The patient was a 20 year-old male who had been diagnosed with purpuric nephritis seven months previously. He had been treated with prednisone which had remitted his condition. However, when he discontinued this treatment, the condition returned. When he again used steroids, there was no good effect. Therefore, the previous doctor treated the man with heat-clearing, blood-cooling medicinals but also without effect. At the time of his examination, there was generalized skin purpura which was relatively worse on the young man's limbs and chest. The color of the lesions was dark red. In addition, there was facial edema, lassitude of the spirit, abdominal distention, torpid intake, occasional nausea, loose stools, common low-grade fever, double plus albuminuria and red blood cells in the urine, normal kidney function, a pale, fat, tender tongue with slightly slimy, white fur, and a deep, moderate (or slightly slow) pulse. Based on these signs and symptoms, the patient's pattern was categorized as spleen-stomach vacuity weakness with non-upbearing of the clear yang resulting in damp heat and loss of containment of the blood. Therefore, *Sheng Yang Yi Wei Tang* was prescribed minus *Bai Shao* (Radix Albus Paeoniae Lactiflorae) and mix-fried *Gan Cao* (Radix Glycyrrhizae Uralensis) but plus 20 grams of stir-fried *Mei Gui Hua* (Flos Rosae Rugosae), 15 grams of carbonized *Pu Huang* (Pollen Typhae), and 10 grams each of *Huo Xiang* (Herba Agastachis Seu Pogostemi) and *Bai Mao Gen* (Rhizoma Imperatae Cylindricae). One packet of these medicinals was decocted in water and administered per day, and, after taking 30 packets,, the low- grade fever had abated, the purpura had dispersed, the young man's appetite had increased, and his urine had turned pale. Albuminuria was plus or minus (±), white blood cells were negative, but there were still RBCs in the urine. The patient continued taking the same formula for another half month to secure and consolidate the treatment effects. On follow-up after six months, there had been no recurrence.

CASE 8: Recalcitrant eczema

The patient was a 42 year-old male who had had eczema on his upper arms, face, neck, and upper back for one month. Prior treatment had been ineffective. At the present time, there was a red maculopapular rash followed by water blisters and ulceration. Bathing this rash in hot water felt good. The man's facial complexion was somber and lusterless, his body was emaciated, and there was lassitude of the spirit. In addition, there was torpid intake, abdominal distention, loose stools, thin, slimy tongue fur, and a fine, slippery pulse. In this case, spleen-stomach vacuity weakness had led to lung qi not being full with resultant loss of security of the defensive exterior. External wind damp heat evil toxins had taken advantage of this vacuity to enter and lodge in the skin. Therefore, the following medicinals were prescribed based on the principles of regulating and rectifying the spleen and stomach, filling the constructive and defensive, upbearing yang, and scattering wind: uncooked *Huang Qi* (Radix Astragali Membranacei), *Dang Shen* (Radix Codonopsitis Pilosulae), and *Fu Ling* (Sclerotium Poriae Cocos), 15g each, *Hu Huang Lian* (Rhizoma Picrorrhizae) and *Chen Pi* (Pericarpium Citri Reticulatae), 5g each, *Bai Zhu* (Rhizoma Atractylodis Macrocephalae) and *Chi Shao* (Radix Rubrus Paeoniae Lactiflorae), 10g each, *Di Fu Zi* (Fructus Kochiae Scopariae), 30g, and *Fang Feng* (Radix Ledebouriellae Divaricatae), *Chai Hu* (Radix Bupleuri), *Qiang Huo* (Radix Et Rhizoma Notopterygii), *Du Huo* (Radix Angelicae Pubescentis), and uncooked *Gan Cao* (Radix Glycyrrhizae Uralensis), 6g each. After taking five packets of these medicinals, the patient's itching had decreased, the maculopapular lesions had receded, and the pustulation had stopped. Another 10 packets of the original formula were prescribed and all the man's symptoms were cured.

CASE 9: Dizziness

The patient was a 50 year-old male who had been dizzy and had had vertigo for more than one year. His blood pressure was 16/9.7kPa and his ECG and blood work were both normal. The patient had been treated with various medicines, but none had been effective. Each time the man got fatigued he would have a bout of dizziness and vertigo. His facial complexion was somber white, his intake was torpid, and there was lassitude of the spirit. Stirring or movement led to shortness of breath. There was also a pale tongue with thin fur and a fine, weak pulse. All this was due to qi vacuity falling downward, non-upbearing of the clear yang, and malnourishment of the brain. Therefore, *Sheng Yang Yi Wei Tang* minus *Ze Xie* (Rhizoma Alismatis Orientalis) and *Huang Lian* (Rhizoma Coptidis Chinensis) but plus one horn or piece of green *He Ye* (Folium Nelumbinis Nuciferae) was prescribed. After 15 packets, the dizziness and vertigo were stabilized. So another 10 packets were administered and all the symptoms were alleviated. On follow-up after one year, there had been no recurrence.

Endnote

[1] *Su Wen*, Ch. 22

5

Rules Concerning Sovereign, Minister, Assistant, & Envoy

The *Zhi Zhen Yao Da Lun (Great Treatise on What is Consummately True & Essential)* states, "It is treatment that governs whether [a medicinal] is toxic or nontoxic."[1] This statement is especially relevant in this day when there is excessive concern over the potential toxicity of Chinese medicinals. Whether an ingredient is toxic or nontoxic depends on how it is used, and this includes its dosage and combinations, not just its indications and contraindications. [The ingredient] which governs the disease is the sovereign. That which assists the sovereign is the minister, and that which responds to [or is at the service of] the minister is the envoy. According to another rule, that which is the biggest in strength is the sovereign.

Regarding the use of medicinals, the ruling [factor] is always their qi and flavor. Qi and *wei* or flavor are a yin/yang dichotomy. Every food or medicinal may be said to possess either more or less of these two qualities. Qi is light and more airy. *Wei* or flavor is denser and heavier. Supplementation and drainage depend on flavor. Qi should be varied in accordance with seasons. The qi that is thin is yin within yang, [while] the qi that is thick is yang within yang. The flavor that is thin is yang within yin, [while] the flavor that is thick is yin within yin. Acrid, sweet, and bland [medicinals] which are hot are yang within yang, [while] acrid, sweet, and bland [medicinals] which are cold are yin within yang. Sour, bitter, and salty [medicinals] which are cold are yin within yin, [while] sour, bitter, and salty [medicinals] which are hot are yang within yin. Acrid, sweet, bland, sour, bitter, and salty are [classified as] yin and yang in terms of flavor and so are they in terms of earth. Warm, cool, cold, and hot are [classified as] yin and yang in terms of qi and so are they in terms of heaven. The mechanism of creation and transformation of yin and yang resides in the [mutual] engenderment and production between qi and flavor. A single substance has simultaneously qi and flavor, and in one medicinal are seen both principle and nature. From these come [a medicinal's] indications and therapeutic effects.

This is a theoretical statement of Jin-Yuan doctors' application of yin-yang, five phase, five transport, and six qi theories to the practice of Chinese herbal medicine. This, in turn, was an outgrowth of Song dynasty Neoconfucianism. For instance, the word *li* or "principle" in the above passage has Neoconfucian connotations. While all this extension of systematic correspondences to the realm of herbal medicine was obviously very important to these Jin-Yuan doctors, it is, in my opinion, the least important of their insights and the most dubious in utility when it comes to clinical practice. Therefore, I caution readers not to make too much of all of this.

For example, *Ma Huang* (Herba Ephedrae) and *Ge Gen* (Radix Puerariae) [for] exterior repletion; *Gui Zhi* (Ramulus Cinnamomi Cassiae) and *Huang Qi* (Radix Astragali Membranacei) [for] exterior vacuity; *Zhi Shi* (Fructus Immaturus Citri Aurantii) and *Da Huang* (Radix Et Rhizoma Rhei) [for] interior repletion; *Ren Shen* (Radix Panacis Ginseng) and *Bai Shao* (Radix Albus Paeoniae Lactiflorae) [for] interior vacuity; *Huang Qin* (Radix Scutellariae Baicalensis) and *Huang Lian* (Rhizoma Coptidis Chinensis) [for] heat; and *Gan Jiang* (dry Rhizoma Zingiberis Officinalis) and *Fu Zi* (Radix Lateralis Praeparatus Aconiti Carmichaeli) [for] cold, serve as sovereigns. The sovereign should be the largest in quantity, the minister is the second largest, and the envoy is again next [in quantity]. The minister should never be allowed to surpass the sovereign [in quantity]. When the sovereign and the minister are balanced to diffuse and contain in cooperation, they are able to resist evils and eliminate disease. Here these two treatment methods, diffusion and containment, are used in a broad sense. They merely imply synergism between yin and yang in treatment. The *Shang Han Lun* (*Treatise on Damage [Due to] Cold*) states, "If the yang pulse is rough [or choppy] and the yin pulse is bowstring, there must be acute abdominal pain." [In this case,] *Bai Shao* (Radix Albus Paeoniae Lactiflorae), which with its sourness drains the liver wood from earth, serves as the sovereign. *Yi Tang* (Maltose) and mix-fried *Gan Cao* (Radix Glycyrrhizae Uralensis), which sweetly and warmly supplement the spleen and nourish the stomach, are the ministers. If, by the strength of wood, water also rebels against earth, the pulse will be bowstring and there will be abdominal pain. [In that case,] *Rou Gui* (Cortex Cinnamomi Cassiae) with its intense acridity and heat can assist *Bai Shao* in beating back cold water. *Jiang* (Rhizoma Zingiberis Officinalis) and *Zao* (Fructus Zizyphi Jujubae), sweet, acrid, and warm, perfuse and dissipate yang qi, making it move in the channels and vessels, the skin and the hair. They also serve as envoys. Thus it is easy to see why this [formula] is named "fortify the center (*jian zhong*)." [Likewise, a formula] may be moderating and intensifying, collecting and dissipating, upbearing and downbearing, floating and sinking, astringing and disinhibiting [at the same time] and also allow for variation. Below is a method for modifying [this formula] in accordance [with the patient's signs].

In fact, Li was a master of composing formulas which combined hot and cold medicinals, supplementing and draining medicinals, ascending and descending medicinals, and moistening and drying medicinals all at the same time. This is exactly what is necessary nine times out of 10 in real-life clinical practice when dealing with the multi-pattern presentations which are the norm in chronic, enduring diseases. And it is to help teach exactly this that I have taken the time and the risk to re-edit and comment on this pre-eminent classic.

[In case of] aching, distended skin and hair, muscles and flesh, absence of great heat, inability to eat, and thirst, add *Ge Gen* (Radix Puerariae), five *qian*. [In case of] dry heat and upsurging of stomach qi, an affection of counterflow of the penetrating vessel or of qi counterflow [symptoms of which include belching and hiccup], plus abdominal urgency, add stir-fried *Huang Bai* (Cortex Phellodendri) and *Zhi Mu* (Rhizoma Anemarrhenae Aspheloidis). [In case of] a sensation of heat in the chest without thirst, add stir-fried *Huang Qin* (Radix Scutellariae Baicalensis). [In case of] binding and inhibited qi in the chest [with symptoms of glomus, fullness, and inhibited breathing] or hot disease, also add this. [In case of] low food intake and scanty urination due to insufficient fluids, do not use disinhibition. Free flow will be naturally reestablished through boosting the qi and supplementing the stomach.

[In case of] weak qi and shortness of breath, add *Ren Shen* (Radix Panacis Ginseng). However, merely using a yang-upbearing formula to assist yang is much better than adding *Ren Shen*. It is possible that there are some misprints in this sentence which might better be understood as follows: Merely using a yang-upbearing formula to assist yang is good, but it is still better if *Ren Shen* is added. For aversion to cold, fever, agitation, and thirst with a large, surging pulse, *Bai Hu Tang* (White Tiger Decoction) is effective.[2] In case of dyspnea, in addition add *Ren Shen* (Radix Panacis Ginseng). In case of incessant thirst, *Han Shui Shi* (Calcitum) and *Shi Gao* (Gypsum Fibrosum) can be used in equal yet small amounts. This in fact is Qian's *Gan Lu San* (Sweet Dew Powder)[3] which is mainly effective against generalized intense fever with frequent urination or urination upon drinking, [a pattern of] dry heat. [In case of] qi dryness [or lung qi vacuity dryness, *i.e.,* upper buner wasting thirst], add *Bai Kui Hua* (white Flos Altheae Roseae). [In case of] blood dryness [or kidney yin vacuity dryness, *i.e.,* lower burner wasting thirst with copious urination], add *Chi Kui Hua* (red Flos Altheae Roseae). In case of bowstring pulse, simply add wind medicinals. Do not use *Wu Ling San* (Five [Ingredients] Poria Powder).[4] If urination is not inhibited but the disease deteriorates, fluids have dried up internally and cannot be collected. [Therefore,] it is necessary to rescue fluids by adding stir-fried *Huang Bai* (Cortex Phellodendri) and *Chi Kui Hua* (red Flos Altheae Roseae).

In case of glomus and oppression below the heart, add *Huang Lian* (Rhizoma Coptidis Chinensis) and *Huang Qin* (Radix Scutellariae Baicalensis) in a ratio of one to three and reduce the various sweet ingredients.

Inability to eat and softness (hardness [later editor]) with glomus below the heart can be cured with *Gan Cao Xie Xin Tang* (Licorice Drain the Heart Decoction).[5] (Glomus is of nine types, for which Zhong-jing's five heart-draining decoctions are the remedies. The five heart-draining decoctions are: *Gan Cao Xie Xin Tang* (Licorice Drain the Heart Decoction), *Ban Xia Xie Xin Tang* (Pinellia Drain the Heart Decoction), *Da Huang Xie Xin Tang* (Rhubarb Drain the Heart Decoction), *Fu Zi Xie Xin Tang* (Aconite Drain the Heart Decoction), and *Sheng Jiang Xie Xin Tang* (Uncooked Ginger Drain the Heart Decoction). [Later editor]) [In case of] dyspnea and fullness, add mixed-fried *Hou Po* (Cortex Magnoliae Officinalis). [In case of] stomach vacuity weakness with glomus, add *Gan Cao* (Radix Glycyrrhizae Uralensis). [In case of] dyspnea with inhibited urination, add bitter *Ting Li Zi* (Semen Lepidii Seu Descurainiae). (This is used if there is inhibited urination but is prohibited if urination is not inhibited. [Later editor]) [In case of] shortness of breath, weak qi, and slight abdominal fullness, do not omit *Ren Shen* (Radix Panacis Ginseng) but remove *Gan Cao* (Radix Glycyrrhizae Uralensis) and add *Hou Po* (Cortex Magnoliae Officinalis). This is, however, not [necessarily] better than draining with bitter medicinals which will not result in loose bowels.

[In case of] slight abdominal fullness with qi not rolling in addition to fullness of the middle, remove *Gan Cao* (Radix Glycyrrhizae Uralensis), double the amount of *Huang Lian* (Rhizoma Coptidis Chinensis), add *Huang Bai* (Cortex Phellodendri) and a small amount of the triplet contained in *Wu Ling San* (Five [Ingredients] Poria Powder). *I.e., Fu Ling* (Sclerotium Poriae Cocos), *Zhu Ling* (Sclerotium Polypori Umbellati), and *Ze Xie* (Rhizoma Alismatis Orientalis). Although this disease calls for upbearing and promoting perspiration, sweating, if profuse, may lead to collapse of yang. In this case, *Huang Qin* (Radix Scutellariae Baicalensis) (*Huang Qi*, Radix Astragali Membranacei [later editor]) should be added. In my opinion, *Huang Qi* is correct here. *Huang Qin* does not make any particular sense clinically.

Distressing heat in the limbs and hot muscles can be cured by administering *Qiang Huo* (Radix Et Rhizoma Notopterygii), *Chai Hu* (Radix Bupleuri), *Sheng Ma* (Rhizoma Cimicifugae), *Ge Gen* (Radix Puerariae), and *Gan Cao* (Radix Glycyrrhizae Uralensis). In case of clear nasal mucus, aversion to wind, or rigidity and pain in the neck, upper back, spine, and paravertebral muscles, *Qiang Huo* (Radix Notopterygii), *Fang Feng* (Radix Ledebouriellae Divaricatae), and *Gan Cao* (Radix Glycyrrhizae Uralensis) in equal amounts and *Huang Qi* (Radix

Astragali Membranacei) in double amount should be taken before sleep. [If there is] high fever with a large, surging pulse and the fever refuses to break despite the use of a bitter, cold formula, add *Shi Gao* (Gypsum Fibrosum).

[If there is] heat in the spleen and stomach, add stir-fried *Huang Lian* (Rhizoma Coptidis Chinensis) and *Gan Cao* (Radix Glycyrrhizae Uralensis). In order to treat such a disease with a rapid pulse, one should use *Huang Bai* (Cortex Phellodendri) or a small amount of *Huang Lian* (Rhizoma Coptidis Chinensis) together with *Chai Hu* (Radix Bupleuri), *Cang Zhu* (Rhizoma Atractylodis), *Huang Qi* (Radix Astragali Membranacei), *Gan Cao* (Radix Glycyrrhizae Uralensis), and particularly *Sheng Ma* (Rhizoma Cimicifugae). As soon as one sweats, the pulse will surely slow down, since depressive fire is dissipated. If the signs are relieved but the pulse remains [persistently] rapid, not surging or large but racing and strong, reduce the bitter ingredients considerably and add *Shi Gao* (Gypsum Fibrosum).

[In case of] soft stools or diarrhea, add *Jie Geng* (Radix Platycodi Grandiflori) and take after meals. Some readers may be puzzled by this use of *Jie Geng*. However, as used in Li-Zhu medicine, *Jie Geng* is an upbearing medicinal, and diarrhea, in this case, is due to lack of upbearing of the clear with the clear falling downward. This medicinal, if misused, can do no small harm. [Therefore,] the physician should deliberate over its use and increase its amount little by little. I have never seen this said before. What I do know is that my teacher, Dr. Yu Min of the Yueyang Hospital in Shanghai, did not like this medicinal and routinely took it out of her formulas unless it was absolutely indicated. When asked why she did this, her reply was that her teacher had not liked this medicinal. Perhaps this dislike of *Jie Geng* by Dr. Yu and her teacher stemmed from Li's opinion expressed here.

[In case of] low food intake, do not use *Shi Gao* (Gypsum Fibrosum). It is strong in mollifying a rapid, racing pulse. If the disease is eliminated but the pulse remains rapid, this indicates incurability. In the absence of great thirst, do not use it either. A bowstring as well as rapid pulse are [due to] yin qi [*i.e.*, effulgent yin fire]. When windy medicinals upbear yang to out-thrust [or perfuse] depressive fire, the rapid pulse will be mollified drastically. The above five rules for additions and subtractions are not [categorically] comprehensive. They are only presented to give a general idea.

The idea that a bowstring, rapid pulse is an indicator of yin fire is an important one. A rapid, bowstring pulse is commonly seen in clinical practice. In standard professional Chinese medicine, it mostly means depressive heat (*i.e.*, liver depression transforming heat). In this case, there commonly is concomitant spleen vacuity. This spleen vacuity may or may not manifest independently on the pulse at the right bar. Therefore, whenever practitioners feel a bowstring, rapid pulse, one should consider the presence of a yin fire scenario.

Endnotes

[1] *Su Wen*, Ch. 74

[2] This formula is composed of *Shi Gao* (Gypsum Fibrosum), *Zhi Mu* (Rhizoma Anemarrhena Aspheloidis), *Gan Cao* (Radix Glycyrrhizae Uralensis), and *Jing Mi* (Semen Oryzae Sativae).

[3] The ingredients of this formula composed by Qian Yi include: *Han Shui Shi* (Calcitum), *Shi Gao* (Gypsum Fibrosum), and *Gan Cao* (Radix Glycyrryhizae Uralensis).

[4] This formula is composed of *Fu Ling* (Sclerotium Poriae Cocos), *Zhu Ling* (Sclerotium Polypori Umbellati), *Bai Zhu* (Rhizoma Atractylodis Macrocephalae), *Ze Xie* (Rhizoma Alismatis Orientalis), and *Gui Zhi* (Ramulus Cinnamomi Cassiae).

[5] This formula is composed of: mix-fried *Gan Cao* (Radix Glycyrrhizae Uralensis), *Huang Qin* (Radix Scutellariae Baicalensis), *Huang Lian* (Rhizoma Coptidis Chinensis), *Gan Jiang* (dry Rhizoma Zingiberis Officinalis), *Ban Xia* (Rhizoma Pinelliae Ternatae), and *Da Zao* (Fructus Zizyphi Jujubae).

6

Composing Formulas [Based on] the Division of Channels & Following the Diseases

The *Mai Jing (Pulse Classic)*[1] states that [contraction of] wind cold with perspiration, pain in the shoulders and back, wind stroke [*i.e.*, cold or flu], and frequent voiding of scanty urine are [due to] wind heat overwhelming the lungs and seriously depressing the lung qi. [In this case,] one should drain wind heat with *Tong Qi Fang Feng Tang* (Free the Flow of the Qi Ledebouriella Decoction).

Tong Qi Fang Feng Tang
(Free the Flow of the Qi Ledebouriella Decoction)

Chai Hu (Radix Bupleuri)
Sheng Ma (Rhizoma Cimicifugae)
Huang Qi (Radix Astragali Membranacei), 1 *liang* for each of the above
Qiang Huo (Radix Et Rhizoma Notopterygii)
Fang Feng (Radix Ledebouriellae Divaricatae)
Chen Pi (Pericarpium Citri Reticulatae)
Ren Shen (Radix Panacis Ginseng)
Gan Cao (Radix Glycyrrhizae Uralensis), 5 *fen* for each of the above
Gao Ben (Radix Et Rhizoma Ligustici Sinensis), 3 *fen*
Qing Pi (Pericarpium Citri Reticulatae Viride)
Bai Dou Kou (Fructus Cardamomi)
Huang Bai (Cortex Phellodendri), 2 *fen* for each of the above

Readers should note the inclusion of *Huang Qi* and *Ren Shen* in the above formula. Although Li makes no mention of any vacuity in the above description of this pattern, he assumes that, if external evils successfully invade, the righteous qi must be vacuous and weak. In this case, he demonstrates no concern over possibly supplementing the evils or, by securing the exterior defensive, "locking" those evils inside the body. This is also very much my own clinical experience.

Slice the above [and take] all as one dose, boiled in two large cups of water down to one cupful. After removing the dregs, take warm after meals. This formula is appropriate for those with exuberant qi. Those with a white facial color [due to] desertion should not take it.

Urinary incontinence indicating lung qi vacuity requires quiet lying down to nurture the qi and does not allow for overtaxation. It can be supplemented with *Huang Qi* (Radix Astragali Membranacei), *Ren Shen* (Radix Panacis Ginseng), and the like. If there is no recovery, this is due to the existence of heat. [In that case,] add *Huang Bai* (Cortex Phellodendri) and *Sheng Di* (uncooked Radix Rehmanniae Glutinosae).

Pain in the shoulder and the back with inability to turn round is [due to] depressed and stagnant qi of the hand tai yang. Dissipate this with windy medicinals. Many contemporary clinicians associate neck and shoulder pain due to emotional stress as liver-gallbladder symptoms. However, it is my experience that treating these symptoms more from the point of view of the hand and foot tai yang achieves better, longer lasting therapeutic results.

Pain in the spine, stiff neck, low back [pain] as if about to break, neck [pain] as if about to be pulled up, and upsurging headache are [due to] the stagnation of the foot tai yang channel. [Therefore,] administer *Qiang Huo Sheng Shi Tang* (Notopterygium Overcome Dampness Decoction) as the main remedy.

Qiang Huo Sheng Shi Tang (Notopterygium Overcome Dampness Decoction)

Qiang Huo (Radix Et Rhizoma Notopterygii)
Du Huo (Radix Angelicae Pubescentis), 1 *qian* each
mix-fried *Gan Cao* (Radix Glycyrrhizae Uralensis)
Gao Ben (Radix Et Rhizoma Ligustici Sinensis)
Fang Feng (Radix Ledebouriellae Divaricatae), 5 *fen* for each of the above
Man Jing Zi (Fructus Viticis), 3 *fen*
Chuan Xiong (Radix Ligustici Wallichii), 2 *fen*

Today, this formula is indicated for wind damp impediment in the exterior and muscle aspects or divisions, generalized aching and pain, a heavy head, aversion to wind, and fever with white tongue fur and a floating pulse. It is also frequently used for the treatment of headaches due to its inclusion of *Gao Ben, Man Jing Zi,* and *Chuan Xiong.* It is sometimes used for the treatment of flus, sinusitis, and allergic rhinitis.

Slice the above ingredients. [Take] all as one dose boiled in two cups of water down to one cupful. After removing the dregs, take warm after meals. Generalized heaviness and heaviness and discomfort in the low back indicate damp heat in the channels. [For this,] add *Huang Bai* (Cortex Phellodendri), one *qian*, *Fu Zi* (Radix Lateralis Praeparatus Aconiti Carmichaeli), 0.5 *qian*, and *Cang Zhu* (Rhizoma Atractylodis), two *qian*.

For heavy, weak legs and feet, add wine-washed *Han Fang Ji* (Radix Stephaniae Tetrandrae), 0.5 *qian*, together with a small amount of *Fu Zi* (Radix Lateralis Praeparatus Aconiti Carmichaeli) in moderate cases or *Chuan Wu* (Radix Aconiti Carmichaeli) in serious cases used as a conductor to move the blood. Today, the addition of *Cang Zhu* (Rhizoma Atractylodis), *Huang Bai* (Cortex Phellodendri), and *Yi Yi Ren* (Semen Coicis Lachryma-jobi) is commonly recommended for wind damp heat impediment with hot, painful joints in the lower extremities, and *Fu Zi* is only recommended in severe cases.

Sleep fraught with fright and urinary dribbling and dripping are due to evils in the [foot] shao yang and jue yin. In this case, the urinary strangury is due to liver depression and the fact that the liver channel network vessels traverse the genitalia, while the fright is due to liver-gallbladder heat causing restlessness of the ethereal soul. In premodern Chinese medicine, sleep disturbances were commonly associated with the ethereal soul and fright was commonly associated with the gallbladder. Nowadays, what is called gallbladder qi timidity or vacuity is actually a combination of liver depression with spleen vacuity leading to nonconstruction and malnourishment of the heart spirit. Use the same formula as for the tai yang channel [*i.e.*, *Qiang Huo Sheng Shi Tang*] with the addition of *Chai Hu* (Radix Bupleuri), 0.5 *qian*. In case of strangury, add *Ze Xie* (Rhizoma Alismatis Orientalis), 0.5 *qian*. This is a combined wind cold disease in two channels in the lower burner. According to the five phases theory, the kidneys are cold water, whereas the liver is wind wood. Therefore, frequently wind is used to represent the liver and cold (*i.e.*, water), the kidneys. The classic explains that kidney and liver diseases are treated by the same method since they both are in the lower burner. They cannot be cured but by moving the channels with windy medicinals.

Whitish pus in the stools or evacuation of nothing but whitish pus is due to damage of the large intestine by overtaxation qi vacuity. [For this,] supplement with *Huang Qi Ren Shen Tang* (Astragalus & Ginseng Decoction).[2] Frequent abdominal urgency is [due to] blood vacuity. [In this case,] add *Dang Gui* (Radix Angelicae Sinensis). Mucus in the stools is considered a sign of damp evils. The implication here is that overtaxation has damaged the spleen qi, not actually the large intestine qi. In modern Chinese medicine, the large intestine qi is largely a manifestation of the spleen, stomach, and/or kidney qi. If the spleen qi is too vacuous and weak to govern the movement and transformation of water fluids, these collect and transform into dampness which then pours downward to the lower burner. One manifestation of this is mucus in the stools. Therefore, treatment is based on fortifying the spleen and boosting the qi, upbearing the clear and eliminating dampness.

Evacuation of whitish pus with a little slippery substance frequently staining the trousers is [due to] qi desertion. Add *Fu Zi Pi* (Cortex Radicis Aconiti Carmichaeli) and, in serious cases, *Ying Su Ke* (Pericarpium Papaveris Somniferi). In case of qi stagnation, administer sweet medicinals alone to supplement the qi. Note that Li says, in case of qi stagnation, to administer sweet-flavored medicinals. This is because the *Nei Jing* says that the sweet flavor is relaxing and qi stagnation is commonly associated with tension. This line also helps underscore the clinical reality that one rarely sees pure qi stagnation as described in undergraduate textbooks. Because of the interrelationship between the spleen and liver, supplementing the spleen in the case of liver depression does not typically cause unwanted side effects but rather renders the coursing of the liver and rectification of the qi all the more efficient. It is also required to lie quietly without speaking to nurture the qi.[3] This is one of the several instances in this book where Li reminds his readers that speaking uses up great quantities of clear qi and that, if we want to recuperate our righteous qi, we need to, in general, speak less.

In case of lung distention and inflation with panting and coughing, an elevated chest with qi fullness, congestion, and exuberance [of qi in the chest] with [qi] up-running, add large quantities of *Wu Wei Zi* (Fructus Schisandrae Chinensis), less of *Ren Shen* (Radix Panacis Ginseng), still less of *Mai Men Dong* (Tuber Ophiopogonis Japonici), and a small amount of *Huang Lian* (Rhizoma Coptidis Chinensis). Qi upsurging in this case refers to rapid dyspneic breathing with the mouth kept open to facilitate respiration.

Serious cases with arms crossed [over the chest] and distorted vision are [due to] great vacuity of the true qi. In case of shortness of breath, add *Huang Qi* (Radix Astragali Membranacei), *Wu Wei Zi* (Fructus Schisandrae Chinensis), and *Ren Shen* (Radix Panacis Ginseng). In case of qi exuberance, add *Wu Wei Zi*, *Ren Shen*, *Huang Qin* (Radix Scutellariae Baicalensis), and *Jing Jie Sui* (Herba Seu Flos Schizonepetae Tenuifoliae). In winter, remove *Jing Jie Sui* but add *Cao Dou Kou* (Semen Alpiniae Katsumadai).

In case of sore throat, submandibular swelling, a large, surging pulse, and red facial complexion, add *Huang Qin*, *Jie Geng* (Radix Platycodi Grandiflori), and *Gan Cao* (Radix Glycyrrhizae Uralensis), five *fen* each. In case of ringing in the ears, yellowing of the eyes, cheek and submandibular swelling, pain in the neck, shoulders, upper arm, elbow, and lateral posterior border of the forearm, a red facial complexion, and large, surging pulse, use *Qiang Huo* (Radix Et Rhizoma Notopterygii), *Fang Feng* (Radix Ledebouriellae Divaricatae), *Gan Cao*, and *Gao Ben* (Radix Et Rhizoma Ligustici Sinensis) to free the flow of channel blood. Use *Huang Qin* and *Huang Lian* (Rhizoma Coptidis Chinensis) to disperse swelling, and use *Ren Shen* and *Huang Qi* to boost the original qi at the same time as draining fire evils. In case of a tight pulse, [which indicates] cold, or a white facial complexion and frequent sneezing or malign and unharmonious facial complexion, [which] also [indicate] cold, add *Qiang Huo* (Radix Et Rhizoma Notopterygii) and the other three ingredients [mentioned above] to drain the foot tai yang. Do not use *Huang Lian* or *Huang Qin*, but do add a small amount of *Fu Zi* (Radix Lateralis Praeparatus Aconiti Carmichaeli) to free the flow of the channel. In case of malign and inharmonious facial complexion, melancholy, and apprehensiveness, add *Rou Gui* (Cortex Cinnamomi Cassiae) and *Fu Zi*.

Today, *Dang Shen* (Radix Codonopsitis Pilosulae) is typically substituted for *Ren Shen* whenever Li calls for the combination of *Huang Qi* and *Ren Shen*. For nasosinusitis with nasal congestion and headache due to externally contracted wind damp evils, add *Cang Er Zi* (Fructus Xanthii Sibirici) to the original formula.

Endnotes

[1] The *Mai Jing (Pulse Classic)* by Wang Shu-he of the Jin dynasty.

[2] This formula is composed of: *Huang Qi* (Radix Astragali Membranacei), *Sheng Ma* (Rhizoma Cimicifugae), *Ren Shen* (Radix Panacis Ginseng), *Chen Pi* (Pericarpium Citri Reticulatae), *Mai Men Dong* (Tuber Ophiopogonis Japonici), *Cang Zhu* (Rhizoma Atractylodis), *Bai Zhu* (Rhizoma Atractylodis Macrocephalae), *Huang Bai* (Cortex Phellodendri), *Shen Qu* (Massa Medica Fermentata), *Dang Gui* (Radix Angelicae Sinensis), mix-fried *Gan Cao* (Radix Glycyrrhizae Uralensis), and *Wu Wei Zi* (Fructus Schisandrae Chinensis).

[3] This paragraph is placed at the end of the volume in the *Yi Tong Zheng Mai* version.

7

Treatise on Medicinal Indications & Prohibitions

To treat disease by administering medication, it is necessary to know the seasonal prohibitions, channel prohibitions, disease prohibitions, and medicinal prohibitions.

Seasonal prohibitions

So-called seasonal prohibitions define the administration of diaphoresis, precipitation, ejection, and disinhibition based on the upbearing and downbearing laws of the four seasons. The general principle [is as follows]: Ejection is appropriate in spring. It is similar to ploughing, weeding, cleaving, and hacking. It allows depressed yang qi to easily reach the tens of thousands of things to help them generate and grow. Diaphoresis is appropriate in summer. It is similar to the floating and superabundance of the tens of thousands of things. Precipitation is appropriate in autumn. It is similar to the collecting and harvesting of the tens of thousands of things — the old giving way to the new, making yang qi easy to collect. Ejection, diaphoresis, and precipitation were the three methods (*san fa*) of treatment advocated by Zhang Zi-he, another of the four great masters of the Jin-Yuan and founder of the School of Attack and Purgation. Closely (tightly [later editor]) compacting [is appropriate] in winter. It is similar to the shutting in and storage of the tens of thousands of things bringing yang qi to a standstill. "Yin and yang in the four seasons float and sink at the [same] gate of birth and growth as the tens of thousands of things." This means that the vicissitudes of yin and yang in the four seasons are in conformity with the laws of growth of living things. "Going counter to its root and felling its root ruins the true."[1] It is also said, "Use warm [medicinals] away from warmth, use hot away from heat, use cool away from cool, and use cold away from cold."[2] This quote implies that it is necessary to avoid employing warm ingredients in warm spring as much as possible, etc. In so doing, that which might overwhelm will not be reinforced. This implies that in spring, for example, when warm qi prevails, if warm medicinals are administered, warm qi will become exaggerated and hence become evil. Based on this, *Bai Hu* [*Tang*, White Tiger Decoction] is not used in winter. *Qing*

Long [*Tang*, Blue-green Dragon Decoction] is not used in summer. This is actually two different formulas, the major (*da*) and minor (*xiao*). *Gui Zhi* [*Tang*, Cinnamon Twig Decoction] is not used in spring and summer. And *Ma Huang* [*Tang*, Ephedra Decoction] is not used in autumn and winter. Thus one does not lose sight of the [seasonal] qi indications. [Whereas, if one] uses precipitation in spring or summer or promoting perspiration in autumn or winter, one loses the regularity of heaven and attacks the harmony of heaven. The regularity of heaven refers to natural law, while heavenly harmony is the harmony within the body insured by heaven. Some interpret heavenly harmony as simply another name for the original qi within the body. [The treatment of specific] diseases allows for makeshift options, but going too far should be corrected.

These seasonal prohibitions are no longer a part of standard professional Chinese medicine. Basically, if a therapy is indicated by the patient's disease plus personal pattern discrimination, then the indicated therapy is used regardless of season. Today, these prohibitions seem overly fastidious.

Channel prohibitions

The foot tai yang urinary bladder channel is the leader of the channels, traveling along the posterior [aspect of the body], the exterior of the exterior. Exterior means yang. Hence the exterior of the exterior is yang within yang. Here it implies that the foot tai yang channel not only travels along the posterior of the body (*i.e.*, yang) but also in the surface which is also yang. If it is damaged by wind cold, sweating is indicated. If [wind cold] transmits into the root, disinhibiting urination is indicated. Root here means the bowel associated with the channel, in this case the urinary bladder. Such transmission leads to bowel pattern yang disease due to cold damage. If precipitation is applied too early, hundreds of transmuted patterns may arise. This is the first prohibition.

The foot yang ming stomach channel, traveling along the anterior of the body, governs abdominal fullness, distention, and difficult defecation. Precipitation is indicated [for its treatment. If] the yang ming transforms dryness and fire and fluids are [consequently] unable to collect, diaphoresis and disinhibiting urination are prohibited for the yang ming since they would cause a double detriment to fluids. This is the second [set of] prohibitions.

The foot shao yang gallbladder channel travels along the side of the body between the tai yang and yang ming. When it is diseased, there occur alternating cold and heat, a bitter [taste in] the mouth, and chest and rib-side pain. The only methods indicated for its treatment are harmonizing and balancing. In addition, since the gallbladder has neither entrance nor exit and governs the engendering and effusing qi, precipitation will infringe on the tai yang, diaphoresis will infringe on the yang ming, and disinhibiting urination will only sink the engendering and effusing qi into the yin. This implies that yang becomes vacuous and yin superabundant. This is the third [set of] prohibitions.

Precipitation is prohibited in the third yin [pattern, *i.e.*, disease of the spleen or the foot tai yin] without stomach repletion since there is no question of transmission [of the disease] to the root with the third yin. Root transmission occurs only in yang disease due to cold damage. Yin disease does not transmit to the root, *i.e.*, the viscus. Precipitation can be used only when the stomach is replete. Administering medicinals based on the channels must be done with justification.

The above channel prohibitions have to do with Zhang Zhong-jing's six yin-yang divisions *vis á vis* cold damage diseases. Personally, I think it is a mistake to conflate Zhang Zhong-jing's six yin-yang divisions describing the progression of disease with the six yin-yang divisions of the 12 regular or main channels. While both use the same model of dividing yin and yang, they are not necessarily one and the same thing.

Disease prohibitions

Foods and medicinals which assist yin and drain yang are prohibited in yang qi insufficiency diseases with superabundance of yin qi. [Hence one should refrain from] the various bland foods and medicinals of bland flavor which drain the upbearing and effusing [of yang qi] and assist [or strengthen] control and contraction. The various bitter medicinals are all sinking and drain the dissipation [or spreading] and floating of yang qi.

It is a central tenet within Li-Zhu medicine that good health is founded on the proper function of the spleen-stomach and that this requires the upbearing and effusing or out-thrusting of clear yang. Therefore, anything which works against this upbearing and effusing is seen as deleterious if yang qi is insufficient, unless there are cogent extenuating circumstances.

Acrid, hot medicinals, such as *Jiang* (Rhizoma Zingiberis Officinalis), *Fu Zi* (Radix Lateralis Praeparatus Aconiti Carmichaeli), and *Guan Gui* (Cortex Tubiformis Cinnamomi Cassiae), as well as sodden wheat foods, wine, and spices all assist fire and drain the original qi.

Once again, Li is saying that heat or fire evils can drain or damage the original qi, remembering that, as Li uses this term, he is referring to the latter heaven orig-inal or source qi. This is a main point within Li-Zhu medicine which we will dis-cuss at more length further on. Sodden wheat food, meaning today's breads, other baked goods, and pasta, especially those made with refined or white flour are not hot by nature. Therefore, they probably should not have been listed with these other foods, all of which are hot in nature. However, sodden wheat foods engender fluids and can cause the engenderment of dampness. Because the spleen is averse to dampness, such foods can damage the spleen and also lead to diminu-tion of the latter heaven source qi. In addition, because dampness impedes and depresses the free flow of yang qi, dampness may cause the transformation of depressive heat and this heat may "eat" and damage the source qi.

Cold and hard foods cause detriment to the yang qi. All these are among the pro-hibited [foods and medicinals]. When yin fire shows a tendency towards being appeased and is about to retreat, for example, there must be a bland taste in the mouth, for the original qi of the triple burner is not yet exuberant. [At this time,] salty foods are also among those prohibited.

A bland taste in the mouth is an indication of spleen qi vacuity. This passage is yet another indication that Li is talking about latter heaven source qi, *i.e.*, the spleen or middle burner qi.

Medicinal prohibitions

If stomach qi, for example, is stagnant with fluids collapsing and drying up in the interior, this must manifest with a desire for boiled water to come to its res-cue. This is not so much [true] thirst as a dry mouth, not so much overwhelm-ing of the warm as a disease of the blood. [For this,] it is appropriate to boost [the stomach] with acrid (sweet [later editor]), sour [medicinals]. Bland, per-colating formulas like *Wu Ling San* (Five [Ingredients] Poria Powder) are justi-fiably among the prohibited. Profuse sweating prohibits disinhibiting urination, while profuse urination prohibits diaphoresis. Sore throat prohibits diaphore-sis and disinhibiting urination. Loose stools should not be made more loose. In case of constipation, *Dang Gui* (Radix Angelicae Sinensis), *Tao Ren* (Semen Pruni Persicae), *Huo Ma Ren* (Semen Cannabis Sativae), *Yu Li Ren* (Semen Pruni), and *Zao Jiao Ren* (Semen Gleditschiae Sinensis) can be used to harmonize the blood and moisten the intestines, whereas drying medicinals are justifiably among the prohibited. Excessive vomiting does not allow ejection. Vomiting and voiding of vacuous, soft stools are [due to] qi congestion and stagnation above. [Therefore,] one should use *Sheng Jiang* (uncooked Rhizoma Zingiberis Officinalis), *Chen Pi* (Pericarpium Citri Reticulatae), and the like to diffuse [the qi. However, in case of] vomiting with constipation, the stools should be disinhibited and the above-mentioned medicinals are justifiably among the prohibited. Solid stools in diseases of various malign sores or after measles in children also require precipitation and *Sheng Jiang* (uncooked Rhizoma Zingiberis Officinalis) and *Chen Pi* (Pericarpium Citri Reticulatae) are justifiably among the prohibited. As another example, administering *Ping Wei San* (Level the Stomach Powder) in the presence of a bowstring pulse and *Huang Qi Jian Zhong Tang* (Astragalus Fortify the Center Decoction) in the presence of a moderate pulse only replenish repletion and evacuate vacuity. Thus they are justifiably among the prohibited.

Humans depend on heaven for the transformation of dampness to engender the stomach. Heaven here means nature, and transformation of dampness refers to those substances produced out of dampness which implies earth. The stomach and dampness, though named differently, can be regarded virtually as the same thing. Dampness is able to enrich and nurture the stomach, but, when dampness becomes superabundant in the stomach, excess dampness should be drained nonetheless. [On the other hand,] stomach insufficiency can be enriched and nourished by nothing but damp substances.

Zhu Dan-xi took this teaching on dampness and the stomach and routinely added stomach yin enriching and nourishing medicinals to Li Dong-yuan type formulas so that their acrid, windy, drying ingredients did not damage stomach fluids.

[Zhang] Zhong-jing explains that a prevailing stomach desires boiled cakes, but taking boiled cakes with a vacuous stomach will, more often than not, exacerbate [the condition]. Boiled cakes refers to steamed breads but also, nowadays, would include oven-baked breads and pastas, all of which tend to be dampening. Dampness can assist fire. Effulgent fire, if depressed and blocked, is responsible for great heat. At the onset of disease, fire is effulgent and, [therefore,] one should not eat food that assists fire. [Instead, one should] observe the seasonal [changes], identify the channels [involved], study the disease, and finally administer medication. If all these four [are performed] in an appropriate way, then [one's practice] will be perfect.

Endnotes

[1] *Su Wen*, Ch. 2
[2] *Ibid.*

8

The Spleen & Stomach According to [Zhang] Zhong-jing's Quotations from the *Nei Jing (Inner Classic)*

Instructions on the composition of formulas have already been given in detail. However, for fear [that practitioners] will not be able to recognize [these instructions'] sources and to facilitate textual research, quotations from the *Huang Di Nei Jing (The Yellow Emperor's Inner Classic)* cited by [Zhang] Zhong-jing explaining the spleen and stomach are given below.

The *Tai Yin Yang Ming Lun (Treatise on the Tai Yin & Yang Ming)* states:

Since the foot tai yin and yang ming, the channels of the spleen and stomach, stand in an exterior/interior relationship, why do they produce different diseases?

Qi Bo answered: Yin and yang are located opposite to each other, [situated in] different phases of repletion and vacuity, and flow in different routes, [and pathogens invade them] via different ways, from the outside or from within. Hence their diseases differ.

The Emperor asked: I would like to know the different forms they take.

Qi Bo answered: The heavenly qi is yang and it governs the exterior. The earthly qi is yin and it governs the interior. Therefore, the yang [*i.e.*, stomach] tract [tends to] repletion, while the yin [spleen] tract [tends to] vacuity. Hence yang suffers from thieving winds and vacuity evils, while yin suffers from dietary irregularity and not keeping regular hours in living. When yang is suffering, [evils] invade the six bowels. When yin is suffering, [evils] invade the five viscera. Invasion of the bowels gives rise to generalized heat with insomnia and causes panting and wheezing above. Invasion of the viscera gives rise to fullness and blockage [in the chest] and causes swill diarrhea below, which, over time, may develop into intestinal afflux. The larynx rules the heavenly qi [*i.e.*, respiration], while the pharynx rules the earthly qi [*i.e.*, digestion]. Hence yang is subject to wind qi, whereas yin to damp qi. The qi of the yin [channels] travels upward from the feet to the head and [then] turns downward to the tips of the fingers along the arms. The qi of the yang [channels] travels upward from the hands to the head and [then] turns downward to the feet. Thus it is said that yang disease turns below after reaching its extreme above, whereas yin disease turns above after reaching its extreme below. For this reason, the upper first suffers from damage by wind and the lower first suffers from damage by dampness.

The fact that the stomach tends to repletion and the spleen tends to vacuity is extremely important in clinical practice. Today, many beginner's textbooks talk about spleen-stomach vacuity weakness. However, spleen and stomach dual vacuity is rare in patients in developed countries. Instead, there is a tendency for the stomach to be hot and dry, while the spleen is vacuous and damp at one and the same time.

The Emperor asked: When the spleen becomes diseased, why does one lose the use of the four limbs?

Qi Bo answered: The four limbs are all supplied by qi from the stomach, but they can only get [this qi] through the spleen, for qi has no [direct] access to the channels. When diseased, the spleen is no longer able to manage fluids and humors for the stomach's sake. [Consequently,] the four limbs lose their supply of qi from water and grains. As the qi becomes diminished day by day, the vessel pathways become inhibited and the sinews, bones, and muscles lack qi for their growth. As a result, use of the four limbs is lost.

The Emperor asked: Why does the spleen not rule a particular season?

Qi Bo answered: The spleen is earth and manages the center. It constantly promotes the growth of the other four viscera throughout the four seasons. With 18 days spared [from each season] for it to manage, it is not allowed to rule one whole season. The spleen constantly carries the essence of the stomach earth. Earth engenders all the tens of thousands of things in accordance with the laws of heaven and earth. Hence [the spleen] reaches up to the head and down to the feet with no whole season for it to rule.[1]

The *Yin Yang Ying Xiang Lun (Treatise on the Mutual Correspondences of Yin & Yang)* states:

Humans have five viscera to transform the five qi and to produce joy, anger, sorrow, worry, and fright. Joy and anger damage the qi. Cold and summerheat damage the form. Intense anger damages yin. Intense joy damages yang. Inverted qi ascends to fill the vessels and carry off the form. Excessive joy and anger and excessive cold and summerheat thus render life insecure.[2]

The *Yu Ji Zhen Zang Lun (Treatise on the Jade Mechanism of the True Visceral [Pulse])* states:

A greatly excess spleen leads to inability to lift the four limbs, [while spleen] insufficiency causes the nine orifices to be blocked. [This disease] is called superimposition disagreement.[3]

Superimposition here means disorders of the five visceral qi overlapping one another, while disagreement is understood to mean disharmony of the stomach qi. Because of the ambiguity of the Chinese, some people interpret this phrase as dual rigidity and have some reason to do so since this pattern is manifested by inability to raise the limbs, *i.e.*, a kind of rigidity, which is homonymous with disagreement in Chinese. What is more, superimposition is also homonymous with dual in Chinese.

Again the *Tong Ping Xu Shi Lun (Comprehensive Treatise on Vacuity & Repletion)* states, "Headache with ringing in the ears and inhibition of the nine orifices is engendered by the spleen and stomach."[4]

The *Tiao Jing Lun (Treatise on Regulating the Channels)* states:

When the form is superabundant, the abdomen is distended and urination and defecation are inhibited. When the form is insufficient, the four limbs lose their use.[5]

Again the *Qi Jiao Bian Lun (Treatise on the Joining & Transmutation of Qi)* states:

If yearly earth is excessive, rain and dampness overflow, kidney water is subjected to evils, and people may become diseased with abdominal pain, clear inversion [*i.e.*, cold inversion], melancholy, generalized heaviness, vexation and depression, and, if extreme, withered muscles, foot wilting and debilitation, tuggings frequently arising in walking, pain in the soles of the feet, [internal] attack of rheum, center fullness, reduced food intake, and inability to raise the four limbs.

The five phases, which represent the five viscera, can also be used to represent the years when doubled to form the 10 heavenly stems. Thus there is a repetitive cycle with the *jia* and *ji* years pertaining to earth, *yi* and *geng* to metal, *bing* and *xin* to water, *ding* and *ren* to wood, and *wu* and *gui* to fire. *Jia* (S1), because it is odd numbered, is yang, and, therefore, earth is believed to be abundant in *jia* years. *Ji* (S6), on the other hand, is even or yin, and thus earth is believed to be insufficient in *ji* years. This is what is referred to as yearly earth which may be abundant or insufficient depending upon whether the year is evenly or oddly numbered.

It further states:

If yearly earth is insufficient, wind moves greatly. [Hence there occur] choleraic disease, generalized heaviness, abdominal pain, rocking of the sinews and bones, twitching and aching pain of the muscles, and a predilection for anger.

It adds:

Everyone may contract disease [due to] a cold center. When the rule of control [or contraction in autumn] is rigorous, there may occur sudden chest and rib-side pain sending a dragging [discomfort] to the lower abdomen and frequent sighing. Insects eat up the sweet yellow, and qi invades the spleen. The people's food [intake] is less with loss of flavor [or taste in the mouth].

In autumn, plants ripen and are then collected or gathered in. Therefore, autumn is believed to be the season when contraction and control prevails. The sweet yellow refers to ripened crops according to the original text of the *Su Wen*. However, as something seems to be missing from this passage, some scholars think this part refers to a pathologic change within the body rather than a natural calamity without. According to this opinion, this phrase should be interpreted as worms gnawing and a dry, yellowish complexion.

It further adds:

When earth is insufficient, if the four linkings see [such natural] events as clouds of dust and moisture, spring will enjoy the rule of whispering twigs and burgeoning leaves and buds. [If,] in the four linkings, there occur shaking, pulling up, blowing off, and soaring, autumn will come back with the bleak and vigorous retaliation of excessive and continual rain. Disasters will occur in the four linkings. This will [affect] the spleen. The disease will settle in the heart and abdomen in the interior and in the muscles and limbs in the exterior.[6]

The four linkings may refer to various things. One interpretation is the four limbs. A second is the four quarters corners — northeast, northwest, southeast, and southwest. A third is four of the twelve months — the 3rd (*chen*, B5), the 6th (*wei*, B8), the 9th (*xu*, B11) and the 12th (*chou*, B2), all of which are ruled by spleen earth as discussed above. Since the rest of the sentence has to do with prognostications based on the weather, the third interpretation is probably the correct one in this case. Dust and moisture is a description of favorable weather. According to five movements and six qi theory, certain weather appearing on the cusps of seasons is indicative of the prevailing influences in that season. Shaking, pulling up, blowing off, and soaring are descriptions of bad or disastrous weather. An example of retaliation is abnormal cold weather in one season followed by abnormal hot weather in another season.

The *Wu Chang Zheng Da Lun (Great Treatise on the Government of the Five Constants)* states:

Adequate earth is called universal availability of the transforming . . . Deficient earth is called abject befalling.

Universal availability of the transforming suggests a favorable condition in which every living thing benefits from the transformation of the thriving spleen earth. Abject befalling implies that, when the spleen is deficient, dampness, which always lies in lowlands, prevails and, therefore, diseases such as diarrhea arise.

It adds:

The pathologic change this causes are sores gushing [with pus], cleaving [of the muscles], ulceration, welling abscesses, and swelling. The [internal] development is moist stagnation . . . When following the pathologic change of wood, the disease it generates is lodging, fullness, glomus, and obstruction, and the disease it generates is swill diarrhea.

Moist stagnation implies that dampness persists on the inside causing malfunction of the spleen and stomach. Pathologic changes of wood implies that liver wood becomes exuberant and the disease presents a picture of liver repletion.

It adds again:

> Excessive earth is called raised mound . . . Its flavor is sweet, salty, and sour. It manifests in long summer. Its channels are the foot tai yin and yang ming.

In this passage, raised means superabundant, while mound implies earth or the spleen. The second line means that, in case of spleen repletion, sweet, salty, and sour should be administered for a cure.

And yet again:

> The disease it generates is abdominal fullness and inability to lift the limbs. This is evils damaging the spleen.[7]

The *Jing Mai Bie Lun (Divergent Treatise on the Channels & Vessels)* states:

> If the tai yin visceral [pulse] beats forcefully, this requires a careful study of the true. If the pulse qi of the five viscera is diminished, the stomach qi is not calm, and the third yin [pattern is indicated], this requires treating the lower transporting points of the third yin, supplementing yang, and draining yin.[8]

True here means the true visceral pulse which suggests a critical disease involving a certain viscus proper. The pulse image is the appearance of a pulse peculiar to the involved viscus, for example, a stone-like pulse for a purely kidney disease. The tai yin is the third yin, thus implying a super-abundant spleen. In this case, draining *Tai Bai* (Sp 3) drains yin, and sup-plementing *Xian Gu* (St 43) supplements yang.

The *Zang Qi Fa Shi Lun (Treatise on the Visceral Qi Following the Seasons)* states:

> The spleen prevails in long summer, [a season] ruled by the foot tai yin and yang ming, and its days are the *wu* and *ji*. The spleen is bitter about [*i.e.*, pained by] dampness and the bitter [flavor] should be administered promptly to dry it.

As mentioned above, the heavenly stems are derived from a doubling of the five phases. In terms of indicating days, each phase corresponds to two out of 10 days which are named for the 10 heavenly stems in the 10 day cycle. The relationships between the phases, days, directions, and viscera are as follows:

Jia (S1), *yi* (S2): wood, liver, east
Bing (S3), *ding* (S4): fire, heart, south
Wu (S5), *ji* (S6): earth, spleen, center
Geng (S7), *xin* (S8): metal, lungs, west
Ren (S9), *gui* (S10): water, kidneys, north

It adds:

> Disease in the spleen will heal in autumn. If not, it will deteriorate in spring. If it does not end in death in spring, it will remain stable in summer and improve in long summer. Warm food, overeating, damp living environments, and sodden clothing are prohibited.

> Disease in the spleen will heal on *geng* and *xin* days. If not, it will deteriorate on *jia* and *yi* days. If it does not end in death on the *jia* and *yi* days, it will remain stable on *bing* and *ding* days and improve on *wu* and *ji* days.

> Disease in the spleen is [characterized by] serenity at the sunset watch, exacerbation at the sunrise watch, and tranquility at the late afternoon watch. When the spleen shows a tendency to relax, promptly take sweet to relax it and use bitter to drain it and sweet to supplement it.

It adds again:

> When the spleen is diseased, [there occurs] generalized heaviness, constant hunger, flesh wilting, debilitated foot with ability to walk but liability to tuggings in walking and pain in the soles of the feet. [Spleen] vacuity leads to abdominal fullness, rumbling of the intestines, swill diarrhea, and untransformed food in the stools. [In that case,] prick and bleed the channels of [foot] tai yin, yang ming, and shao yin.[9]

The *Jing Mai Bie Lun (Divergent Treatise on the Channels & Vessels)* explains:

> Food qi, having entered the stomach, spreads essence to the liver and diffuses qi into the sinews. Having entered the stomach, the food qi, the turbid of which gathers at the heart, diffuses essence into the vessels. With the vessel qi flowing in the channels, the channel qi gathers in the lungs.

The lungs, facing the hundreds of vessels, transport essence to the skin and hair. The minute vessels, taking in essence, move qi to the bowels. With the bowel essence and the spirit brightness maintained in the four viscera, qi tends towards balance. To examine this balance, the qi mouth [pulse] is the gauge which can tell life and death.

Having entered the stomach, fluids float the essence qi and transport it up to the spleen. The spleen qi spreads essence which gathers in the lungs and frees the flow of the water passageways, transporting [water essence] down to the urinary bladder. Water essence spreads in the four directions and the five channels run side by side in agreement with the four seasons, the five viscera, and the measurements of yin and yang. Thus normalcy is kept.[10]

The *Wu Chang Zheng Da Lun (Great Treatise on the Government of the Five Constants)* explains:

There are excess and deficiency. What is excess oppresses its restraining and overwhelms its restrained [organs] . . . Whatever fails to arrive when it ought will lead to deficiency. [Then] the restrained will move frenetically, the generated will suffer from disease, and the restraining will overwhelm it.[11]

[Zhang] Zhong-jing explains:

Humans receive qi from water and grains to nourish the spirit. Therefore, spirit departs when water and grains run out. Hence it is said that entertainment with grains leads to prosperity, while deprivation of grains leads to death . . . Loss of water leads to dissipated constructive [qi], while dispersion of grains leads to collapse of defensive [qi]. With the constructive dissipated [or scattered] and the defensive collapsing, the spirit has nothing on which to rely. (This quotation can be found in the notes in the 43rd Difficulty in the *Nan Jing*. [Later editor])

He adds:

Not until water has entered the channels, can blood be formed. Not until grain has entered the stomach, can the vessel passageways move. (*Ping Mai Fa, Methods of Examining the Pulse; Shang Han Lun, Treatise on Damage [Due to] Cold* [Later editor])

It follows that blood must be nurtured by all means and the defensive must be warmed by all means. With blood warm and the defensive in harmony, [one will] live out one's heaven[-decreed] years.

Personally, I do not find all this five transport and six qi theory very useful in clinical practice. When some Chinese doctors, such as those in the *Han Xue Pai* (School of Studying the Han), criticize(ed) Jin-Yuan medicine, they typically attack(ed) this highly speculative and theoretical aspect of this medicine. However, it would be a shame if these, I believe, valid criticisms were to lead to a dismissal or lack of recognition of the valuable parts of Li-Zhu medicine.

Endnotes

[1] *Su Wen*, Ch. 29
[2] *Su Wen*, Ch. 5
[3] *Su Wen*, Ch. 19
[4] *Su Wen*, Ch. 28
[5] *Su Wen*, Ch. 62
[6] *Su Wen*, Ch. 69
[7] *Su Wen*, Ch. 70
[8] *Su Wen*, Ch. 21
[9] *Su Wen*, Ch. 22
[10] *Su Wen*, Ch. 21
[11] *Su Wen*, Ch. 70

脾胃論

Book Two

1

Diagrams & Explanations on the
Waxing & Waning of the Movement of Qi

Concerning the interchange of function and substance between heaven and earth, there are four theories by which one can observe the subtle mechanisms of disease.

Dampness, stomach, transformation [This terse phrase implies that dampness prevails in long summer, which corresponds to the stomach, and that the stomach is responsible for the engenderment and transformation to promote the development of everything. The meaning of the parallel phrases following should be understood in a similar way]; heat, small intestine, growth [The small intestine (and heart) are fire, and fire prevails in summer. Therefore, they promote growth.]; wind, gallbladder, engendering. The gallbladder and liver are wood and wood prevails in spring, a season when everything is budding. Therefore, these two organs are responsible for engenderment within the body. If all of these have sunken and are insufficient, one should give priority to supplementation. *Huang Qi* (Radix Astragali Membranacei), *Ren Shen* (Radix Panacis Ginseng), *Gan Cao* (Radix Glycyrrhizae Uralensis), *Dang Gui* (Radix Angelicae Sinensis), *Chai Hu* (Radix Bupleuri), and *Sheng Ma* (Rhizoma Cimicifugae) are acrid, sweet, effusing, and dissipating [medicinals which can] be used to promote engendering and growth in spring and summer.

Earth, spleen, form [This terse phrase implies that the spleen is earth, responsible for transforming essence to nourish the form. The meaning of the parallel phrases following should be understood in a similar way.]; fire, heart, spirit; wood, liver, blood. If all of these are immensely exuberant, [going up] to overwhelm the qi of engendering and growth, one should apply drainage later. This implies that the draining of yin fire should follow the supplementation of the spleen and stomach. *Gan Cao Shao* (Extremitas Radicis Glycyrrhizae Uralensis), which is sweet and cold, drains fire. Fire expresses itself in the lungs and counterflows in the chest. It damages the qi. *Huang Qin* (Radix Scutellariae Baicalensis), which is bitter and cold, drains heat in the chest [to treat] qi ascent panting. *Hong Hua* (Flos Carthami Tinctorii) breaks malign blood. Together with *Huang Qin* (Radix

Scutellariae Baicalensis), it greatly supplements kidney water and boosts the qi of the lungs to drain fire dryness from the blood.

Cold, urinary bladder, storing qi [This terse phrase implies that the channel of the urinary bladder is cold water, responsible for the storage of qi in winter. The parallel phrase following should be understood in a similar way.]; dryness, large intestine, harvesting qi. The large intestine and the lungs are metal and prevail in autumn, a season when every living thing is gathered in and collected. Therefore, the large intestine is responsible for harvesting qi. If both are immensely efful-gent, one should apply drainage later. *Huang Qi* (Radix Astragali Membranacei), which is sweet and warm, can check spontaneous perspiration and replenish exterior vacuity to protect [the exterior] from cold evils. *Dang Gui* (Radix Angelicae Sinensis), which is acrid and warm, moistens dryness. With the help of *Tao Ren* (Semen Pruni Persicae), it can relieve the dark gate [or pylorus] of blockage, dis-inhibit the secret passageway [or the lower section of the large intestine], and resolve difficult voiding of dry stools.

Water, kidneys, essence; metal, lungs, qi. If both of these are vacuous, debilitated, and insufficient, one should first supplement. *Huang Bai* (Cortex Phellodendri), which is bitter and cold, can eliminate damp heat that has caused wilting and is overwhelming the kidneys. It relieves weakness of the feet and knees, resolves genital sweating and impotence, and boosts the essence. Today, we no longer say that *Huang Bai* boosts the essence. However, clearing and eliminating damp heat from the lower burner may allow the kidneys to recuperate. *Gan Cao Shao* (Extremitas Radicis Glycyrrhizae Uralensis) and *Huang Qin* (Radix Scutellariae Baicalensis) supplement the lung qi and drain and downbear yin fire. The lungs are bitter about qi ascent counterflow. [Thus] take bitters promptly to drain [this qi]. This is not a makeshift but a conventional treatment method for the begin-nings of heat in the center. So-called makeshift [treatments] are only stopgap measures for a particular illness. The division of treatments into makeshift and stopgap as opposed to conventional ones is a distinction that has been lost in contemporary Chinese medicine but one which, I think, might profitably be rein-troduced. For instance, simple, single-pattern formulas, such as *Dao Chi San* (Abduct the Red Powder) and *Long Dan Xie Gan Tang* (Gentiana Drain the Liver Decoction) can be used as stopgap measures to treat the tip or branches of acute conditions. However, one should be absolutely clear that this is only a makeshift or stopgap measure which is intentionally ignoring the root condition. If one wants to treat the condition more comprehensively and insure that it does not recur or transmute into some other manifestation, then one should treat the root and branch at the same time. Typically, this means draining and supplementing at the same time. If one is clear about a treatment being only a stopgap meas-ure, then they will also be clear about its short-term, temporary use.

Normalcy is the law [or rule], and disease is a breach [of this law]. Spring and summer are heaven in function on the substance of earth. Autumn and winter are earth in function on the substance of heaven.

This expression suggests interchange between yin and yang or earth and heaven. In spring and summer, qi ascends from the earth to heaven. Therefore, earth can be considered the substance from which qi is produced. In autumn and winter, cold descends from heaven to earth. Thus heaven can be considered the substance from which it is produced. Spring and summer imply a picture of everything flourishing, presumably as a result of yang or heavenly qi. Because of this, these two seasons embody the action or function of heaven. Conversely, the same logic implies that autumn and winter embody the function of earth. The reader should note that such terse expressions in Chinese medicine often imply much more than what is explicitly said. Therefore, to grasp the rich meanings of these terms, one should keep in mind all the pertinent correspondences in weather, the body, viscera, etc. It is also important to note that this statement implies that, in spring, yang is working vigorously and, therefore, should be particularly well protected. While in autumn and winter, yin is working vigorously and, therefore, should be particularly well protected.

However, there is also another interpretation. This chapter implies that the five phases — metal, wood, water, fire and earth — are substances. While the six qi — wind, heat, summerheat, dampness, dryness, and fire — are functions or actions. Spring and summer are wood and fire, which resonate with the earth, and, in these seasons, wind and heat prevail, which resonate with heaven. Autumn and summer are metal and water, which resonate with heaven, and, in these seasons, dryness and cold prevail, which resonate with earth. This is the constant law of heaven and earth. When [this law] is violated, there is disease. Spring and summer are heaven in function. Humanity corresponds with this. After a meal, the limbs become nimble. Essence, qi, and spirit all emanate. The nine orifices are freely flowing and uninhibited. The breath through the mouth and nose becomes noiseless and the voice resonants like a bell. Spring and summer are earth in substance. Humanity corresponds with this too. After a meal, the skin, flesh, sinews, bones, and blood vessels all become smooth and uninhibited, flexible and pliant, and the bones become strong and powerful with inexhaustible energy.

The only thing I have to say about this chapter is that Miriam Lee, the famous Palo Alto, CA acupuncturist, used to teach that most people have deep-lying heat in their lungs and that this heat has to be drained before one can successfully supplement the lung qi. The lungs are the florid canopy at the top of the torso, covering like a tent all the other viscera and bowels. Heat is yang and, therefore, has an innate tendency to rise upward. Thus any heat evils engendered in the body, no matter what their original location, tend to float upward to accumulate in the heart and/or lungs. Since *Huang Qin* is an extremely effective medicinal for clearing heat from the lungs, I believe this is the underlying principle when Li says that *Huang Qin* combined with *Gan Cao Shao* can supplement the lung qi.

Treatise On Initiation of Heat in the Center Due to Damage by Food & Drink and Taxation Fatigue

To me, this is the most important chapter in the *Pi Wei Lun*. It is where Li defines yin fire and also presents his most famous formula, *Bu Zhong Yi Qi Tang* (Supplement the Center & Boost the Qi Decoction).

The consummate ancient one [*i.e.*, Huang Di] comprehensively researched the vicissitudes of yin and yang and deeply studied life and death. In the works he compiled, the *Nei Jing (Inner Classic)* and the *Wai Jing (Outer Classic)*,[1] he explained at length that the stomach qi is the root of humans. To live, humans must receive qi from water and grains. So-called clear qi, constructive qi, conveying qi, defensive qi, and the upbearing qi of spring are all synonymous with stomach qi. Stomach is the sea of water and grains. Having entered the stomach, food and drink float the essence qi and transport it up to the spleen. The spleen qi spreads essence which gathers in the lungs and frees the flow of the water passageways, transporting [water fluids] down to the urinary bladder. Water essence spreads in the four directions and the five channels run side by side in agreement with the four seasons, the five viscera, and the measurements of yin and yang. Thus, normalcy is kept.

Dietary irregularity and immoderate [eating of] cold and warm [foods] damage the spleen and stomach. Joy, anger, worry, and fright consume and bring detriment to the original qi. Once again, Li is emphasizing the role of diet and the emotions as disease causes as opposed to externally contracted wind evils. If spleen and stomach qi become decrepit and original qi becomes insufficient, heart fire becomes effulgent on its own. This heart fire is a yin fire. It starts from the lower burner and its ligation links to the heart. These are, perhaps, the most important and most often quoted lines in the *Pi Wei Lun*. What these lines mean is that, if for any reason, the spleen and stomach become vacuous and weak, heat may arise in the heart. Li calls this evil heat yin fire. It is a pathological man-ifestation of ministerial or life-gate fire which counterflows upward to accumulate in the heart. **The heart does not reign [personally. Rather,] ministerial fire is its deputy.** Ministerial fire is also known as the small fire. This is stored in the kidneys and engenders the original qi. Here it also implies the pericardium. The kidney channel ascends to link with the pericardium channel in the chest. **Ministerial fire is the fire of the pericardium developing from the lower burner. It is a foe to the original qi. [This yin] fire and the original qi are irreconcilable to each other. When one is victorious, the other must be the loser. When spleen and stomach qi becomes vacuous and (their qi) consequently runs down into the kidneys, yin fire is given a chance to overwhelm the earth phase.** Ministerial/life-gate fire is only physiologically healthy and correct when it remains level or calm in its lower source, *i.e.*, the lower burner. If ministerial/life-gate fire stirs frenetically and counterflows upward, it damages the spleen or latter heaven original qi. Because the ministerial/life-gate fire is connected to the heart and pericardium, when it counterflows upward, it tends to eventually accumulate in the heart.

Within the *Pi Wei Lun*, Li identifies five disease mechanisms which can give rise to yin fire or pathological upward stirring of ministerial/life-gate fire. These are 1) spleen qi vacuity, 2) liver depression, 3) damp heat, 4) yin-blood vacuity, and 5) stirring of ministerial fire. Although I must explain these one after the other in a linear fashion, the reader should understand that these five disease mechanisms are all mutually interdependent. This means that any one of these mechanisms can result in the creation of any of the others. Because of this, real-life patients do not typically exhibit only one or another of these five, but rather three, four, or all five at one time. However, Li begins his explanation of yin fire with the spleen, and that is where we will also begin.

If, due to overthinking, anxiety and worry, underexercise, overtaxation, faulty diet, or erroneous medical treatment, the spleen qi is damaged and becomes vacuous and weak, then the spleen will not be able to do its various duties and functions. One function of the spleen is to control water liquids in the body, moving and transforming these. If the spleen qi becomes vacuous and weak and, thus, cannot move and transform water liquids, these may gather and accumulate and transform into dampness. This dampness may then hinder and obstruct the free flow of yang qi. Because yang qi is inherently warm, it too becomes stagnant and depressed. The yang qi backs up and transforms into depressive heat. If this depressive heat mutually binds with accumulated dampness, this will give rise to damp heat. Although this damp heat may be engendered in the middle burner, dampness, being turbid and heavy, typically seeps or percolates downward to the lower burner. If the heat of damp heat mutually combines and inflames ministerial/life-gate fire, the combination tends to counterflow upward. It is also possible for central qi falling downward to result in depressive heat in the lower burner which also inflames and stirs up ministerial/life-gate fire. Yet another scenario involving spleen vacuity is enduring blood vacuity due to the spleen's nonengenderment and nontransformation of new blood. In that case, blood vacuity may evolve into yin vacuity, yin vacuity may fail to control yang, and ministerial/life-gate fire may ascend hyperactively.

If, due to unfilled desires or anger damaging the liver, the liver loses its command over coursing and discharge, the liver will become depressed and the qi become stagnant. Once again, because the qi is inherently yang and, therefore, warm, qi depression may transform into depressive heat in the lower burner. If this depressive heat in the lower burner mutually inflames ministerial/life-gate fire, it may give rise to yin fire surging upward. Further, because liver depression is a repletion and replete liver wood may counterflow horizontally to assail the spleen, liver depression typically results in concomitant spleen qi vacuity. Therefore, spleen vacuity mechanisms for yin fire may add to those of liver depression/depressive heat. Even more, because the liver can only perform its function of governing, coursing, and discharging if it obtains sufficient blood to nourish it, blood vacuity due to spleen qi vacuity may cause or aggravate liver depression.

As we have just seen above, damp heat may be engendered internally by a combination of spleen vacuity induced dampness and depressive heat. Damp heat may also be due to overeating foods which engender fluids and heat. Foods which engender fluids include anything which is markedly sweet, such as sugar, honey, molasses, malt, and many fruits. Other foods which strongly engender fluids are dairy products, such as milk and cheese, as well as specifically the grain wheat. Food which engender heat in the body include anything whose nature is hot, such as cayenne pepper, black pepper, dry ginger, and many other culinary spices. Then there are foods which tend to produce both dampness and heat simultaneously. These are mainly greasy, fatty foods, such as fatty meals and oils, but also include alcohol. In addition, damp heat may invade the body from the outside due to living in a damp, hot environment or due to seasonal summerheat.

The process of life is a process of transforming yin substance into yang function. As we live, we are constantly consuming yin. Up until the mid-30s, most of us make more qi and blood every day than we consume by that day's activities (functions). When we sleep at night, that surplus qi and blood is stored for future use in the form of latter heaven essence. However, some time in the mid-30s or early 40s, the pendulum swings and the spleen begins to become vacuous and weak. Now it no longer makes as much qi and blood. Eventually, we begin running a deficit, dipping into our former heaven reserves of essence. Thus the *Nei*

Jing (Inner Classic) says, "At 40 years, yin [is] automatically half." As Zhu Dan-xi later expounded, the rate of this transformation of yin is also dependent on how much we stir, in other words, how active we are. The more yang function and activity, the quicker we consume yin. In terms of stirring or activity, there is physical stirring, verbal stirring, and mental-emotional stirring. Therefore, one may "burn through" their yin more quickly than someone else because of excessive stirring. Additionally, certain therapeutic and recreational drugs, such as steroids in the former case and opioids in the latter, may also damage and consume yin essence. In any case, if yin becomes too vacuous and weak to control yang, then yang may become hyperactive and ascend or float upward in the form of yin fire.

And finally, ministerial/life-gate fire may stir all on its own. For instance, at puberty, kidney yang becomes mature and this results in a temporary frenetic stirring of ministerial/life-gate fire due to the maturing of yin not taking place at the same pace. This then explains the excessive sexual stirring, physical stirring, and mental-emotional stirring of adolescents. Because the ministerial/life-gate fire is so closely associated to kidney yang and kidney yang is the root of our libido, sexual stirring or activity especially easily stirs ministerial/life-gate fire as do most, if not all, recreational drugs. Nevertheless, any excessive stirring, mental, verbal, or physical stirring can directly lead to stirring of ministerial/life-gate fire. The following diagram graphically shows how these five basic causes of yin fire are all mutually engendering and bidirectional.

THE FIVE BASIC MECHANISMS OF YIN FIRE

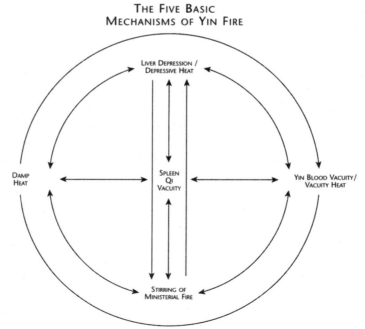

While Li only talks about the above five basic mechanisms for the engenderment of yin fire, there is a sixth. Because ministerial/life-gate fire ramifies throughout the entire body, the viscera and bowels, bones and sinews, muscles and flesh, and skin and hair, it is connected to all other parts of the body. That being said, the ministerial/life-gate fire has an especially close connection with the liver-gall-bladder, stomach, heart, pericardium, and triple burner. If heat is either externally contracted or internally engendered in any of these special viscera or bowels, it may mutually engender inflammation in the ministerial/life-gate fire. In other words, the relationship of ministerial/life-gate and the organ and tissues with which it communicates is bidirectional. Therefore, depending on how habitually (*i.e.*, constitutionally) hot one's ministerial/life-gate fire is, any heat evils in the body may cause it to become inflamed, and especially any heat evils in the liver-gallbladder, stomach, heart, pericardium, and/or triple burner.

In modern professional Chinese medicine, there is no single pattern called yin fire. Instead, yin fire is a general description for a multi-pattern presentation that includes internally engendered heat plus spleen vacuity at the very least. If there is spleen vacuity and damp heat, spleen vacuity and depressive heat, spleen vacuity and yin vacuity heat, spleen vacuity and ascendant liver yang hyperactivity, spleen vacuity and liver fire flaming upward, or spleen vacuity and heart fire effulgence, any and all of these multi-pattern presentations can be spoken of as yin fire scenarios.

Because of this, at the outset of a spleen pathocondition, there occurs raised qi with dyspnea, generalized fever with vexation, a large, surging pulse, headache, or incessant thirst. The skin, unable to stand wind or cold, generates (alternating) cold and heat. As yin fire surges upward, there occurs raised qi and dyspnea with distressing fever, headache, thirst, and a surging pulse. According to Li, a surging pulse is also indicative of yin fire. A surging pulse is defined as a floating, slippery, forceful pulse. Its floating character indicates the yang qi of the ministerial/life-gate fire is counterflowing upward and outward. As spleen and stomach qi run down, grain qi is deterred from rising and floating. Because the ministerial/life-gate fire is counterflowing upward, the spleen qi is damaged (or further damaged) and, therefore, failing to upbear the clear. While this may appear contradictory at first, it is an extremely important point. There can most definitely be pathological ascendency, stirring, hyperactivity, counterflow, surging, and floating at exactly the same time as there is non-upbearing of the clear and downward falling of the central qi. In fact, such pathological ascendency and hyperactivity result in non-upbearing of the central or spleen qi, and non-upbearing of the spleen qi results in failure of the ministerial/life-gate fire to remain calm and level in its lower source. Thus spleen qi vacuity promotes the upward counterflow of yin fire, and the upward counterflow of yin fire promotes spleen qi vacuity. Hence a self-perpetuating negative feedback loop is created. This is the engendering government of spring failing to work. This figurative statement implies that the spleen and stomach fail to convey and transform. In addition, it implies confined or lack of yang qi. Consequently, there is no yang [meaning insufficient spleen yang qi] to sustain the constructive and defensive. As they are unable to stand wind and cold, cold and heat are generated. Because the spleen is the latter heaven root of the engenderment and transformation of the qi and the source of both the constructive and the defensive, the defensive qi becomes vacuous and insufficient and fails to secure the exterior. Thus external evils are easily contracted and, once contracted, are difficult to thrust out from the body again. This helps explain why patients suffering from yin fire often have lowered immunity. All this is due to insufficient qi of the spleen and stomach.

However, although they look quite the same, this differs essentially from the pattern of external contraction of wind cold. Internal damage of the spleen and stomach is a damage of the qi. While external contraction of wind cold is a damage of the form [or physical body]. External damage is a superabundance. It requires drainage. Internal damage is an insufficiency. It requires supplementation. If an insufficiency disease of internal damage is mistaken for a superabundance disease of external contraction and subsequently [treated with] drainage, this is evacuating vacuity. Death caused by replenishing repletion or evacuating vacuity is murder committed by the physician. Here, Li is talking about the specific pattern of qi vacuity fever, and it is this fever which may be easily misdiagnosed as an external contraction of wind cold. In this case, typically due to enduring disease, the spleen qi falls downward to become depressed in the lower burner. Because qi is yang and inherently warm, this depressed, non-upbearing and non-extending qi transforms heat. This pathological depressive heat then inflames the ministerial/life-gate fire which has its source in the lower burner. Heat added to heat causes this ministerial/life-gate fire to counterflow upward and outward. However, this is a vacuity heat. Not yin vacuity, but a qi vacuity heat. Therefore, the correct method for its remedy is supplementation, specifically the fortification of the spleen and the upbearing of the clear. To try to clear and drain this heat as if it were a species of replete heat evil will only make this condition worse.

Then how to treat this? The only choice is to employ acrid, sweet, warm ingredients to supplement the center and upraise yang along with sweet, cold [ingredients] to drain fire. Care should be taken to note that Li does not say one should never, in the case of yin fire, use bitter, cold medicinals. In fact, as we will see, most Li Dong-yuan formulas contain a combination of sweet, acrid, warm and bitter, cold medicinals. Thus a cure is affected. The classic instructs, "Taxation should be warmed; what has been reduced should be warmed."[2] It adds, "Warm [medicinals] can eliminate intense heat." The use of bitter, cold medicinals which might damage the spleen and stomach is absolutely prohibited. Although uses the words "absolutely prohibited," in clinical practice, this is actually not the case as mentioned above. At their outset, pathoconditions involving the spleen and stomach [always] involve heat in the center. Below is a treatment designed for the outset of such a pattern.

Bu Zhong Yi Qi Tang
(Supplement the Center & Boost the Qi Decoction)

Huang Qi (Radix Astragali Membranacei), increase to 1 *qian* for diseases with overtaxation or serious heat

mix-fried *Gan Cao* (Radix Glycyrrhizae Uralensis), 5 *fen* each

Ren Shen (Radix Panacis Ginseng), stemmed, remove in case of coughing, 3 *fen*; the above three ingredients are divine medicinals for eliminating damp heat and distressing heat

Dang Gui (Radix Angelicae Sinensis), baked dry with wine or sun-dried for harmonizing the blood, 2 *fen*

Chen Pi (Pericarpium Citri Reticulatae), with the inner white skin preserved in order to conduct qi and boost the original qi as well; all right used in combination with sweet medicinals; if used alone, capable of draining the spleen and stomach; 2-3 *fen*

Sheng Ma (Rhizoma Cimicifugae), able to lead the stomach qi to soar up and return to position, *i.e.*, to exercise the government of upbearing spring; 2-3 *fen*

Chai Hu (Radix Bupleuri), able to conduct the clear qi and move the upbearing qi of the shao yang; 2-3 *fen*

Bai Zhu (Rhizoma Atractylodis Macrocephalae), able to eliminate heat in the stomach and disinhibit the blood around the lumbar spine (umbilicus [later editor]), 3 *fen*

Slice the above ingredients [and take] all as one dose boiled in two cups of water down to one cup, the size of the cup depending on whether qi is weak or exuberant. Remove the dregs and take while moderately hot between meals. For serious damage, two doses at the most will affect a cure. For enduring cases, vary the composition in accordance [with the signs].

In this source text, Li is recommending *Bu Zhong Yi Qi Tang* for the treatment of center heat resulting in a qi vacuity fever. Today, this formula is the standard formula for central qi falling downward. However, it can be used whenever there is a marked spleen qi vacuity accompanied by fatigue whether or not there is qi vacuity fever or specific signs and symptoms of central qi downward falling, such as chronic hemorrhoids or prolapsed uterus. In addition, it can also be used for the treatment of a liver-spleen disharmony. By increasing the dosage of *Chai Hu* (Radix Bupleuri), one can alter its functions from upbearing yang to coursing the liver and more powerfully rectifying the qi. Once one understands that *Bu Zhong Yi Qi Tang* can be used as a harmonizing formula, its scope becomes extremely wide, much wider in fact, than many practitioners erroneously assume.

[In case of] abdominal pain, add *Bai Shao* (Radix Albus Paeoniae Lactiflorae), five *fen*, and mix-fried *Gan Cao* (Radix Glycyrrhizae Uralensis), three *fen*. This results in adding the ingredients of *Shao Yao Gan Cao Tang* (Peony & Licorice Decoction), Zhang Zhong-jing's classic formula for the treatment of cramping pain. In case of aversion to cold and cold [abdominal] pain, add debarked *Gui Zhi* (Ramulus Cinnamomi Cassiae, *i.e.*, core of Ramulus Cinnamomi Cassiae), 1-3 *fen*. [In case of] aversion to heat and liking for cold with abdominal pain, add uncooked *Huang Qin* (Radix Scutellariae Baicalensis), 2-3 *fen*, plus *Bai Shao* and the other. "The other" refers to mixed-fried *Gan Cao* (Radix Glycyrrhizae Uralensis). [In case of] abdominal pain without aversion to heat in the summer months, also add [the above]. This is a remedy for seasonal heat. In the cool season, in case of aversion to heat with [abdominal] pain, add a small amount of *Gui Zhi* besides *Bai Shao*, *Gan Cao*, and *Huang Qin*. In the cold season, [in case of] abdominal pain, delete *Bai Shao*, since it is of sour flavor and cold, [but] add *Yi Zhi Ren* (Fructus Alpiniae Oxyphyllae), 2-3 *fen*, or *Ban Xia* (Rhizoma Pinelliae Ternatae), five *fen*, and *Sheng Jiang* (uncooked Rhizoma Zingiberis Officinalis), three slices. [In case of] headache, add *Man Jing Zi* (Fructus Viticis), 2-3 *fen*. [In case of] severe headache, add *Chuan Xiong* (Radix Ligustici Wallichii), two *fen*. [In case of] pain in the top of the head and in the brain, add *Gao Ben* (Radix Et Rhizoma Ligustici Sinensis), 3-5 *fen*. [In case of] tormenting headache, add *Xi Xin* (Herba Asari Cum Radice), two *fen*, produced in Huayin [a county in Shanxi province famous for good quality *Xi Xin*]. For various types of headache, the above four medicinals suffice. For heat in the head, the above are not effective. This should be treated by another formula, *Qing Kong Gao* (Clear the Cavity Paste).[3]

[In case of] pain below the umbilicus, add *Shu Di* (cooked Radix Rehmanniae Glutinosae), five *fen*, and the pain will be relieved instantly. If not, this proves it to be due to intense cold. In that case, add debarked *Rou Gui* (Cortex Cinnamomi Cassiae), 2-3 *fen*. It is stated in the *Nei Jing (Inner Classic)* that all kinds of lower abdominal pain are cold patterns derived from revengeful retaliation. If spleen earth is vacuous, its restraining phase, liver wood, will conquer it. But the phase it engenders, lung metal, will wreak vengeance upon liver wood, causing it to be diseased. This is called revengeful retaliation. The classic explains that great victory incurs fierce retaliation. This cold pattern is transmuted from a hot disease. It is not the jue yin pattern of cold damage. [Zhang] Zhong-jing treated this with *Di Dang Tang* (Dead-on Decoction) and the *Di Dang Wan* (Dead-on Pills).[4] This is blood being bound in the urinary bladder of the lower burner. The signs and symptoms of bound blood in the bladder are jaundice, fever, a tight, full lower abdomen, uninhibited urination, and manic behavior. Here Li is warning against the use of Zhang Zhong-jing's formulas in this case, that the situation is not the same as described by Zhang Zhong-jing.

[In case of] qi congestion and stagnation in the chest, add *Qing Pi* (Pericarpium Citri Reticulatae Viride), two *fen*; [however, in case of] distressed rapid breathing or diminished qi, delete this. Diminished qi here means shortness of breath. Clearly this addition, shows that Li assumed this formula could be used for a liver-spleen disharmony, not just a simple vacuity. For pain in the body due to dampness and generalized heaviness also due to dampness, add one *qian* of *Wu Ling San* (Five [Ingredients] Poria Powder) from which *Gui Zhi* (Ramulus Cinnamomi Cassiae) has been deleted. If wind and dampness are locked in contention, giving rise to generalized pain, add *Qiang Huo* (Radix Et Rhizoma Notopterygii), *Fang Feng* (Radix Ledebouriellae Divaricatae), and *Ga Ben* (Radix Et Rhizoma Ligustici Sinensis), five *fen* each, and *Sheng Ma* (Rhizoma Cimicifugae) and *Cang Zhu* (Rhizoma Atractylodis), 1.5 *qian* each. [In that case,] do not use *Wu Ling San*. These windy medicinals are quite capable of overcoming dampness, and they form a distinctive formula. Once the disease is relieved, [however,] do not administer these further since the various windy medicinals [are liable to] cause detriment to the body's original qi and deteriorate the [patient's] condition.

[In case of] dry, bound stools, add *Dang Gui Wei* (Extremitas Radicis Angelicae Sinensis), one *qian*. [In case of] constipation, boil the standard formula [*i.e., Bu Zhong Yi Qi Tang*]. Take a [big] mouthful of the decoction with five *fen* or one *qian* of *Xuan Ming Fen* [a compound of Glauber's salt and *Gan Cao*, Radix Glycyrrhizae Uralensis]. Once the bowels move, stop administering [this formula]. Precipitation is prohibited in this disease. Precipitation may well give rise to precarious transmuted patterns.

[In case of] coughing with phlegm in a chronic disease, delete *Ren Shen*. For [coughing] at the initial stage of a disease, do not delete it. Winter months, cold spring weather, or cool autumn weather call for the addition of *Ma Huang* (Herba

Ephedrae) without root or joint, five *fen*. In very warm weather in spring, merely add *Fo Er Cao* (Herba Saxifragae), three *fen*, and *Kuan Dong Hua* (Flos Tussilaginis Farfarae), one *fen*. In case of cough contracted in summer months, add *Wu Wei Zi* (Fructus Schisandrae Chinensis), 32 pieces, and *Mai Men Dong* (Tuber Ophiopogonis Japonici), cored, 2-3 *fen*. White, glossy tongue fur indicates cold in the chest. [In that case,] do not use these.

In the absence of cough during the summer months, add *Ren Shen*, 2-3 *fen*, nonetheless together with *Wu Wei Zi* and *Mai Men Dong* in equal amounts to rescue the lungs from fire evils. If the patient is able to take in food but has glomus below the heart, add *Huang Lian* (Rhizoma Coptidis Chinensis), 1-3 *fen*. [In case of] glomus below the heart with inability to take in food, do not add *Huang Lian*. For rib-side pain or acute spasm, add *Chai Hu* (Radix Bupleuri), three *fen* or five *fen* in serious cases.

These variations of the above formula [*i.e., Bu Zhong Yi Qi Tang*] are applicable for [spleen] disease with heat in the center due to dietary irregularity and taxation fatigue or [excessive] joy and anger before this has transmuted into center cold. [After that,] sweet and sour [ingredients], such as *Huang Qi, Ren Shen, Gan Cao*, and *Wu Wei Zi*, may exacerbate the disease. The details of center heat and center cold are illustrated below [by the following cites] from the *Nei Jing (Inner Classic)* and *Wai Jing (Outer Classic)*.

The *Tiao Jing Lun (Treatise on Regulating the Channels)* states:

> When blood is confined in the yang and qi is confined in the yin, center heat develops. When blood is confined in the upper and qi is confined in the lower, there occurs vexation and depression of the heart and irascibility.

It adds, "That which arises in the yin is ascribed to the diet and lifestyle, yin and yang, joy and anger." Here yin and yang refer to excessive indulgence in sexual intercourse. It says, [this manifests by]

> . . .all the [symptoms of] taxation fatigue, decrepit and diminished form qi, meager grain qi, obstructed upper burner, and blocked lower duct. Stomach qi becomes hot and hot qi steams the chest causing internal heat . . . Exuberant yin engenders internal cold. With ascending counterflow of reversed qi, cold qi accumulates in the chest without being drained. [With the cold qi] not drained, warm qi has to depart and what is left is nothing but cold. With cold left alone, blood congeals and stagnates. With congealed, stagnated blood, the vessels are blocked. The pulse is large, exuberant, and rough (or choppy). This is, therefore, called center cold.

The following are *Bu Zhong Yi Qi Tang's* contemporary indications: 1) spleen-stomach qi vacuity, 2) qi vacuity downward falling, 3) qi vacuity fever. Debility after prolonged disease, common cold in a person with bodily vacuity, chronic bronchitis, prolapsed uterus, prolapsed rectum, chronic hemorrhoids, gastroptosis, hernia, chronic gonorrhea, diarrhea, persistent malaria, habitual miscarriage, functional uterine bleeding and other hemorrhagic disorders, abnormal vaginal discharge, various postpartum problems, such as urinary incontinence, lochioschesis, and agalactia, chronic hepatitis, peritonitis, tuberculosis, neurasthenia, impotence, corneal ulcers, cerebral arteriosclerosis, pernicious anemia, leukopenia, chronic nephritis, and myasthenia gravis

The main contemporary signs and symptoms of the three main indicated patterns include: 1) Fatigue, lack of strength, poor appetite, spontaneous sweating, shortness of breath, disinclination to speak, dizziness standing up, an ashen white or sallow yellow facial complexion, loose stools, a pale tongue with thin, white fur, and a short; flooding, vacuous; or large, vacuous pulse; 2) anal prolapse, first and second degree uterine prolapse, prolonged diarrhea, prolonged dysentery, and other such complaints due to downward falling of clear yang; 3) fever associated with fatigue, thirst with a desire for warm drinks, possible lack of warmth in the hands and feet, enduring malaria-like diseases.

Besides the above additions and subtractions originally suggested by Li, there are many others which have become relatively standard in contemporary professional Chinese medicine. The following are a selection of these.

If blood vacuity is prominent, increase the dosage of *Dang Gui* (Radix Angelicae Sinensis).

For prolapse, increase the dosage of *Huang Qi* (Radix Astragali Membranacei) and add *Zhi Shi* (Fructus Immaturus Citri Aurantii).

For uterine prolapse, add *Yi Zhi Ren* (Fructus Alpiniae Oxyphyllae), *Ai Ye* (Folium Artemisiae Argyii), and *Wu Wei Zi* (Fructus Schisandrae Chinensis).

For headache with vertigo and dizziness, add *Chuan Xiong* (Radix Ligustici Wallichii) and *Ban Xia* (Rhizoma Pinelliae Ternatae).

For vertigo and vomiting, add *Ge Gen* (Radix Puerariae) and *Ze Xie* (Rhizoma Alismatis Orientalis).

For bodily heaviness, joint pain, irritability, loss of appetite, chest oppression, shortness of breath, etc. due to qi stagnation and damp accumulation, replace *Bai Zhu* (Rhizoma Atractylodis Macrocephalae) with *Cang Zhu* (Rhizoma Atractylodis), subtract *Dang Gui* (Radix Angelicae Sinensis), and add *Bai Shao* (Radix Albus Paeoniae Lactiflorae). This results in *Tiao Zhong Yi Qi Tang* (Regulate the Center & Boost the Qi Decoction), another of Li's famous formulas.

For myasthenia gravis, increase the dosages of *Huang Qi* (Radix Astragali Membranacei) and *Sheng Ma* (Rhizoma Cimicifugae).

For diarrhea due to excessive thinking and worry resulting in liver-spleen disharmony, add *Mu Xiang* (Radix Auklandiae Lappae).

For diarrhea due to dampness, subtract *Dang Gui* (Radix Angelicae Sinensis) and add *Fu Ling* (Sclerotium Poriae Cocos), *Cang Zhu* (Rhizoma Atractylodis), and *Yi Zhi Ren* (Fructus Alpiniae Oxyphyllae).

Prolonged diarrhea with intestinal qi loss of securing and astringency, add *He Zi* (Fructus Terminaliae Chebulae), *Rou Dou Kou* (Semen Myristicae Fragrantis), *Wu Wei Zi* (Fructus Schisandrae Chinensis), and *Wu Mei* (Fructus Pruni Mume).

For dysentery with tenesmus, subtract *Dang Gui* (Radix Angelicae Sinensis) and add *Mu Xiang* (Radix Auklandiae Lappae).

For dysentery after the blood and pus have resolved but there is still foamy mucus, add *Pao Jiang* (blast-fried Rhizoma Zingiberis Officinalis) and *Chi Shi Zhi* (Hallyositum Rubrum).

After dysentery when there is still tenesmus and mucus in the stools but constipation, add *Fang Feng* (Radix Ledebouriellae Divaricatae).

For cold stomach with qi stagnation, add *Qing Pi* (Pericarpium Citri Reticulatae Viride), *Sha Ren* (Fructus Amomi), *Mu Xiang* (Radix Auklandiae Lappae), and *Yi Zhi Ren* (Fructus Alpiniae Oxyphyllae).

For ringing in the ears or loss of hearing due to spleen-kidney qi vacuity, add *Shan Zhu Yu* (Fructus Corni Officinalis) and *Yi Zhi Ren* (Fructus Alpiniae Oxyphyllae).

For diminished eyesight or blurred vision due to spleen qi and liver blood vacuity, add *Gou Qi Zi* (Fructus Lycii Chinensis) and *Chuan Xiong* (Radix Ligustici Wallichii).

For habitual miscarriage due to spleen-kidney dual vacuity, add *Du Zhong* (Cortex Eucommiae Ulmoidis) and *Tu Si Zi* (Semen Cuscutae Chinensis).

For restless fetus and threatened abortion, add *E Jiao* (Gelatinum Corii Asini) and *Ai Ye* (Folium Artemisiae Argyii). This modification can then be made even stronger by adding *Xu Duan* (Radix Dipsaci) and *Sang Ji Sheng* (Ramulus Loranthi Seu Visci).

For abnormal vaginal discharge, add *Er Miao San* (Two Wonders Powder), *i.e.*, *Cang Zhu* (Rhizoma Atractylodis) and *Huang Bai* (Cortex Phellodendri).

For abdominal distention, add *Zhi Shi* (Fructus Immaturus Citri Aurantii), *Hou Po* (Cortex Magnoliae Officinalis), *Mu Xiang* (Radix Auklandiae Lappae), and *Sha Ren* (Fructus Amomi).

For mounting disorders, add *Ju He* (Semen Citri Reticulatae), *Xiao Hui Xiang* (Fructus Foeniculi Vulgaris), and *Li Zhi He* (Semen Litchi Chinensis).

For constipation, add processed *Da Huang* (Radix Et Rhizoma Rhei).

For constipation due to spleen vacuity, add honey and sesame oil.

For painful urinary strangury in the elderly due to fallen yang qi, add *Ze Xie* (Rhizoma Alismatis Orientalis) and *Mu Tong* (Caulis Akebiae).

For taxation strangury with heat, add *Zhi Bai Di Huang Wan* (Anemarrhena & Phellodendron Rehmannia Pills), *i.e.*, *Zhi Mu* (Rhizoma Anemarrhenae Aspheloidis), *Huang Bai* (Cortex Phellodendri), *Shu Di* (cooked Radix Rehmanniae Glutinosae), *Shan Yao* (Radix Dioscoreae Oppositae), *Shan Zhu Yu* (Fructus Corni Officinalis), *Fu Ling* (Sclerotium Poriae Cocos), *Ze Xie* (Rhizoma Alismatis Orientalis), and *Dan Pi* (Cortex Radicis Moutan).

Also for taxation strangury without heat, add *Liu Wei Di Huang Wan* (Six Flavors Rehmannia Pills), *i.e.*, *Shu Di* (cooked Radix Rehmanniae Glutinosae), *Shan Yao* (Radix Dioscoreae Oppositae), *Shan Zhu Yu* (Fructus Corni Officinalis), *Fu Ling* (Sclerotium Poriae Cocos), *Ze Xie* (Rhizoma Alismatis Orientalis), and *Dan Pi* (Cortex Radicis Moutan), plus *Mai Men Dong* (Tuber Ophiopogonis Japonici) and *Wu Wei Zi* (Fructus Schisandrae Chinensis).

For frequent urination aggravated by exertion, add *Shan Yao* (Radix Dioscoreae Oppositae) and *Wu Wei Zi* (Fructus Schisandrae Chinensis).

For dark yellow, concentrated urination after diarrhea due to damaged fluids, add *Mai Men Dong* (Tuber Ophiopogonis Japonici) and *Wu Wei Zi* (Fructus Schisandrae Chinensis).

For premenstrual diarrhea, add *Pao Jiang* (blast-fried Rhizoma Zingiberis Officinalis) and *Huang Lian* (Rhizoma Coptidis Chinensis).

For pediatric bed-wetting, add *Sang Piao Xiao* (Ootheca Mantidis) and *Yi Zhi Ren* (Fructus Alpiniae Oxyphyllae).

For chronic rhinitis, add *Cang Er Zi* (Fructus Xanthii Sibirici) and *Xin Yi Hua* (Flos Magnoliae).

For corneal ulcers, add *Gu Jing Cao* (Scapus Eriocaulonis Buergeriani), *Jue Ming Zi* (Semen Cassiae Torae), and *Shan Yao* (Radix Dioscoreae Oppositae).

If there is concomitant yin vacuity, either subtract *Chai Hu* (Radix Bupleuri) and *Sheng Ma* (Rhizoma Cimicifugae) or reduce their dosages and add *Zhi Mu* (Rhizoma Anemarrhenae Aspheloidis) and *Huang Bai* (Cortex Phellodendri).

Also for yin vacuity, subtract *Chai Hu* (Radix Bupleuri) and *Sheng Ma* (Rhizoma Cimicifugae) and add *Shan Zhu Yu* (Fructus Corni Officinalis), *Shan Yao* (Radix Dioscoreae Oppositae), and *Shu Di* (cooked Radix Rehmanniae Glutinosae).

For qi vacuity fever, add *Zhi Mu* (Rhizoma Anemarrhenae Aspheloidis) and *Di Gu Pi* (Cortex Radicis Lycii Chinensis).

Also for qi vacuity fever, increase the dosage of *Chai Hu* (Radix Bupleuri) and add *Huang Qin* (Radix Scutellariae Baicalensis) and *Ge Gen* (Radix Puerariae).

For coronary heart disease with exertional angina pectoris due to concomitant blood stasis, add *Dan Shen* (Radix Salviae Miltiorrhizae), *Chuan Xiong* (Radix Ligustici Wallichii), *Chi Shao* (Radix Rubrus Paeoniae Lactiflorae), *Hong Hua* (Flos Carthami Tinctorii), and *Jiang Xiang* (Lignum Dalbergiae Odoriferae).

For chronic sore throat, add *Jie Geng* (Radix Platycodi Grandiflori).

For profuse menstruation, add wine-fried *Bai Shao* (Radix Albus Paeoniae Lactiflorae). If there is liver heat, also add *Huang Qin* (Radix Scutellariae Baicalensis).

For flooding and leaking, add *Di Yu* (Radix Sanguisorbae) for damp or replete heat, *Ai Ye* (Folium Artemisiae Argyii) and *E Jiao* (Gelatinum Corii Asini) for qi vacuity, *Sheng Di* (uncooked Radix Rehmanniae Glutinosae) for vacuity heat, and *Hai Piao Xiao* (Os Sepiae Seu Sepiellae) for loss of securing and astringing.

For profuse menstruation or uterine bleeding with pale, watery blood accompanied by heart palpitations, shortness of breath, faint, forceless speech, fatigue, and a sagging, dragging feeling in the lower abdomen, subtract *Dang Gui* (Radix Angelicae Sinensis), *Chai Hu* (Radix Bupleuri), and *Chen Pi* (Pericarpium Citri Reticulatae). This results in *Ju Yuan Jian* (Lift the Source Decoction). This formula can then be augmented by adding *Hai Piao Xiao* (Os Sepiae Seu Sepiellae), *Qian Cao* (Radix Rubiae Cordifoliae), and *Wu Mei* (Fructus Pruni Mume). If there is liver heat, also add *Huang Qin* (Radix Scutellariae Baicalensis).

For numbness of the fingers and face due to qi vacuity with exuberant wind, subtract *Dang Gui* (Radix Angelicae Sinensis), *Bai Zhu* (Rhizoma Atractylodis Macrocephalae), and *Chen Pi* (Pericarpium Citri Reticulatae), and add *Bai Shao* (Radix Albus Paeoniae Lactiflorae) and *Wu Wei Zi* (Fructus Schisandrae Chinensis).

For numbness accompanying bodily weakness, dry, flaky skin, and itching, add *Shu Di* (cooked Radix Rehmanniae Glutinosae) and *Bai Shao* (Radix Albus Paeoniae Lactiflorae) to nourish the blood.

For concomitant restlessness of the heart spirit, add *Long Gu* (Os Draconis), *Mu Li* (Concha Ostreae), and *Ye Jiao Teng* (Caulis Polygoni Multiflori).

These recommendations do not come close to exhausting the possibilities of modifying this hugely important formula. This formula is one of my five most commonly used formulas.

The pattern of center heat disease at the onset arises because the fire of the penetrating vessel attaches to that inside the two yin [*i.e.*, that contained within the perineum] and is transmitted to the governing vessel. What is known as the governing vessel [begins at] *Chang Qiang* (GV 1) under the twenty-first vertebra and is a channel that mutually attaches with the foot tai yang urinary bladder cold qi. The kidneys govern cold water or cold qi. This coldness does not imply any abnormality. Because it is coupled with the urinary bladder, this sentence may also be rendered: " . . . with the foot *tai yang* urinary bladder channel." The governing vessel, when exuberant, runs like a great river or like a rapidly galloping horse with an uncheckable tremendous momentum. [But] tai yang cold qi is as thin as a thread. When [fire] travels upwards against the current of the tai yang cold qi, [it] surges into the top of the head, turns down the tip of the nose, and enters the hand tai yang in the chest. The hand tai yang is *bing* which is hot qi. The foot urinary bladder [channel] is *ren* which is cold qi. *Ren* is able to overwhelm *bing*. According to five phases theory, *jia* (S1) and *yi* (S2) are wood, *bing* (S3) and *ding* (S4) are fire, *wu* (S5) and *ji* (S6) are earth, *geng* (S7) and *xin* (S8) are metal, and *ren* (S9) and *gui* (S10) are water. This implies that a generating phase, the kidneys for instance, if diseased, can make the generated phase, the liver, contract an illness of repletion. But as cold and heat counterflow in the chest, the pulse becomes large and exuberant. Since the hot qi of the hand tai yang small intestine [channel] cannot join and enter the urinary bladder channel, the qi of the other 11 channels [becomes] exuberant and gathers in the chest. Therefore, the pulse is large and exuberant. The urinary bladder counterflows and is extremely exuberant. The child is capable of making the mother replete. Cold water (the urinary bladder or foot tai yang channel) is engendered by metal (the large intestine or hand yang ming channel). The hand yang ming channel, metal, is just the mother. This corresponds to effulgent dryness. By the strength of the son, this dry qi results in a rough [or choppy] pulse and constipation. From this point of view, this large, exuberant, rough pulse is due to the hand yang ming large intestine channel.

This is, in my mind, an extremely interesting passage. It explains how yin fire engendered internally can spill over into the channels and vessels. Li begins by saying that yin fire is associated with the penetrating vessel. The penetrating vessel is the vessel which connects the kidneys and the heart by way of the reproductive organs. Although Li does not say so, this is the pathway by which ministerial/life-gate fire stirs upward, moving out of the lower burner to eventually arise at the heart-pericardium. The penetrating vessel connects with the governing vessel at *Chang Qiang* (GV 1). The governing vessel is the sea of all yang, and heat evils are yang in nature. Therefore, it is not surprising that these heat evils might shift or move into the governing vessel. In the mid-thoracic region the governing vessel also connects with the inner line of the foot tai yang bladder channel. If these heat evils spill over into the bladder channel, they may also spill over into the hand tai yang small intestine channel. In this case, they surge into the yin and yang channels of the chest where they cause chaos and counterflow. Hence congestion and accumulation may occur in the shoulders, back of the neck, head, face, throat, and/or chest and breast regions. Zhu Dan-xi used a slight variation of this same theory to help explain chronic neck and shoulder tension as well as breast cancer. As Zhu points out in the case of neck and shoulder tension, although this obstruction and accumulation of yang qi eventually spills over into the gallbladder and triple heater channels, it does not originate there (or at least not entirely). This helps explain why treatment of these channels rarely produces lasting relief of chronic neck and shoulder pain and also why points on the hand tai yang small intestine channel are so effective for treating a variety of breast disorders.

The *Huang Di Zhen Jing* (*Yellow Emperor's Acupuncture Classic*) states, "For stomach disease with abdominal distention, pain of the duct in the cardiac region propping up against the rib-side regions, obstructed diaphragm, and a throat which does not allow food and drink to pass downward, treat [*Zu*] *San Li* (St 36) with supplementation."[5]

If any of the above patterns is observed, which are all ascribed to great cold, no sweet or sour medicinals should be used. This is already obvious from the above discussion.

REPRESENTATIVE CASE HISTORIES:

The following case histories are presented to help demonstrate the huge scope of practice of *Bu Zhong Yi Qi Tang* and the clinical utility of the theories on which it is based. They primarily come from the Chinese medical journal literature from the People's Republic of China.

From "New Uses of *Bu Zhong Yi Qi Tang*," by Qiu Li-ming appearing in Si Chuan Zhong Yi (Sichuan Chinese Medicine), #6, 2000, p. 57

CASE 1: Recurrent oral apthae

The patient was a 34 year-old male cadre who was first examined on Oct. 25, 1998. The man had had recurrent oral ulcers for five years. For the last two months, the number of these oral sores had increased and they were both burning hot and peppery painful. Due to this, the man was not able to eat. The patient had already taken various Chinese medicinals to clear heat and drain fire as well as vitamin B complex and several Western medicines, all without effect. Accompanying the oral sores were venter and abdominal glomus and fullness, torpid intake, loose stools, lassitude of the spirit, lack of strength, a dry throat, somnolence, a pale, fat tongue with teeth-marks on its edges and thin, white fur, and a deep, fine, rapid pulse. On examination, there were ulcers on the man's upper and lower lips and mucus membranes on both sides of his cheeks. The tip of his tongue also had many ulcerated sores whose bases were concave and depressed. The color of these sores was ashen white, and pressure pain was pronounced.

Based on the above signs and symptoms, the man's pattern was categorized as spleen-stomach vacuity weakness with clear yang not being upborne and yin fire ascending and flaming, steaming and burning the mouth and tongue. Thus treatment should supplement the center and boost the qi, subdue and downbear yin fire. The formula used was *Bu Zhong Yi Qi Tang* with additions and subtractions: *Huang Qi* (Radix Astragali Membranacei), 30g, *Dang Shen* (Radix Codonopsitis Pilosulae) and *Bai Zhu* (Rhizoma Atractylodis Macrocephalae), 15g each, *Sheng Ma* (Rhizoma Cimicifugae), *Chai Hu* (Radix

Bupleuri), *Dan Zhu Ye* (Herba Lophatheri Gracilis), and *Wu Zhu Yu* (Fructus Evodiae Rutecarpae), 10g each, *Chen Pi* (Pericarpium Citri Reticulatae) and mix-fried *Gan Cao* (Radix Glycyrrhizae Uralensis), 6g each, and *Rou Gui* (Cortex Cinnamomi Cassiae), 3g. After administering seven packets of this formula, the ulcers had shrunk and become smaller and eating was no longer painful. All the man's symptoms were greatly reduced. Ten more packets were administered continuously and the ulcers were cured as well as all other symptoms. On follow-up in 2000, there had been no recurrence.

CASE 2: Chronically chilled limbs

The patient was a 29 year-old female teacher who was first examined on Dec. 2, 1997. This woman had caught cold two years earlier after having given birth and had lost her regular nourishment. This resulted in the emission of chill in both her lower extremities. Initially this was not serious. However, during the last year, this condition had gradually worsened to the point that all four limbs emitted chill. This was especially bad during the cold and chilly seasons. The woman had already seen several doctors and had been diagnosed with cold lodged in her blood vessels resulting in uneasy flow of the qi and blood. For this, she had been given yang-warming, cold-scattering, blood-quickening, and network vessel freeing Chinese medicinals, after which there was slight improvement. The coldness and chilling were most severe below her elbows and knees. Her facial complexion was lusterless, and her stools were loose. Intake was torpid, there was bodily fatigue, and she lacked strength. The use of her body and limbs was normal, and there was no numbness, pain, or itching. Her tongue was pale with thin, white fur, and her pulse was deep and fine.

Based on the above signs and symptoms, the patient's Chinese medical pattern was categorized as middle burner vacuity cold with spleen qi unable to upbear, emit, and spread clear yang to the four extremities. The treatment principles were to supplement the center and boost the qi, upbear and emit clear yang. The formula used was *Bu Zhong Yi Qi Tang* with added flavors: *Huang Qi* (Radix Astragali Membranacei), 50g, *Dang Shen* (Radix Codonopsitis Pilosulae), 30g, *Dang Gui* (Radix Angelicae Sinensis), *Bai Zhu* (Rhizoma Atractylodis Macrocephalae), and *Gui Zhi* (Ramulus Cinnamomi Cassiae), 15g each, and *Sheng Ma* (Rhizoma Cimicifugae), *Chai Hu* (Radix Bupleuri), *Chen Pi* (Pericarpium Citri Reticulatae), dry *Gan Jiang* (Rhizoma Zingiberis Officinalis), and mix-fried *Gan Cao* (Radix Glycyrrhizae Uralensis), 6g each. Ten packets of these medicinals were administered orally, after which her four limbs were already warm, her intake of food had improved, and her loose stools had disappeared. Therefore, these same medicinals were administered for another half month when all her symptoms were eliminated. On follow-up after one year, there had been no recurrence.

CASE 3: Postpartum urinary incontinence

The patient was a 30 year-old female cadre who was first examined on Mar. 5, 1998. One year previously she had caught cold after giving birth. This had resulted in her leaking urine whenever she coughed. Initially this was not severe, and she did not seek treatment for it. However, two months ago, this condition had become more pronounced and her urination had become incontinent. Whenever the patient was fatigued, this incontinence was worse. Other symptoms included low back soreness, weak lower limbs, lassitude of the spirit, shortness of breath, dizziness, blurred vision, occasional stomach duct distention and fullness, a fat body, a pale red tongue which was also slightly fat with thin, white fur, and a vacuous, fine, forceless pulse.

Based on these signs and symptoms, the woman's Chinese medical pattern was categorized as spleen-kidney qi vacuity with the bladder not doing its duty. The treatment principles were to supplement the center and boost the qi, regulate the qi, secure and gather. The formula used was modified *Bu Zhong Yi Qi Tang*: *Huang Qi* (Radix Astragali Membranacei), 30g, *Dang Shen* (Radix Codonopsitis Pilosulae), *Bai Zhu* (Rhizoma Atractylodis Macrocephalae), and *Dang Gui* (Radix Angelicae Sinensis), 20g each. *Chen Pi* (Pericarpium Citri Reticulatae), *Sheng Ma* (Rhizoma Cimicifugae), *Chai Hu* (Radix Bupleuri), and *Du Zhong* (Cortex Eucommiae Ulmoidis), 10g each, *Shan Zhu Yu* (Fructus Corni Officinalis), 15g, and *Gui Zhi* (Ramulus Cinnamomi Cassiae) and mix-fried *Gan Cao* (Radix Glycyrrhizae Uralensis), 6g each. After taking 10 packets of this formula, the urinary incontinence disappeared. This prescription was then administered for another month, after which all her symptoms disappeared. On follow-up after two years, there had been no recurrence.

From "New Uses of *Bu Zhong Yi Qi Tang*" by Luo Chang-yi & Wang Shu-ying, *Si Chuan Zhong Yi (Sichuan Chinese Medicine)*, #10, 2001, p. 74-75

CASE 4: Chronic nephritis

The patient was a 32 year-old female who was first seen on Jul. 18, 1996. The patient had had generalized edema for the past year. This was worse in the lower half of her body. In the last two months, this condition had gotten even worse and was accompanied by low back soreness and pain, torpid intake, abdominal distention, and loose stools. Her urine tested 4-plus positive for protein, and she was diagnosed as suffering from chronic nephritis, for which she was treated with Prednisone and diuretics for two months. However, her symptoms did not markedly improve. Instead, her edema had gotten worse day by day and she returned to the hospital for re-examination, at which time, her blood pressure was 18/12KPa. The patient's tongue was pale with white fur and her pulse was deep and fine. Urine protein was still 4-plus positive.

Based on the above, the authors categorized this woman's pattern as central qi insufficiency with spleen loss of fortification and movement, kidney vacuity not managing, qi stagnation and blood stasis, and water dampness internally collecting. Therefore, their treatment principles were to supplement the center and boost the qi, bank earth and disinhibit water. The formula used was modified *Bu Zhong Yi Qi Tang* which consisted of: *Huang Qi* (Radix Astragali Membranacei), 60g, *Dang Gui* (Radix Angelicae Sinensis), *Bai Zhu* (Rhizoma Atractylodis Macrocephalae), *Fu Ling* (Sclerotium Poriae Cocos), *Shi Wei* (Herba Pyrossiae), and *Da Fu Pi* (Pericarpium Arecae Catechu), 15g each, *Chen Pi* (Pericarpium Citri Reticulatae), *Chai Hu* (Radix Bupleuri), *Sheng Ma* (Rhizoma Cimicifugae), and mix-fried *Gan Cao* (Radix Glycyrrhizae Uralensis), 10g each, *Dang Shen* (Radix Codonopsitis Pilosulae), 30g, *Bai Mao Gen* (Rhizoma Imperatae Cylindricae), 50g, and *Yi Mu Cao* (Herba Leonuri Heterophylli), 40g. One packet of these medicinals was decocted in water and administered per day, and, after five packets, all the patient's symptoms were greatly reduced. Her appetite had improved, her urination had increased, her abdominal distention was less, albuminuria was 2-plus positive, and the edema had gradually receded. Another 50 packets of this formula were administered with additions and subtractions following her condition and her symptoms completely disappeared. Numerous re-examinations of her urine were normal, and there had been no recurrence on follow-up after one year.

CASE 5: Digestive ulcers

The patient was a 46 year-old female who was first seen on Oct. 25, 1998. The patient had had recurrent stomach duct pain for five years which had gotten worse in the preceding month. Gradually, work had become more taxing and fatiguing and her mood had become depressed. Her facial complexion was somber white and she had duct and abdominal aching and pain which was lessened with warmth. Her eating and drinking were devitalized and her abdomen became distended after meals along with repeated burping and belching. Her tongue fur was white and glossy, and the woman's pulse was fine, rapid, and forceless. Hemafecia was triple-plus positive, and gastrointestinal examination revealed duodenal ulcers. Her Western medical diagnosis was chronic superficial gastritis.

Based on the above, the authors categorized this woman's pattern was spleen-stomach qi vacuity with qi not managing the blood. The treatment principles were to boost the qi to manage the blood, supplement the center and bank earth. The medicinals prescribed were a modification of *Bu Zhong Yi Qi Tang* which included: *Huang Qi* (Radix Astragali Membranacei), 60g, *Hong Shen* (red Radix Panacis Ginseng), *Fu Ling* (Sclerotium Poriae Cocos), and *Bai Zhu* (Rhizoma Atractylodis Macrocephalae), 15g each, *Bai Ji* (Radix Bletillae Striatae) and stir-fried *Di Yu* (Radix Sanguisorbae), 20g each, *Chai Hu* (Radix Bupleuri), *Chen Pi* (Pericarpium Citri Reticulatae), and mix-fried *Gan Cao* (Radix Glycyrrhizae Uralensis), 10g each, *Hai Piao Xiao* (Os Sepiae Seu Sepiellae) and *Huang Qin* (Radix Scutellariae Baicalensis), 30g each, and *Sheng Ma* (Rhizoma Cimicifugae), 6g. In addition, *Yun Nan Bai Yao* (Yunnan White Medicine) was swallowed with each dose. After three packets, the hemafecia had turned negative and all the symptoms had decreased. However, there was still a feeling of bodily fatigue and lack of strength. Therefore, *Hong Shen* was changed to *Dang Shen* (Radix Codonopsitis Pilosulae). Treatment was given for two more months with appropriate modifications, at which time all the patient's symptoms were eliminated and her mood had improved. Repeat gastrointestinal examination showed no abnormalities.

CASE 6: Urolithiasis

The patient was a 38 year-old male who was first seen on Feb. 15, 1998. For the past 10 days, due to overtaxation and fatigue, the man had had left-sided low back pain accompanied by massive sweating and a somber white facial complexion. After receiving 50ml of *leng ding* (an unidentified Western medicine) via intramuscular injection, the pain remitted. However, the patient continued to have left-sided, lower abdominal pain, he was diagnosed with urinary tract stones, and was treated with 30 packets of *Ba Zheng San* (Eight [Ingredients] Correcting Powder) and *Shi Wei San* (Pyrossia Powder). However, the man continued to have the pain from time to time even though it was less. Therefore, he returned to the hospital where ultrasound confirmed the continued presence of a left-sided urinary tract stone. In addition, the patient was thin, his intake was torpid, and his spirit was listless. There was lower abdominal fullness and cramping and difficult-to-bear urinary tract piercing pain. His urination was short, red, and choppy. His pulse was bowstring, fine, and rapid, and his tongue was red with thin, yellow, slightly slimy fur.

Based on the above, the man was diagnosed as suffering from stone strangury and his pattern was categorized as enduring dampness and heat brewing and binding along with qi and yin vacuity. Thus there was a righteous vacuity and an evil repletion. The treatment principles Luo and Wang advanced were to boost the qi and free the flow of strangury, clear heat, nourish yin, and disinhibit dampness, support the righteous and dispel evils. The formula they prescribed consisted of the following modification of *Bu Zhong Yi Qi*

Tang: *Huang Qi* (Radix Astragali Membranacei), 80g, *Tai Zi Shen* (Radix Pseudostellariae Heterophyllae), *Bai Shao* (Radix Albus Paeoniae Lactiflorae), and *Jin Qian Cao* (Herba Desmodii Seu Lysimachiae), 30g each, *Chai Hu* (Radix Bupleuri), *Chen Pi* (Pericarpium Citri Reticulatae), and *Sheng Ma* (Rhizoma Cimicifugae), 10g each, *Bai Zhu* (Rhizoma Atractylodis Macrocephalae), *Dang Gui* (Radix Angelicae Sinensis), mix-fried *Gan Cao* (Radix Glycyrrhizae Uralensis), and *Shi Wei* (Herba Pyrossiae), 15g each, and *Hai Jin Sha* (Spora Lygodii Japonici), 25g. After two packets, the man felt the stone moving downward with urination and all his symptoms gradually resolved. Therefore, *Bai Mao Gen* (Rhizoma Imperatae Cylindricae), 50g, and *Yan Hu Suo* (Rhizoma Corydalis Yanhusuo), 15g, were added to the formula. After another five packets of these medicinals, the man passed a stone 0.8 x 0.7 x 0.6cm and all his symptoms disappeared. He was then given medicinals to boost the qi and nourish yin for several days to continue regulating and rectifying and everything was fine after that.

CASE 7: Geriatric constipation

The patient was a 75 year-old female who was initially seen on Oct. 15, 1998. The woman had been constipated for half a month without a movement. This was accompanied by duct and abdominal glomus, fullness, aching, and pain for the last two days as well as repeated belching, toprid intake, and lassitude of the spirit. A previous doctor had treated the woman with two *ji* of *Zeng Jin Cheng Qi Tang* (Increase Fluids & Order the Qi Decoction) with no result. When examined by Drs. Luo and Wang, the patient appeared anxious. Her voice was low and her speech was faint. Her eating and drinking were devitalized and she had attacks of abdominal pain. The woman's tongue fur was thin and slightly yellow. Her pulse was bowstring, fine, and rapid. Her urination was yellow and slightly hot.

Based on the above, Drs. Luo and Wang categorized this woman's pattern as spleen-stomach vacuity weakness with central qi downward falling, stomach loss of harmony and downbearing, and non-free flow of the bowel qi. Therefore, the treatment principles were to boost the qi and supplement the center, regulate upbearing and downbearing, and free the flow of the bowel qi. To accomplish these principles, they prescribed another modification of *Bu Zhong Yi Qi Tang*: *Huang Qi* (Radix Astragali Membranacei) and *Sha Shen* (Radix Glehniae Littoralis), 30g each, *Chai Hu* (Radix Bupleuri), 12g, *Dang Gui* (Radix Angelicae Sinensis), *Bai Zhu* (Rhizoma Atractylodis Macrocephalae), *Bai Shao* (Radix Albus Paeoniae Lactiflorae), *Mai Men Dong* (Tuber Ophiopogonis Japonici), *Shi Hu* (Herba Dendrobii), *Lai Fu Zi* (Semen Raphani Sativi), *Sheng Di* (uncooked Radix Rehmanniae Glutinosae), and *Zhi Shi* (Fructus Immaturus Citri Aurantii), 15g each, *Sheng Ma* (Rhizoma Cimicifugae), 8g, and *Gan Cao*

(Radix Glycyrrhizae Uralensis), 10g. One packet of these medicinals promoted free flow and increased the woman's eating and drinking. After three more packets, the woman's mood improved.

CASE 8: Enduring, nonhealing sores

The patient was a 73 year-old male who was first seen on Oct. 21, 1998. The man had had an ulcerated, purulent sore on his left elbow for half a month. The mouth of this sore was two inches in diameter. It was red, swollen, and burning hot. When pressed, it was concave and the skin did not stand back up again. This condition had been treated at the local hospital but had steadily gotten worse. Therefore, the man had come to see Drs. Luo and Wang. The patient's facial complexion was sallow yellow and lusterless. His intake was torpid and his spirit was listless. His tongue was pale with white fur, and his pulse was fine and rapid. The man was hospitalized and treated with Western anti-inflammatory medicines. At the same time, he was given Chinese medicines adjunctively to boost the qi and support the righteous, expel pus and engender flesh. The formula consisted of the following modification of *Bu Zhong Yi Qi Tang*: *Huang Qi* (Radix Astragali Membranacei), 100g, *Dang Gui* (Radix Angelicae Sinensis), 20g, *Tai Zi Shen* (Radix Pseudostellariae Heterophyllae), *Lian Qiao* (Fructus Forsythiae Suspensae), *Yi Yi Ren* (Semen Coicis Lachryma-jobi), and *Pu Gong Ying* (Herba Taraxaci Mongolici Cum Radice), 30g each, *Bai Zhu* (Rhizoma Atractylodis Macrocephalae), *Bai Zhi* (Radix Angelicae Dahuricae), *Zao Jiao Ci* (Spina Gleditschiae Sinensis), and *Chai Hu* (Radix Bupleuri), 15g each, and *Chen Pi* (Pericarpium Citri Reticulatae), *Gan Cao* (Radix Glycyrrhizae Uralensis), and *Sheng Ma* (Rhizoma Cimicifugae), 10g each. Fifteen packets of these medicinals were given with additions and subtractions and the man stayed in the hospital for 20 days. At the end of that time, the sore had healed well, the man was able to flex and extend his elbow normally, and all his symptoms were completely eliminated.

CASE 9: Urethral syndrome

The patient was a 52 year-old female who was initially examined on Sept. 20, 1998. The patient had had frequent, urgent, burning urination for half a month. Numerous urine examinations had all been negative, and she had been administered Chinese and Western medical heat-clearing, anti-inflammatory medicinals without effect. Instead, her disease had become worse. The woman's voice was low and her speech was faint. Her facial complexion was sallow yellow, her intake was torpid, and her spirit was listless. The woman's tongue was pale with white fur, and her pulse was fine and forceless. In addition, her stools were dry. Drs. Luo and Wang categorized this woman's Chinese medical pattern as spleen-stomach qi vacuity and thus lack of force for qi transformation.

The treatment principles were to supplement the center and boost the qi, warm yang and transform the qi by administering modified *Bu Zhong Yi Qi Tang*: *Huang Qi* (Radix Astragali Membranacei), 50g, *Dang Gui* (Radix Angelicae Sinensis), *Mai Men Dong* (Tuber Ophiopogonis Japonici), *Bai Shao* (Radix Albus Paeoniae Lactiflorae), *Bai Zhu* (Rhizoma Atractylodis Macrocephalae), and *Chai Hu* (Radix Bupleuri), 15g each, *Sheng Ma* (Rhizoma Cimicifugae), mix-fried *Gan Cao* (Radix Glycyrrhizae Uralensis), *Gui Zhi* (Ramulus Cinnamomi Cassiae), and *Chen Pi* (Pericarpium Citri Reticulatae), 10g each, and *Dang Shen* (Radix Codonopsitis Pilosulae), 30g. After five packets of these medicinals, all the patient's symptoms were greatly decreased and her stools were freely and smoothly flowing. The patient's eating and drinking had increased, her affect had markedly improved, and her complexion was red and moist. Another five packets were administered with additions and subtractions to secure the treatment effects. There was no recurrence on follow-up after half a year.

From "Lifting the Borders of *Bu Zhong Yi Qi Tang* in the Treatment of Knotty, Difficult Miscellaneous Diseases." by Zhang Xian-bin, *Hu Nan Zhong Yi Za Zhi (Hunan Journal of Chinese Medicine)*, #5, 2003, p. 49

CASE 10: Continuous fever

The patient was a 43 year-old female who was first seen by Dr. Zhang on Jul. 13, 1999. The patient complained of intermittent fever, cough, and lack of strength for six months. The patient's body was habitually depleted and vacuous. Six months previous she had contracted a chill and developed a cough, nasal congestion, fever, and lack of strength. She had received treatment with both Western antibiotics and antiviral medicines, but there had been no obvious improvement in her condition. One week after stopping these medications, her body temperature was still elevated, and various medications did nothing to help this. When examined by Dr. Zhang, the woman's facial complexion was somber white with decreased luster. There was disinclination to speak and/or a faint, weak voice, cough, a body temperature of 38.6 degrees Centigrade, heart palpitations, and shortness of breath, but normal urination and defecation. Her tongue was pale with thin, white fur, and her pulse was rapid and forceless. Therefore, her condition was categorized as qi vacuity fever and the treatment principles were to use sweet, warm medicinals to eliminate heat as well as to bank earth to engender metal.

The formula Dr. Zhang prescribed consisted of *Bu Zhong Yi Qi Tang* with added flavors: *Huang Qi* (Radix Astragali Membranacei), 30g, *Hong Shen* (red Radix Panacis Ginseng), 15g, stir-fried *Bai Zhu* (Rhizoma Atractylodis Macrocephalae), 15g, *Dang Gui* (Radix Angelicae Sinensis), 10g, uncooked *Gan Cao* (Radix Glycyrrhizae Uralensis), 6g, *Chai Hu* (Radix Bupleuri), 6g, *Sheng Ma* (Rhizoma

Cimicifugae), 6g, *Di Gu Pi* (Cortex Radicis Lycii Chinensis), 10g, *Yu Xing Cao* (Herba Houttuyniae Cordatae Cum Radice), 20g, and *Lu Gen* (Rhizoma Phragmitis Communis), 10g. After taking seven packets of these medicinals, the patient's body temperature was markedly lower and there was no apparent cough. Also the patient said her heart palpitations and shortness of breath were markedly better. After another three continuous weeks of taking these herbs, the patient was switched to a combination of *Bu Zhong Yi Qi Tang* and *Liu Wei Di Huang Wan* (Six Flavors Rehmannia Pills) with modifications. On follow-up three months later, there had been no recurrence.

CASE 11: Post-surgical nonhealing of wound

The patient was a 61 year-old female. On Oct. 6, 2001, the patient had had a right-sided mastectomy for breast cancer and was discharged from the hospital on Nov. 3. However, the surgical wound was still suppurating and had not healed. Therefore, on Nov. 15, 2001, the patient came to see Dr. Zhang. At that time, there was an incision 10 x 0.5cm wide on her right chest wall that had not completely closed. There was no redness or swelling, but there was also no healthy granulation tissue. The wound weeped a small amount of blood. In addition, there was a lusterless, sallow yellow facial complexion, torpid intake, lassitude of the spirit, a pale tongue with white fur, and a weak, forceless pulse. Therefore, in order to boost the qi and support the righteous, Dr. Zhang prescribed the following modification of *Bu Zhong Yi Qi Tang*: *Huang Qi* (Radix Astragali Membranacei), 30g, *Bai Zhu* (Rhizoma Atractylodis Macrocephalae), 15g, *Chen Pi* (Pericarpium Citri Reticulatae), 6g, *Chai Hu* (Radix Bupleuri), 6g, *Tai Zi Shen* (Radix Pseudostellariae Heterophyllae), 15g, *Gan Cao* (Radix Glycyrrhizae Uralensis), 10g, *Sheng Ma* (Rhizoma Cimicifugae), 6g, *Dang Gui* (Radix Angelicae Sinensis), 10g, *Bai Zhi* (Radix Angelicae Dahuricae), 10g, *Pu Gong Ying* (Herba Taraxaci Mongolici Cum Radice), 20g, and *Yi Yi Ren* (Semen Coicis Lachryma-jobi), 30g. After 20 packets of these medicinals with additions and subtractions, the wound had healed satisfactorily and all the woman's other symptoms had been eliminated.

CASE 12: Dizziness

The patient was a 58 year-old male who was first seen by Dr. Zhang on Aug. 9, 2000. This patient had a history of high blood pressure and commonly experienced dizziness, blurred vision, generalized weakness, and poor appetite. A half year before, his dizziness had gotten suddenly worse. This was accompanied by heart palpitations and vomiting. The man received *Sheng Mai Zhu She Ye* (Engender the Pulse Injectable Fluid) intravenously as well as several Western heart medications orally. However, there was no obvious improvement in his symptoms. When the man was seen by Dr. Zhang, he had a sallow yellow facial complexion, torpid intake, a pale tongue with white fur, and a deep, weak pulse. His Chinese medical disease diagnosis was dizziness and his pattern was categorized as qi and blood depletion and vacuity. Thus the treatment principles were to supplement the qi and boost the blood. *Bu Zhong Yi Qi Tang* with added flavors consisted of: *Huang Qi* (Radix Astragali Membranacei), 30g, *Dang Shen* (Radix Codonopsitis Pilosulae), 15g, *Gui Ban* (Plastrum Testudinis), 10g, *Bai Zhu* (Rhizoma Atractylodis Macrocephalae), 15g, *Chen Pi* (Pericarpium Citri Reticulatae), 10g, *Sheng Ma* (Rhizoma Cimicifugae), 6g, *Chai Hu* (Radix Bupleuri), 6g, *Gan Cao* (Radix Glycyrrhizae Uralensis), 9g, *Dang Gui* (Radix Angelicae Sinensis), 12g, *Shu Di* (cooked Radix Rehmanniae Glutinosae), 30g, *Bai Shao* (Radix Albus Paeoniae Lactiflorae), 15g, *Yi Mu Cao* (Herba Leonuri Heterophylli), 15g, *Nu Zhen Zi* (Fructus Ligustri Lucidi), 10g, *Han Lian Cao* (Herba Ecliptae Prostratae), 10g, and *Xian Mao* (Rhizoma Curculiginis Orchioidis), 10g. Three packets of these medicinals were prescribed, one packet to be decocted in water and taken per day. After this, the patient's dizziness was markedly improved. Thus he was prescribed another 10 packets, after which his body returned to normal.

From "New Uses of *Bu Zhong Yi Qi Tang*," by Wei Chang-peng & Zhang Lei, *Xin Zhong Yi (New Chinese Medicine)*, #10, 2003, p. 67-68

CASE 13: Urethral syndrome

The patient was a 26 year-old female who was initially seen on Jan. 16, 2003. The patient reported that she had had recurrent urinary frequency for three years. Urine cultures were negative, but she had taken numerous courses of antibiotics without effect. Her facial complexion was somber white and she reported shortness of breath, lack of strength, decreased appetite, torpid intake, and a cold body and chilled limbs. Each day she urinated 10 times, while she urinated 5-8 times each night. Her tongue was pale with white fur, and her pulse was fine and weak. Therefore, her pattern was categorized as central qi downward falling and the treatment principles were to fortify the spleen and supplement the qi, raise and lift the central qi, assisted by securing the essence and restraining urination. The formula used was *Bu Zhong Yi Qi Tang* with additions and subtractions: *Huang Qi* (Radix Astragali Membranacei), 30g, *Shan Yao* (Radix Dioscoreae Oppositae), 20g, *Chen Pi* (Pericarpium Citri Reticulatae), *Sheng Ma* (Rhizoma Cimicifugae), and *Chai Hu* (Radix Bupleuri), 10g each, *Tu Si Zi* (Semen Cuscutae Chinensis), *Dang Shen* (Radix Codonopsitis Pilosulae), and *Bai Zhu* (Rhizoma Atractylodis Macrocephalae), 15g each, *Jiu Cai Zi* (Semen Allii Fistulosi), *Yi Zhi Ren* (Fructus Alpiniae Oxyphyllae), and *Sang Piao Xiao* (Ootheca Mantidis), 10g each. One packet of these medicinals was decocted in water and administered per day.

After taking a continuous seven packets, the number of times of urination was decreased and the patient's appetite was increased. Therefore, another 10 packets were administered and the patient was cured.

CASE 14: Galactorrhea

The patient was a 23 year-old female who was first seen on Oct. 28, 2002. Ten days previous the patient had given birth to her first child. Due to breast-feeding, sometimes her milk leaked and her blouse was continuously damp. This resulted in her child not getting enough breast milk. When examined, the patient's facial complexion was somber white. She reported dizziness, heart palpitations, spontaneous perspiration, torpid intake, and constipation. Her tongue was pale with teeth-marks on its edges and thin, white fur. Her pulse was fine and weak. Therefore, her pattern was categorized as central qi insufficiency and the treatment principles were to boost the qi and secure and restrain assisted by engendering fluids and moistening the intestines. The formula used was *Bu Zhong Yi Qi Tang* with added flavors: *Huang Qi* (Radix Astragali Membranacei) and *Dang Shen* (Radix Codonopsitis Pilosulae), 30g each, stir-fried *Bai Zhu* (Rhizoma Atractylodis Macrocephalae), 15g, *Chen Pi* (Pericarpium Citri Reticulatae), *Sheng Ma* (Rhizoma Cimicifugae), and *Chai Hu* (Radix Bupleuri), 9g each, *Dang Gui* (Radix Angelicae Sinensis), 12g, *Mai Ya* (Fructus Germinatus Hordei Vulgaris), *Wu Wei Zi* (Fructus Schisandrae Chinensis), mix-fried *Gan Cao* (Radix Glycyrrhizae Uralensis), and *Huo Ma Ren* (Semen Cannabis Sativae), 10g each, *Da Zao* (Fructus Zizyphi Jujubae), 6 pieces, and honey, 30g. One packet of these medicinals was decocted in water and administered per day in three divided doses. After taking four packets of these medicinals, the patient was judged cured.

From "Experiences in the Treatment of Three Cases with *Bu Zhong Yi Qi Tang* (Supplement the Center & Boost the Qi Decoction)," by Wang Shi-chun & Yang Li-hua, *Jiang Xi Zhong Yi Yao (Jiangxi Chinese Medicine & Medicinals)*, #11, 2003, p. 35-36

CASE 15: Yellow vaginal discharge

The patient was a 14 year-old female student who was initially examined on August 7, 1999. This young woman had not yet experienced menarche. However, she had a profuse, watery yellow discharge from her vaginal tract which had continued for more than three months. Ultrasonography showed that her uterine development was ok. Microscopic examination of the discharge revealed WBC 0-2/Hp. Doctors at her local hospital had prescribed antibiotics for half a month, but her symptoms had not improved. Thereafter, she was treated with heat-clearing, dampness disinhibiting Chinese medicinals which caused her vaginal discharge to become thick and sticky but not stop. At the time of the current examination, the patient had a profuse, yellow-colored, clear, thin liquid discharge. Her body was slightly emaciated and her facial complexion was sallow yellow. She was not digesting her foods well and her stools were yellow and soft. Her urine was clear, her tongue was pale red with thin fur, and her pulse was deep. Based on these signs and symptoms, her pattern was categorized as qi vacuity downward falling. Therefore, the treatment principles were to supplement the center and boost the qi, upbear yang and lift the fallen. The medicinals prescribed consisted of *Bu Zhong Yi Qi Tang* with added flavors: *Huang Qi* (Radix Astragali Membranacei), 20g, *Dang Shen* (Radix Codonopsitis Pilosulae), 15g, *Bai Zhu* (Rhizoma Atractylodis Macrocephalae) and *Dang Gui* (Radix Angelicae Sinensis), 10g each, *Chen Pi* (Pericarpium Citri Reticulatae), *Sheng Ma* (Rhizoma Cimicifugae), and *Chai Hu* (Radix Bupleuri), 6g each, calcined *Long Gu* (Os Draconis) and *Mu Li* (Concha Ostreae), 30g each, *Che Qian Zi* (Semen Plantaginis), 10g, *Shan Yao* (Radix Dioscoreae Oppositae), 12g, and mix-fried *Gan Cao* (Radix Glycyrrhizae Uralensis), 6g. One packet of these medicinals was decocted in water and 200ml of the resulting medicinal liquid was administered warm internally in two divided doses per day.

After taking five packets of the above medicinals, all the patient's accompanying signs and symptoms had improved, but yellow water still flowed from her vaginal meatus. However, after another seven packets, the yellow vaginal discharge was markedly decreased. On August 16, the patient was examined for the second time. At that time, the young woman's facial complexion was red and moist and her affect and appetite were obviously improved. Again the same formula was prescribed for another seven days, at the end of which there was no longer any yellow vaginal discharge. To secure and consolidate the treatment effects, the patient was prescribed *Bu Zhong Yi Qi Wan* (Supplement the Center & Boost the Qi Pills) and *Gui Pi Wan* (Restore the Spleen Pills). On follow-up after one half year, there had been no recurrence and all her symptoms had been cured.

CASE 16: Urinary incontinence

The patient was a 63 year-old male retired cadre who had had a stroke due to embolism five years previously. The man's mind was clear, but his right side was paralyzed. If he lay for a long time, he could not stand back up. The patient had undergone numerous prior treatments at one of the authors' hospitals. For the last half year, the man had suffered from urinary incontinence. He had already taken one hundred packets of kidney-supplementing, securing and astringing prescriptions but without obvious effect. If the man lay in bed for a long time, he was then not able to control his urination, and this caused him a lot of suffering. The man's affect was comparatively poor, his voice was low and weak, and his facial complexion was sallow yellow. His tongue was pale and fat with thin, white fur, and his bar pulses were deep and weak. Based on the foregoing signs and symptoms, the man's pattern was categorized as central qi downward falling with clear yang not being upborne. Based on the saying, "To treat disease, search out the root," he was prescribed the following modification of *Bu Zhong Yi Qi Tang*: mix-fried *Huang Qi* (Radix Astragali Membranacei), 30g, *Dang Shen* (Radix Codonopsitis Pilosulae), 15g, mix-fried *Gan Cao* (Radix Glycyrrhizae Uralensis), *Dang Gui* (Radix Angelicae Sinensis), and stir-fried *Bai Zhu* (Rhizoma Actractylodis Macrocephalae), 10g each, *Chen Pi* (Pericarpium Citri Reticulatae), *Sheng Ma* (Rhizoma Cimicifugae), and *Chai Hu* (Radix Bupleuri), 6g each, *Tu Si Zi* (Semen Cuscutae Chinensis) and *Mai Ya* (Fructus Germinatus Hordei Vulgaris), 15g each, and *Ji Nei Jin* (Endothelium Corneum Gigeriae Galli), 10g. One packet of these medicinals were decocted in water and administered per day. After taking 10 packets, the man's affect had improved, his speech was more forceful, and his appetite had increased. In addition, his urinary incontinence had improved. After another 20 packets of the same formula, the man was able to control his urination and his incontinence was basically cured. His facial complexion was red and moist and, over the month, the man's body had become stronger and more robust. Therefore, the patient was prescribed *Bu Zhong Yi Qi Wan* for another month to consolidate the treatment effects. On follow-up after one half year, there had been no recurrence.

CASE 17: Oral apthae

The patient was a 41 year-old male who was first examined on Nov. 16, 2000. This man had had recurrent mouth sores for at least six years, for which he had been prescribed a number of standard heat-clearing formulas, such as *Zhi Bai Di Huang Wan* (Anemarrhena & Phellodendron Rehmannia Pills) as well as antibiotics for numerous days. However, every half to one month, the sores would recur. both sides of the man's oral mucosa and his tongue had four mung bean sized ulcerations which were only slightly painful. The patient's tongue was pale with thin, white fur, and his pulse was deep and weak. Accompanying signs and symptoms included devitalized appetite, lack of strength, fatigue, borborygmus, loose stools, and frequent, profuse urination. Accordingly, the man's pattern was discriminated as spleen-stomach suffering detriment with central qi vacuity weakness and qi and blood insufficiency. The treatment principles proposed by the authors were to regulate and supplement the spleen and stomach, support the righteous and dispel evils. The man's initial formula consisted of modified *Bu Zhong Yi Qi Tang*:

uncooked *Huang Qi* (Radix Astragali Membranacei), 30g, stir-fried *Bai Zhu* (Rhizoma Atractylodis Macrocephalae), 10g, *Chen Pi* (Pericarpium Citri Reticulatae), *Sheng Ma* (Rhizoma Cimicifugae), and *Chai Hu* (Radix Bupleuri), 6g each, *Dang Gui* (Radix Angelicae Sinensis), *Sha Shen* (Radix Glehniae Littoralis), *Dang Shen* (Radix Codonopsitis Pilosulae), and *Yu Zhu* (Rhizoma Polygonati Odorati), 10g each, *Da Zao* (Fructus Zizyphi Jujubae), 3 pieces, and mix-fried *Gan Cao* (Radix Glycyrrhizae Uralensis), 6g. One packet of these medicinals was decocted in water and administered per day.

After taking three packets of these medicinals, the man was re-examined and his mouth pain had been eliminated and the ulcerous sores had shrunk. His appetite had also improved. Therefore, he was prescribed another six packets of the same medicinals, after which his mouth sores were cured. In order to secure and consolidate the treatment effects and prevent the condition from recurring, the man was prescribed 30 packets of *Bu Zhong Yi Qi Tang* plus 10 grams of *Bai Bian Dou* (Semen Dolichoris Lablab) and 15 grams of *Fu Ling* (Sclerotium Poriae Cocos) and *Bu Zhong Yi Qi Wan* all at the same time. On follow-up after one year, there had been no recurrence of the mouth sores.

"Two Case Histories on the New Uses of *Bu Zhong Yi Qi Tang* (Supplement the Center & Boost the Qi Decoction)" by Hu Fang-bo, *Shan Xi Zhong Yi (Shanxi Chinese Medicine)*, #12, 2003, p. 6

CASE 18: Shedding of the gastric mucosa

The patient was a 42 year-old female who was initially seen by Dr. Hu on May 8, 2002. This patient had had upper abdominal pain for two years which had gotten worse in the last one month. The pain was located in the upper right and center parts of the epigastrium, and mostly it was continuous, insidious pain. There was no accompanying vomiting or black hemafecia. The affected region was painful to pressure. Barium x-ray of the stomach and intestines showed shedding of the gastric mucosa and superficial gastritis. The patient's tongue tended to be pale and her pulse was bowstring and fine. Therefore, her Chinese medical pattern was categorized as spleen-stomach vacuity detriment with loss of duty of upbearing and downbearing, and the treatment principles proposed by Dr. Hu were to fortify the spleen and boost the qi, upbear the clear and downbear the turbid. The formula she selected was *Bu Zhong Yi Qi Tang* with additions and subtractions: *Huang Qi* (Radix Astragali Membranacei), *Gu Ya* (Fructus Germinatus Oryzae Sativae), *Mai Ya* (Fructus Germinatus Hordei Vulgaris), and *Pu Gong Ying* (Herba Taraxaci Mongolici Cum Radice), 30g each, *Dang Shen* (Radix Codonopsitis Pilosulae), *Bai Zhu* (Rhizoma Atractylodis Macrocephalae), *Dang Gui* (Radix Angelicae Sinensis), and *Yan Hu Suo* (Rhizoma Corydalis Yanhusuo), 15g each, *Sheng Ma* (Rhizoma

Cimicifugae), *Chai Hu* (Radix Bupleuri), and *Chen Pi* (Pericarpium Citri Reticulatae), 10g each, and mix-fried *Gan Cao* (Radix Glycyrrhizae Uralensis), 5g. One packet of these medicinals was decocted in water and administered orally per day. After taking five packets, the upper, middle epigastric pain was markedly decreased and the woman's appetite had improved. Minor additions and subtractions were made following the woman's symptoms for the next month. At the end of that time, all her signs and symptoms were completely cured. Repeat barium GI x-ray on June 10 showed that she no longer had gastritis and that her gastric mucosa had healed.

CASE 19: Still's disease

The patient was a 30 year-old female who Dr. Hu saw for the first time on Oct. 18, 2002. The patient had suffered from recurrent fevers for four years. Four years previous, she had caught a cold with which she had developed fever, sore throat, and generalized erythmatous macules. This had been accompanied by joint distention, soreness, and pain. The woman had been treated at her local hospital with penicillin with no effect. The next year in June, she went to a hospital affiliated with a university medical college, was diagnosed with Still's disease, and was prescribed 75mg of prednisone per day. This controlled her temperature between 37-38.5C.

When examined by Dr. Hu, the patient had a fever of 37.8C which was worse after noon. Both cheeks were flushed but there was no sweating and no chill. The woman's facial complexion was sallow yellow and her skin was sticky, but there were no apparent macules. Her hands and feet were not warm. In the affected areas, her skin was dark and purplish. She said that, if her joints of her fingers and toes got cold, they were painful. Her body was skinny or emaciated and weak. Other signs and symptoms included fatigue, lack of strength, torpid intake, a pale but purplish tongue with white fur, and a deep, fine, forceless pulse. Blood analysis showed her WBCs at 8.6 x 10^9/L, N at 0.73, HB at 89g/L, ESR at 30mm/h, TP at 60g/L, A at 31g/L, G at 29g/L, rheumatoid factor negative, c-reactive protein negative, ASO negative, and antitubercular antibodies negative. X-rays of her hands and feet showed slight osteoporosis and sklight deformation of her joints. Ultrasonography of her liver and spleen showed a slight degree of enlargement.

Based on all of the above, Dr. Hu categorized this case as internal damage emission of heat due to qi vacuity effusing heat. The woman was told to stop taking the Western medications and was prescribed the following sweet, warm Chinese medicinals in the form of modified *Bu Zhong Yi Qi Tang* to eliminate heat: *Huang Qi* (Radix Astragali Membranacei) and *Dang Shen* (Radix Codonopsitis Pilosulae), 30g each, *Bai Zhu* (Rhizoma Atractylodis

Macrocephalae), *Dang Gui* (Radix Angelicae Sinensis), and *Long Yan Rou* (Arillus Euphoriae Longanae), 20g each, *Sheng Di* (uncooked Radix Rehmanniae Glutinosae), 15g, *Sheng Ma* (Rhizoma Cimicifugae) and mix-fried *Gan Cao* (Radix Glycyrrhizae Uralensis), 10g each. One packet of these medicinals was decocted in water and administered per day. After one month of this treatment, the woman's body temperature had reduced. However, she still had chilled limbs and lack of strength. Therefore, the *Sheng Di* was removed from the original formula and 30 grams of cooked Radix Rehmanniae Glutinosae (*Shu Di*) and 15 grams of *Bai Shao* (Radix Albus Paeoniae Lactiflorae) were added. After another two months of treatment with this prescription, the woman's temperature was normal, there was no joint pain, her hands and feet were warm, and she had regained her strength. In addition, her tongue was pale red with white fur and her pulse was merely deep.

From "New Uses of *Bu Zhong Yi Qi Tang* (Supplement the Center & Boost the Qi Decoction)" by Sun Hong-li & Zhao Zhi-hua, *Xin Zhong Yi (New Chinese Medicine)* #4, 2003, p. 67

CASE 20: Urticaria

The patient was a 24 year-old female who was first examined on Jun. 19, 2000. This patient had suffered from recurrent bouts of generalized skin rash for 10 years. These lesions were light red in color. The smallest were the size of flax seeds and the largest were the size of beans. When really severe, these lesions could form plaques. These lesions were slightly raised above the skin and were itchy. They would last 2-3 days and then disappear. The patient had gone to many doctors and tried various treatments. Her diagnosis was urticaria or hives. She had been treated with prednisone and vitamin C. She had been tested for allergies to 40 different common allergens, but she was not positive to any of these. Accompanying signs and symptoms included bodily heaviness, lack of strength, decreased intake of food, a pale tongue with thin, white fur, and a floating, forceless pulse. Therefore, her pattern was discriminated as qi vacuity with insecurity of the defensive qi allowing for repeated contraction of wind evils. Based on this pattern discrimination, the treatment principles were to fortify the spleen and boost the qi, dispel wind and secure the exterior, and regulate and harmonize the constructive and defensive. The formula used consisted of *Bu Zhong Yi Qi Tang* with added flavors: *Huang Qi* (Radix Astragali Membranacei), 15g, *Dang Shen* (Radix Codonopsitis Pilosulae), *Bai Zhu* (Rhizoma Atractylodis Macrocephalae), *Dang Gui* (Radix Angelicae Sinensis*)*, and *Fang Feng* (Radix Ledebouriellae Divaricatae), 10g each, *Gui Zhi* (Ramulus Cinnamomi Cassiae), *Bai Shao* (Radix Albus Paeoniae Lactiflorae), and *Sheng Jiang* (uncooked Rhizoma Zingiberis Officinalis),

9g each, *Chen Pi* (Pericarpium Citri Reticulatae), 6g, mix-fried *Gan Cao* (Radix Glycyrrhizae Uralensis), 5g, and *Sheng Ma* (Rhizoma Cimcifugae) and *Chai Hu* (Radix Bupleuri), 3g each.Three packets were prescribed, with one packet decocted in water and administered per day in divided doses. At the second examination, the skin rash had disappeared. There was still lack of strength and torpid intake. Therefore, *Fang Feng, Gui Zhi*, and *Sheng Jiang* were removed and 15 grams of *Fu Ling* (Sclerotium Poriae Cocos) were added. The patient took 12 packets of these medicinals continuously. On follow-up after two years, there had been no recurrence.

CASE 21: Chilling & heaviness on one half of the body

The patient was a 59 year-old male who was first seen on Aug. 21, 1999. Last year, the patient had caught cold. This had been accompanied by nasal congestion, sneezing, itchy, sore throat, and left-sided bodily chilling and heaviness, aching and pain, and discomfort. The man had taken an unspecified cold remedy (or remedies) and all the symptoms had resolved except for the left-sided chilling and heaviness which did slowly go away over the course of half a month. Recently, the man had caught cold again and again he experienced left-sided chilling and heaviness which did not get better. The man had a CT scan and other examinations of his head, but no one was able to make a clear diagnosis. Therefore, the man was treated with medicines to regulate his autonomic nervous system, but this treatment was ineffective. The patient then took 10 packets of channel-warming, network vessel flow-freeing Chinese medicinals, but again there was no improvement. When examined by the author of this case history, the man's tongue was pale red with thin, white fur and his pulse was deep and moderate (or slightly slow). Therefore, his pattern discrimination was qi vacuity with wind damp assailing and taking advantage and the treatment principles were to boost the qi and fortify the spleen, dispel wind and eliminate dampness. The formula used for these purposes was *Bu Zhong Yi Qi Tang* with added flavors: *Huang Qi* (Radix Astragali Membranacei), 15g, *Qiang Huo* (Radix Et Rhizoma Notopterygii) and *Du Huo* (Radix Angelicae Pubescentis), 12g each, *Dang Shen* (Radix Codonopsitis Pilosulae), *Bai Zhu* (Rhizoma Atractylodis Macrocephalae), *Dang Gui* (Radix Angelicae Sinensis), and *Fang Feng* (Radix Ledebouriellae Divaricatae), 10g each, *Chen Pi* (Pericarpium Citri Reticulatae), 6g, mix-fried *Gan Cao* (Radix Glycyrrhizae Uralensis), 5g, and *Sheng Ma* (Rhizoma Cimicifugae) and *Chai Hu* (Radix Bupleuri), 3g each. Five packets of these medicinals were prescribed with one packet decocted and administered per day in divided doses. When examined the second time, the one-sided chilling, heaviness, pain, and discomfort were less by more than half and the man said that his mood was better than before. Therefore, another five packets of the above formula was prescribed to consolidate the therapeutic results. On the third visit, the man said his left side now felt warm and had strength. In order to prevent a relapse, he was prescribed 10 more packets without *Sheng Ma* and *Chai Hu*. On follow-up after one half year, there had been no recurrence.

CASE 22: Edema

The patient was a 69 year-old male who was initially examined on Jun. 21, 2001. Three months previously the man had developed bilateral lower extremity pitting edema. Electrocardiogram showed a sinus heart rhythm of 75 BPM and that the man had slight myocardial ischemia. His liver and kidney function were examined and these were found to be within normal parameters. When the man took diuretics, the edema resolved. However, as soon as he stopped these, the edema reappeared. Therefore, the man was prescribed 10 packets of kidney-warming, water-disinhibiting Chinese medicinals. Again the edema decreased. However, the man developed a dry, painful throat and mouth sores, and, when he stopped these herbs, his edema again came right back. When examined by the author of this case, the man not only had pitting edema of his lower extremities but bodily heaviness, lack of strength, disinclination to speak and/or weak voice, a fat, pale tongue with teeth-marks on its edges and white, slimy fur, and a deep pulse. These symptoms were differentiated as spleen vacuity loss of strength of movement and transformation with water dampness collecting internally. Therefore, the treatment principles were to boost the qi and fortify the spleen, disinhibit dampness and disperse swelling. The formula used was *Bu Zhong Yi Qi Tang* with added flavors: *Huang Qi* (Radix Astragali Membranacei), *Ze Xie* (Rhizoma Alismatis Orientalis), and *Fu Ling* (Sclerotium Poriae Cocos), 15g each, *Dang Shen* (Radix Codonopsitis Pilosulae), *Bai Zhu* (Rhizoma Atractylodis Macrocephalae), *Dang Gui* (Radix Angelicae Sinensis), and *Da Fu Pi* (Pericarpium Arecae Catechu), 10g each, *Chen Pi* (Pericarpium Citri Reticulatae), 6g, mix-fried *Gan Cao* (Radix Glycyrrhizae Uralensis), 5g, and *Sheng Ma* (Rhizoma Cimicifugae) and *Chai Hu* (Radix Bupleuri), 3g each. Five packets of these medicinals were prescribed with one packet decocted in water and administered per day in divided doses. On the second visit, the patient reported that the edema had markedly decreased and that his mood had improved. Therefore, another three packets were prescribed. On the third visit, the edema had disappeared. However, the man still had a feeling of bodily heaviness and lack of strength. Therefore, *Ze Xie*, *Da Fu Pi*, and *Chai Hu* were removed and 15 grams each of *Niu Xi* (Radix Achyranthis Bidentatae) and *Xu Duan* (Radix Dipsaci) were added. The man took another 10 packets of these medicinals continuously, and, on follow-up after one half year, there had been no recurrence.

From "New Uses of *Bu Zhong Yi Qi Tang* (Supplement the Center & Boost the Qi Decoction)" by He Hong-quan, *Xin Zhong Yi (New Chinese Medicine)*, #2, 2003, p. 68

CASE 23: Renal vein compression syndrome

The patient was a 33 year-old male who was initially examined on Mar. 6, 2000. The patient's body was long and thin and he had had hematuria for five years. This was accompanied by weakness of the extremities, bodily fatigue, lassitude of the spirit, lack of strength, loose stools, and a pale, pur-plish tongue with thin, white fur. Red blood cells in the urine were double-plus to triple-plus positive. Ultrasonography showed left renal vein compression. The patient's pattern was, therefore, categorized as spleen-stomach qi vacu-ity with central qi falling downward complicated by blood stasis. Thus treat-ment was in order to supplement the center and boost the qi, quicken the blood and transform stasis, and the formula prescribed consisted of *Bu Zhong Yi Qi Tang* with added flavors: *Huang Qi* (Radix Astragali Membranacei), 20g, *Ren Shen* (Radix Panacis Ginseng), *Dang Gui* (Radix Angelicae Sinensis), *Sheng Ma* (Rhizoma Cimicifugae), *Chuan Xiong* (Radix Ligustici Wallichii), *Bai Zhu* (Rhizoma Atractylodis Macrocephalae), uncooked *Pu Huang* (Pollen Typhae), and *Liu Ji Nu* (Radix Angelicae Anomalae), 10g each, *Chen Pi* (Pericarpium Citri Reticulatae) and mix-fried *Gan Cao* (Radix Glycyrrhizae Uralensis), 6g each, and *Chai Hu* (Radix Bupleuri), powdered *San Qi* (Radix Pseudoginseng), and *Shui Zhi* (Hirudo Seu Whitmania), 3g each. These medicinals were decocted in water and administered at one packet per day for two weeks. At the end of that time, the patient reported his symptoms were markedly improved and his urine examination showed RBCs at 1-plus. Therefore, the same prescrip-tion was continued for another month. At that point, RBCs were extremely few. The man was advised to continue taking *Bu Zhong Yi Qi Wan* (Supplement the Center & Boost the Qi Pills) for another half year. On follow-up after one year, there had been no recurrence.

CASE 24: Cough with urinary incontinence

The patient was a 54 year-old female who was initially examined on Apr. 21, 2001. One month previous, the woman had caught a chill which had resulted in a fever, sore throat, nasal congestion, runny nose, and cough with scanty phlegm. The patient was diagnosed with an upper respiratory tract infection, and, after one week of treatment, all her symptoms disappeared except for a cough with no phlegm. Whenever the woman coughed, she discharged urine. The patient had a lusterless facial complexion, dizziness, lack of strength, torpid intake, loose stools, a pale tongue with thin, white fur, and a fine, weak, forceless pulse. Therefore, her pattern was categorized as central qi down-ward falling with kidney qi not securing. The treatment principles were to supplement the center and boost the qi, secure, astringe, and shrink urina-tion, and the formula prescribed consisted of *Bu Zhong Yi Qi Tang* with addi-tions and subtractions: *Huang Qi* (Radix Astragali Membranacei), 20g, *Ren Shen* (Radix Panacis Ginseng), *Dang Gui* (Radix Angelicae Sinensis), *Bai Zhu* (Rhizoma Atractylodis Macrocephalae), and *Sang Piao Xiao* (Ootheca Mantidis), 10g each, and *Yi Zhi Ren* (Fructus Alpiniae Oxyphyllae), *Chai Hu* (Radix Bupleuri), *Chen Pi* (Pericarpium Citri Reticulatae), *Wu Wei Zi* (Fructus Schisandrae Chinensis), and mix-fried *Gan Cao* (Radix Glycyrrhizae Uralensis), 6g each. One packet of these medicinals was decocted in water and administered per day. After seven days, the condition was completely cured.

From "New Uses of *Bu Zhong Yi Qi Tang* (Supplement the Center & Boost the Qi Decoction)" by Lin Jin- hong, *Xin Zhong Yi (New Chinese Medicine)*, #2, 2002, p. 67-68

CASE 25: Headache

The patient was a 65 year-old male who was first seen on Sept. 6, 1998. This man had acute pain at the vertex which had been recurring for a half year. Initially the pain had been slight and would come and go. For the last two months, the pain had gradually gotten worse to the point where he was never without it. This pain was worse at night and was slightly less when pressed. In the last day, the patient had caught a cold with sneezing and pain in the nuchal region and vertex. His appetite was ok as were his two excretions. The man was diagnosed with external wind headache and treated via the princi-ples of coursing wind, freeing the flow of the network vessels, dispelling sta-sis, and stopping pain with *Chuan Xiong Cha Tiao San* (Ligusticum Wallichium Mixed with Tea Powder) plus *Wu Gong* (Scolopendra Subspinipes), *Dang Gui* (Radix Angelicae Sinensis), *Man Jing Zi* (Fructus Viticis), and *Tian Ma* (Rhizoma Gastrodiae Elatae) in a water-based decoction. After taking three packets of these medicinals, there was no improvement in the headache or other symp-toms. Additionally, the man complained of lack of strength in the four limbs and somnolence. Therefore, the previous treatment was stopped and the man was re-examined. At this time, the patient's facial complexion was white and there was lassitude of the spirit, a pale tongue with thin, white fur, and a large, forceless pulse. CT scan showed slight brain atrophy and shrinkage.

Based on the above, the man's pattern was categorized as qi vacuity down-ward falling and the treatment principles were changed to mainly boosting the qi and upbearing the clear assisted by dispelling stasis. The formula pre-scribed consisted of *Bu Zhong Yi Qi Tang* with added flavors: *Huang Qi* (Radix

Astragali Membranacei), 40g, *Dang Shen* (Radix Codonopsitis Pilosulae), 30g, *Dang Gui* (Radix Angelicae Sinensis), *Bai Zhu* (Rhizoma Atractylodis Macrocephalae), *Chen Pi* (Pericarpium Citri Reticulatae), *Sheng Ma* (Rhizoma Cimicifugae), *Chai Hu* (Radix Bupleuri), and *Chuan Xiong* (Radix Ligustici Wallichii), 10g each, *Bai Shao* (Radix Albus Paeoniae Lactiflorae) and *Dan Shen* (Radix Salviae Miltiorrhizae), 20g each, and mix-fried *Gan Cao* (Radix Glycyrrhizae Uralensis), 9g. One packet of these medicinals was decocted in water and administered per day. After two packets, the headache was markedly decreased and the man's mood was improved. After another three packets, the headache was eliminated. Therefore, *Chuan Xiong* was removed from the formula and 30 grams of *Shu Di* (cooked Radix Rehmanniae Glutinosae) were added. Each week, the man took one packet of these medicinals. On follow-up after two years, there had been no recurrence.

CASE 26: Lochiorrhea

The patient was a 36 year-old female who was initially examined on Sept. 14, 1998. Recently the woman had surgery for an ectopic pregnancy. Two weeks later and she was still bleeding from her vaginal orifice. She had taken *Yi Mu Cao* (Herba Leonuri Heterophylli) both orally and intravenously and was treated with several other formulas. However, her symptoms recurred. The day before, her vaginal bleeding had increased, so she came in for an examination. At this time, the woman's facial complexion was lusterless and there was a torpid affect, lack of strength in the four limbs, dizziness, blurred vision, and bleeding from the vaginal orifice which was pale in color but sometimes also dark red and contained clots. The patient was nauseous, had a torpid appetite, a bland taste in her mouth, and her stools were loose. There was slight lower abdominal distention but no abdominal pain. Her tongue was pale and fat with white fur, and her pulse was deep and fine. Based on these signs and symptoms, the patient's pattern was categorized as the chong and ren having suffered detriment with qi vacuity and blood stasis. Therefore, the treatment principles were to supplement the qi and contain the blood assisted by dispelling stasis. The formula used consisted of modified *Bu Zhong Yi Qi Tang*: *Huang Qi* (Radix Astragali Membranacei), 40g, *Dang Shen* (Radix Codonopsitis Pilosulae), *E Jiao* (Gelatinum Corii Asini), and *Yi Mu Cao* (Herba Leonuri Heterophylli), 30g each, *Bai Zhu* (Rhizoma Atractylodis Macrocephalae), *Chen Pi* (Pericarpium Citri Reticulatae), *Sheng Ma* (Rhizoma Cimicifugae), and *Chai Hu* (Radix Bupleuri), 10g each, *Dang Gui* (Radix Angelicae Sinensis) and *Shan Zha* (Fructus Crataegi), 15g each, and *Pao Jiang* (blast-fried Rhizoma Zingiberis Officinalis), 1 small piece.

One packet of these medicinals was decocted in water and administered per day warm, morning and evening. After taking one packet, the patient expelled lots of clots from her vagina and her dizziness and blurred vision decreased. After taking two packets, the vaginal bleeding lessened and all her other symptoms markedly improved. There was no nausea, but she did still have lack of strength, fear of chill, and a bland taste in the mouth. The woman's tongue and pulse were the same as before. Therefore, 60 grams of *Fu Long Gan* (Terra Flava Usta) was added to the formula and the amount of *Pao Jiang* was doubled. After three packets of these medicinals, the vaginal bleeding disappeared and all the other symptoms were eliminated. The *Fu Long Gan, Yi Mu Cao*, and *Pao Jiang* were removed from the patient's formula and another three packets were administered, after which the patient was cured.

CASE 27: Dizziness

The patient was a 68 year-old female who was first seen on Dec. 3, 1999. Three months previously, the woman had had surgery for right-sided breast cancer. Happily, no affected lymph nodes were found. Two weeks after surgery the wound healed and the woman's condition gradually improved. However, she commonly was dizzy and had blurred vision as well as generalized lack of strength and poor appetite. The woman was readmitted to the hospital where she received an intravenous drip of *Bu Xue Kang* (Supplement Blood Health) as well as several different types of medications and formulas, including multivitamins for two months. After this, although the woman felt she had regained her strength, her dizziness had not decreased, her appetite was still poor, and she had a pale tongue with white fur and a deep, fine pulse. Based on these signs and symptoms, the patient's pattern was categorized as qi and blood dual depletion, and the treatment principles were to supplement the qi and boost the blood, quicken the blood and foster essence. The formula used for these purposes consisted of modified *Bu Zhong Yi Qi Tang*: *Huang Qi* (Radix Astragali Membranacei), *Dang Shen* (Radix Codonopsitis Pilosulae), *Gui Ban* (Plastrum Testudinis), and *Shu Di* (cooked Radix Rehmanniae Glutinosae), 30g each, *Dang Gui* (Radix Angelicae Sinensis) and *Bai Zhu* (Rhizoma Atractylodis Macrocephalae), 12g each, *Chen Pi* (Pericarpium Citri Reticulatae), *Sheng Ma* (Rhizoma Cimicifugae), *Chuan Xiong* (Radix Ligustici Wallichii), and *Chai Hu* (Radix Bupleuri), 9g each, and *Bai Shao* (Radix Albus Paeoniae Lactiflorae), 15g. After taking three packets of these medicinals, the dizziness was markedly improved as was the lack of appetite. Therefore, the prescribing practitioner added 30 grams of *Gu Ya* (Fructus Germinatus Oryzae Sativae) and prescribed another 14 packets. After this, the patient's condition had returned to the same as before undergoing surgery. She then took *Bu Zhong Yi Qi Wan* (Supplement the Center & Boost the Qi Pills) for a half year and was judged cured.

From "New Uses of *Bu Zhong Yi Qi Tang* (Supplement the Center & Boost the Qi Decoction)" by Zheng Ya-lan & Wang Su-min, *Xin Zhong Yi (New Chinese Medicine)*, #3, 2002, p. 70-71

CASE 28: Oral apthae

The patient was a 63 year-old female who was initially examined on Oct. 12, 1998. This woman had had oral sores and pain for several years with recurrent outbreaks. The surface of the sores was greyish white and eating or drinking stimulating foods made the pain worse. Accompanying symptoms included dizziness, shortness of breath, generalized lack of strength, a bland taste in the mouth, torpid intake, and loose stools. The woman had already undergone several treatments in the stomatology department with vitamin B complex tablets and external applications, but the effects were not good. Therefore, she decided to try Chinese medicine. At the time of examination, the patient had ulcers on both cheeks and the tip of her tongue. These were the size of a soybean or a mung bean. Her tongue was pale red with thin, white fur, and her pulse was deep and fine. Based on these signs and symptoms, her pattern was categorized as spleen-stomach qi vacuity with blood not nourishing the tongue. Therefore, the treatment principles were to supplement the qi and fortify the spleen, and the formula consisted of modified *Bu Zhong Yi Qi Tang*: *Huang Qi* (Radix Astragali Membranacei) and *Bai Zhu* (Rhizoma Atractylodis Macrocephalae), 30g each, *Sheng Ma* (Rhizoma Cimicifugae) and *Chai Hu* (Radix Bupleuri), 10g each, *Chen Pi* (Pericarpium Citri Reticulatae), mix-fried *Gan Cao* (Radix Glycyrrhizae Uralensis), and *Rou Gui* (Cortex Cinnamomi Cassiae), 6g each, *Dang Gui* (Radix Angelicae Sinensis), 9g, *Dang Shen* (Radix Codonopsitis Pilosulae) and *Shan Zha* (Fructus Crataegi), 20g each, and *Bai Dou Kou* (Fructus Cardamomi) and *Shen Qu* (Massa Medica Fermentata), 15g each. One packet of these medicinals was decocted in water and administered per day for seven days, after which, the oral sores were markedly decreased in number and the size of the lesions had shrunk. The patient's mood had also improved as well as her other signs and symptoms. She still had 3-4 mung bean sized lesions on the tip of her tongue. Her tongue and pulse were the same as before. Therefore, she was prescribed the same formula plus 20 grams of *Fu Ling* (Sclerotium Poriae Cocos) for half a month. By then, all this patient's symptoms had disappeared. She was prescribed *Bu Zhong Yi Qi Wan* (Supplement the Center & Boost the Qi Pills) plus *Gui Pi Wan* (Restore the Spleen Pills) to consolidate the treatment effect. On follow-up after one half year, there had been no recurrence.

CASE 29: Tinnitus

The patient was a 75 year-old female who was initially examined on Aug. 12,

1999. This woman had had tinnitus, ear pain, and decreased auditory acuity for two months. Two months previous she had caught a cold with nasal congestion and runny nose for which she had received treatment at the ENT department. These treatments as well as Chinese herbal medicine had not been effective for the tinnitus and decreased hearing. These symptoms were accompanied by dizziness, lassitude of the spirit, and lack of strength which were made worse by taxation, torpid intake, encumbered, heavy limbs, and slightly loose stools. Her tongue was pale red with thin, white fur, and her pulse was deep and fine. Based on these signs and symptoms, the patient's pattern was categorized as spleen-stomach vacuity weakness with clear qi not being upborne. Therefore, the treatment principles were to supplement the center and boost the qi, upbear and lift the clear qi, and the formula prescribed consisted of modified *Bu Zhong Yi Qi Tang*: *Huang Qi* (Radix Astragali Membranacei), 30g, *Bai Zhu* (Rhizoma Atractylodis Macrocephalae) and *Dang Shen* (Radix Codonopsitis Pilosulae), 20g each, *Sheng Ma* (Rhizoma Cimicifugae), *Chai Hu* (Radix Bupleuri), and *Dang Gui* (Radix Angelicae Sinensis), 10g each, *Shi Chang Pu* (Rhizoma Acori Graminei), *Cang Er Zi* (Fructus Xanthii Sibirici), and *Bai Shao* (Radix Albus Paeoniae Lactiflorae), 15g each, and *Chen Pi* (Pericarpium Citri Reticulatae) and mix-fried *Gan Cao* (Radix Glycycrrhizae Uralensis), 6g each. After taking seven packets of these medicinals, the patient's mood had improved as had her dizziness, lassitude of the spirit, lack of strength, heavy, encumbered limbs, and torpid intake. However, there was still tinnitus like chirping cicadas and her hearing was only slightly better. Therefore, the same formula was represcribed with the addition of 15 grams each of *Tian Ma* (Rhizoma Gastrodiae Elatae), *Du Zhong* (Cortex Eucommiae Ulmoidis), and *Ba Ji Tian* (Radix Morindae Officinalis). The patient took these medicinals for three months and her tinnitus and hearing improved and all her other symptoms were cured. On follow-up after one year, the patient was healthy and well.

CASE 30: Ulcers

The patient was a 68 year-old male who was initially examined on Jun. 8, 1998. In 1997, this man had undergone surgery and chemotherapy for stomach cancer. Due to chemotherapy caused vasculitis, he had developed a sore on the ventral surface of his upper arm just above the elbow joint. The skin in this area was red and swollen. External applications were made to this sore, but they were without effect. Gradually, this condition worsened and eventually the skin ulcerated. The ulcer was 20 x 12cm in size and, within its depression had a shiny or glossy head. The surrounding tissue was white although the immediate edge of the lesion was dark. The lesion leaked a watery fluid, the skin was hard, and there was pressure pain. Accompanying symptoms included lassitude of the spirit, somnolence, shortness of breath,

lack of strength, insidious pain in the stomach duct region, an occasional distended feeling, acid regurgitation, and loose stools once per day. The man's
tongue was pale yet dark with thin, white fur, and his pulse was deep and fine.
Based on this, his pattern was categorized as spleen-stomach qi vacuity with
qi and blood depletion and scantiness. Therefore, the treatment principles
were to boost the qi and nourish the blood, supplement the spleen and nourish the stomach.

The formula used consisted of modified *Bu Zhong Yi Qi Tang*: *Huang Qi* (Radix
Astragali Membranacei), 40g, *Bai Zhu* (Rhizoma Atractylodis Macrocephalae),
Dang Shen (Radix Codonopsitis Pilosulae), and *Bai Hua She She Cao* (Herba
Oldenlandiae Diffusae Cum Radice), 20g each, *Sheng Ma* (Rhizoma
Cimicifugae), *Chai Hu* (Radix Bupleuri), *Chen Pi* (Pericarpium Citri Reticulatae),
and mix-fried *Gan Cao* (Radix Glycyrrhizae Uralensis), 10g each, *Sha Ren*
(Fructus Amomi), *Dang Gui* (Radix Angelicae Sinensis), and *Fo Shou* (Fructus
Citri Sacrodactylis), 15g each, *Yi Yi Ren* (Semen Coicis Lachryma-jobi), 30g,
and *E Zhu* (Rhizoma Curcumae Zedoariae), 12g. One packet of these medicinals was decocted in water and administered per day. After seven days, the
patient's mood had improved as did his shortness of breath, lack of strength,
and somnolence. There was still some stomach duct discomfort and distention as well as some sticky phlegm in his throat. Therefore, 15 grams of *Ban
Xia* (Rhizoma Pinelliae Ternatae) was added to the above formula. After a half
month of treatment, the man came back for his third visit. His mood was
good, his abdominal distention was less, and all his other symptoms had disappeared. In addition, the leakage from the upper arm ulcer was less. The
man continued taking *Bu Zhong Yi Qi Tang* combined with *Shen Ling Bai Zhu
San* (Ginseng, Poria & Atractylodes Powder) with additions and subtractions
for half a year. At this point, the ulcer had basically healed. The skin around
the edges was réd and moist and the tissue had turned soft. The man continued treatment with Chinese medicinals to regulate and rectify his spleen
and stomach and to combat cancer.

From "New Uses of *Bu Zhong Yi Qi Tang* (Supplement the Center & Boost the
Qi Decoction)" by Jun Wen-yan, *Xin Zhong Yi (New Chinese Medicine)*, #3,
2001, p. 68

CASE 31: External auditory meatus granuloma

The patient was a 39 year-old male who was initially seen on Apr. 21, 1999.
This man's left ear hurt and had been leaking blood for two months. When
examined, a granuloma was found inside the auditory meatus which was the
size of a mung bean. Its surface was shiny and smooth and it easily bled. The
man had already been treated with antibiotics and *Long Dan Xie Gan Tang*

(Gentiana Drain the Liver Decoction) without result. In addition, the man habitually ate sweet, fatty, thick-flavored foods. The patient's facial complexion was a somber, lusterless white. He also had shortness of breath, lack of strength, sweating, a bitter taste in the mouth, heart vexation, yellow urination, a pale red tongue with thin, slimy fur, and a deep, fine, forceless pulse. Based on the foregoing, the man's pattern was categorized as spleen-stomach vacuity weakness with the spleen not transforming dampness. The formula prescribed consisted of *Bu Zhong Yi Qi Tang* with additions and subtractions: *Huang Qi* (Radix Astragali Membranacei), 30g, *Fu Ling* (Sclerotium Poriae Cocos) and *Dang Shen* (Radix Codonopsitis Pilosulae), 20g each, and *Chen Pi* (Pericarpium Citri Reticulatae), *Bai Zhu* (Rhizoma Atractylodis Macrocephalae), *Sheng Ma* (Rhizoma Cimicifugae), *Chai Hu* (Radix Bupleuri), *Zhe Bei Mu* (Bulbus Fritllariae Thunbergii), *Ze Xie* (Rhizoma Alismatis Orientalis), stir-fried *Huang Qin* (Radix Scutellariae Baicalensis), *Xia Ku Cao* (Spica Prunellae Vulgaris), *and Zao Jiao Ci* (Spina Gledistchiae Chinensis), 10g each. One packet of these medicinals was decocted in water and administered per day. After taking five packets of these medicinals, the ear pain had decreased and the bleeding had stopped, while the granuloma had shrunk to the size of a grain of rice. The patient's mood was better and all his symptoms had improved. Therefore, *Huang Qin* and *Ze Xie* were removed and 20 grams of *Yi Yi Ren* (Semen Coicis Lachryma-jobi) and 15 grams of *Dong Gua Zi* (Semen Benincasae Hispidae) were added. After taking 10 packets of these medicinals, the ear pain disappeared and the auditory meatus had returned to normal. The man was advised to adopt a clear, bland diet. On follow-up after half a year, there had been no recurrence.

CASE 32: Epistaxis

The patient was a 52 year-old male who was initially examined on Jan. 12, 1999. The man had left-sided nose-bleeding which had been recurring for the last five days. The amount of blood was profuse and its color was pale. He had already tried large doses of heat-clearing, blood-cooling medicinals to no effect. Accompanying symptoms included shortness of breath, lack of strength, a somber white facial complexion, decreased appetite, loose stools, a pale tongue with thin, white fur, and a fine, weak pulse. Based on this, the man's pattern was discriminated as spleen-stomach vacuity weakness with the qi not containing the blood. The formula prescribed consisted of *Bu Zhong Yi Qi Tang* with additions and subtractions: *Dang Shen* (Radix Codonopsitis Pilosulae), 20g, *Huang Qi* (Radix Astragali Membranacei), *Dang Gui* (Radix Angelicae Sinensis), and *Sheng Ma* (Rhizoma Cimicifugae), 15g each, *Bai Zhu* (Rhizoma Atractylodis Macrocephalae), *Da Zao* (Fructus Zizyphi Jujubae), *Chen Pi* (Pericarpium Citri Reticulatae), *Bai Shao* (Radix Albus Paeoniae Lactiflorae),

Bai Ma Gen (Rhizoma Imperatae Cylindricae), carbonized *Ce Bai Ye* (Cacumen Biotae Orientalis), and *Ou Jie* (Nodus Rhizomatis Nelumbinis Nuciferae), 10g each. One packet of these medicinals was decocted in water and administered per day. After 10 packets of these medicinals, the bleeding had stopped. There were now only small threads of blood in the nasal mucus. All the other signs and symptoms had disappeared and there was no longer any ulceration within the nose. To consolidate the treatment effect, *Bu Zhong Yi Qi Wan* (Supplement the Center & Boost the Qi Pills) were prescribed at nine grams each time, two times per day. On follow-up after three months, there had been no recurrence.

CASE 33: Parapharyngeal cysts

The patient was a 57 year-old female who was first seen on Aug. 22, 1997. This patient had had a sore throat for 20 days. The pain was continuous and it involved the right side of the ear region. This pain was accompanied by difficulty swallowing. CT scan showed the tonsil on the right side had a cystic growth 5.5cm x 3.1cm x 4.4cm. The Western MDs first tried treating this condition with large doses of intravenous antibiotics, such as penicillin, but without effect. Then they wanted to excise this growth with surgery. The patient declined and decided to try Chinese medicine instead. At that time, the patient's tongue was pale red with thin, white fur, and her pulse was vacuous, large, and forceless. Therefore, her pattern was discriminated as a central qi vacuity weakness, and the formula prescribed consisted of modified *Bu Zhong Yi Qi Tang*: *Huang Qi* (Radix Astragali Membranacei), *Dan Shen* (Radix Salviae Miltiorrhizae), *Fu Ling* (Sclerotium Poriae Cocos), and *Dang Shen* (Radix Codonopsitis Pilosulae), 20g each, *Bai Zhu* (Rhizoma Atractylodis Macrocephalae), *Si Gua Luo* (Fasciculus Vascularis Luffae Cylindricae), *Chen Pi* (Pericarpium Citri Reticulatae), *Sheng Ma* (Rhizoma Cimicifugae), and *Chai Hu* (Radix Bupleuri), 10g each, *Dang Gui* (Radix Angelicae Sinensis), *Zhe Bei Mu* (Bulbus Fritillariae Thunbergii), and *Kun Bu* (Thallus Algae), 15g each, and *Hong Hua* (Flos Carthami Tinctorii), 6g. One packet of these medicinals was decocted in water and administered per day. After taking six packets, the patient's mood was better and her appetite had increased. The difficulty swallowing had lessened and the swelling in the throat had shrunk by half. After taking yet another 15 packets, the throat pain had disappeared and the throat had visually returned to normal. CT scan showed the right tonsil was normal. There was no recurrence on follow-up after half a year.

From "New Uses of *Bu Zhong Yi Qi Tang* (Supplement the Center & Boost the Qi Decoction)" by Ding Xiao-hong, *Xin Zhong Yi (New Chinese Medicine)*, #6, 2003, p. 51

CASE 34: Recalcitrant geriatric constipation

The patient was a 69 year-old female who was initially examined in October 1999. The patient had been constipated for several years, she usually took laxatives, and her symptoms were sometimes lighter and sometimes worse. Three months previously she had developed a cough and asthma. She was treated at her local hospital and the cough and asthma remitted. However, her constipation was as always. The hospital could not find any organic reason for this constipation. Therefore, the woman came for treatment with Chinese medicine. At the time of examination, the patient was obese, fatigued, had lack of strength, sweated easily, had shortness of breath, and was even more fatigued and weak after defecation. This woman's stools were not either hard or dry. She had a white facial complexion, torpid intake, a pale red tongue with thin, white fur, and a deep, fine pulse. Therefore, her pattern was categorized as spleen vacuity and qi weakness. Thus the clear was not upborne and conduction and conveyance lacked power. The treatment principles were to fortify the spleen and supplement the center, boost the qi and upbear yang, and the formula prescribed consisted of modified *Bu Zhong Yi Qi Tang*: *Huang Qi* (Radix Astragali Membranacei), 30g, *Dang Shen* (Radix Codonopsitis Pilosulae) and *Bai Zhu* (Rhizoma Atractylodis Macrocephalae), 15g each, *Sheng Ma* (Rhizoma Cimicifugae), mix-fried *Gan Cao* (Radix Glycyrrhizae Uralensis), and *Chai Hu* (Radix Bupleuri), 6g each, *Dang Gui* (Radix Angelicae Sinensis), *Chen Pi* (Pericarpium Citri Reticulatae), *Rou Cong Rong* (Herba Cistanchis Deserticolae), and *Tao Ren* (Semen Pruni Persicae), 10g each. Three packets of these medicinals were prescribed, with one packet decocted in water and administered per day. After taking these medicinals, the patient said her bowel movements had markedly improved. So she continued taking the same basic formula with additions and subtractions for half a month. At the end of that time, the woman's appetite was good and her bowel movements were normal. The same formula as above was made into honey pills and administered for another three months to consolidate the treatment effects. On follow-up after one year, there had been no recurrence.

CASE 35: Headache

The patient was a 41 year-old male who was initially examined on Mar. 12, 2000. The patient said he had had headaches for 10 years. He took a lot of different pain-killing medications, and sometimes his condition was better and sometimes it was worse. The man said he had an empty or hollow pain in his brain which liked to be rubbed. This headache commonly occurred in the morning and was worse after fatigue or taxation. When severe, this pain was accompanied by a dry cough. There was lassitude of the spirit, spontaneous perspiration, a white facial complexion, limp limbs, scanty intake, and loose stools. His tongue was pale red with thin, white fur, and his pulse was fine and weak. Therefore, his pattern was discriminated as spleen-lung qi vacuity with the clear yang not being upborne. The treatment principles were to fortify the spleen and supplement the lungs, upbear yang and boost the qi, and the formula prescribed consisted of *Bu Zhong Yi Qi Tang* with added flavors: *Huang Qi* (Radix Astragali Membranacei), 30g, *Bai Zhu* (Rhizoma Atractylodis Macrocephalae) and *Dang Shen* (Radix Codonopsitis Pilosulae), 15g each, *Sheng Ma* (Rhizoma Cimicifugae), mix-fried *Gan Cao* (Radix Glycyrrhizae Uralensis), *Chai Hu* (Radix Bupleuri), and *Dang Gui* (Radix Angelicae Sinensis), 6g each, *Chen Pi* (Pericarpium Citri Reticulatae), *Man Jing Zi* (Fructus Viticis), and *Fang Feng* (Radix Ledebouriellae Divaricatae), 10g each. Three packets of these medicinals were prescribed with one packet decocted in water and administered per day. After taking these medicinals, the headaches were markedly decreased. After taking another seven packets of the above formula, the headaches had disappeared. The man took *Bu Zhong Yi Qi Wan* (Supplement the Center & Boost the Qi Pills) for another month to consolidate the therapeutics effects. On follow-up after one year, there had been no recurrence.

CASE 36: Chyluria

The patient was a 45 year-old male who was first seen on Aug. 24, 2000. This man had recurrent bouts of turbid urination for the past five years. His urine was cloudy like rice-washing water. He had taken *Long Dan Xie Gan Wan* (Gentiana Drain the Liver Pills) and other medications without effect. When examined, the man had had turbid urination for days. This was accompanied by lower abdominal sagging and distention which was worse with exertion, lassitude of the spirit, bodily fatigue, lack of strength in the four limbs, devitalized appetite, a dry mouth but reduced drinking, a pale, tender tongue with thin, white fur, and a deep, fine pulse. Therefore, the man's pattern was categorized as spleen qi vacuity weakness with the clear yang falling downward. Hence the treatment principles were to supplement the spleen and boost the qi, upbear yang and secure and contain. The medicinals prescribed consisted of modified *Bu Zhong Yi Qi Tang*: *Huang Qi* (Radix Astragali Membranacei), 30g, *Dang Shen* (Radix Codonopsitis Pilosulae) and *Bai Zhu* (Rhizoma Atractylodis Macrocephalae), 15g each, *Sheng Ma* (Rhizoma Cimicifugae), *Chai Hu* (Radix Bupleuri), *Chen Pi* (Pericarpium Citri Reticulatae), *Xiao Hui Xiang* (Fructus Foeniculi Vulgaris), *Dang Gui* (Radix Angelicae Sinensis), and *Cang Zhu* (Rhizoma Atractylodis), 10g each, calcined *Long Gu* (Os Draconis), 30g, and *Gan Cao* (Radix Glycyrrhizae Uralensis), 6g. Three packets were prescribed, and one packet was decocted in water and administered per day. After taking these medicinals, the urination was a little bit clearer and the man's affect and appetite gradually improved. After taking another 10 packets of the same formula, one packet every two days, the urine was now clear and all his other symptoms were markedly improved. Therefore, he took *Bu Zhong Yi Qi Wan* (Supplement the Center & Boost the Qi Pills) for another three months to consolidate the therapeutic effects, after which time he was judged completely cured.

From "New Clinical Uses of *Bu Zhong Yi Qi Tang* (Supplement the Center & Boost the Qi Decoction)" by Ma Rong-hua, *Jiang Xi Zhong Yi Yao (Jiangxi Chinese Medicine & Medicinals)*, #5, 2003, p. 33

CASE 37: Chronic atrophic gingivitis

The patient was an 11 year-old female who was first seen on Sept. 20, 2000. This little girl had had purplish red, swollen upper and lower gums for three years. This had been accompanied by moderate atrophy and shrinkage during the last half year. The Western medical diagnosis was chronic gingivitis, and the patient had undergone a number of treatments with Western drugs to no effect. She had also taken Chinese medicinals to clear heat, disperse swelling, and cool the blood which had made the condition worse. The little girl had a lusterless facial complexion, torpid intake, loose stools, nighttime drooling, lower extremity cramps, lack of strength, spontaneous perspiration, easily caught cold, and had a pale, fat tongue with teeth-marks on its edges and white fur, and a fine, moderate (*i.e.*, slightly slow), forceless pulse. Therefore, her Chinese medical pattern was categorized as spleen vacuity with the central qi insufficient to lift and raise and, therefore, lack of nourishment of the gums. The treatment principles were to fortify the spleen and supplement the center, lift and raise and harmonize the blood. The medicinals prescribed consisted of modified *Bu Zhong Yi Qi Tang*: *Huang Qi* (Radix Astragali Membranacei), *Dang Shen* (Radix Codonopsitis Pilosulae), *Bai Zhu* (Rhizoma Atractylodis Macrocephalae), *Chen Pi* (Pericarpium Citri Reticulatae), *Dang Gui* (Radix Angelicae Sinensis), and *Fu Ling* (Sclerotium Poriae Cocos), 6g each, *Sheng Ma* (Rhizoma Cimicifugae) and *Chai Hu* (Radix Bupleuri), 6g each, *Tao Ren* (Semen Pruni Persicae), 8g, *Shen Qu* (Massa Medica Fermentata), 10g, and *Gan Cao* (Radix Glycyrrhizae Uralensis), 3g. One packet of these medicinals was decocted in water and administered per day. After taking six packets, the swelling of the upper gums had disappeared but the upper gums were still red. The lower gums were now completely normal, the drooling was less, and stools were formed. The patient reported she felt she had more strength in general. Her tongue was pale red with thin, white fur, and her pulse had more strength. Therefore, she continued to take another 20 packets of the above medicinals, after which all her symptoms had disappeared.

CASE 38: Periodic numbness

The patient was a 34 year-old male who was first seen on Apr. 17, 1999. For the last two years, whenever the patient became extremely taxed and then contracted a wind chill, he developed generalized muscle limpness, paralysis, and lack of strength. Each year this would happen 2-3 times and last three days or so each time. However, each episode was getting worse and now each attack lasted 10 days to a month. When these attacks occurred, the man was not able to take care of himself even though his mind was clear and alert and he felt normal. The patient had a thin body, lack of strength, a yellow facial complexion, low back pain, scanty intake of food, loose stools, a pale tongue with white fur, and a moderate (i.e., slightly slow), forceless pulse. The Western medical diagnosis was hypokalemia leading to periodic numbness. When the man was treated with supplemental calcium, his condition would remit. However, before long it would recur again. After being paralyzed for three days, he decided to come for Chinese medical treatment. His Chinese medical diagnosis was wilting condition and his pattern was categorized as spleen-stomach qi vacuity. Therefore, the finest essence of water and grains lacked a source for its transformation and thus the muscles and flesh of the four limbs were malnourished. The treatment principles were to fortify the spleen and harmonize the stomach, supplement the center and boost the qi. The medicinals prescribed consisted of *Bu Zhong Yi Qi Tang* with added flavors: *Huang Qi* (Radix Astragali Membranacei), 60g, *Dang Gui* (Radix Angelicae Sinensis), 15g, *Dang Shen* (Radix Codonopsitis Pilosulae), 30g, *Bai Zhu* (Rhizoma Atractylodis Macrocephalae), 15g, *Chen Pi* (Pericarpium Citri Reticulatae), 12g, *Sheng Ma* (Rhizoma Cimicifugae) and *Chai Hu* (Radix Bupleuri), 6g each, mix-fried *Gan Cao* (Radix Glycyrrhizae Uralensis), 6g, *Xian He Cao* (Herba Agrimoniae Pilosae), 30g, *Yi Yi Ren* (Semen Coicis Lachryma-jobi), 30g, scorched *San Xian* (Three Immortals, three food-abducting medicinals), 15g, and *Da Zao* (Fructus Zizyphi Jujubae), 3 pieces. One packet of these medicinals was decocted in water and administered per day. After taking three packets, the man's four limbs had strength. After six more packets, he was able to move his lower extremities and walk around. After yet another 10 packets, everything had returned to normal.

CASE 39: Atrial fibrillation

The patient was a 62 year-old female who had coronary heart disease. Three days previous, due to a sore, swollen throat, the woman had taken unspecified Chinese and Western medicines. Afterwards, she developed heart fluster, heart palpitations, sweating, and shortness of breath. She was given an ECG which found that her P wave had disappeared and that she had atrial fibrillation at 480 beats per minute and a heart rate of 92 bpm. Her Western medical diagnosis was coronary heart disease resulting in atrial fibrillation. The woman hospitalized on Mar. 10, 2001 and treated to restore normal heart rhythm. However, the results were not marked and the woman was referred for Chinese medical treatment. At this point, the woman's facial complexion was lusterless and movement resulted in perspiration. She had no appetite. Her stools were formed but she defecated 6-8 times per day and their amount was small. After defecation, her heart palpitations were worse. Her tongue was dark yet pale with thin, white fur, and her pulse was bound and regularly irregular. Therefore, the woman's Chinese medical pattern was categorized as heart qi insufficiency with central qi falling downward, and the treatment principles were to fortify the spleen and boost the qi, upbear yang and lift the fallen. The medicinals prescribed consisted of *Bu Zhong Yi Qi Tang* with added flavors: *Huang Qi* (Radix Astragali Membranacei), 30g, *Ren Shen* (Radix Panacis Ginseng), 10g, *Wu Wei Zi* (Fructus Schisandrae Chinensis), *Bai Zhu* (Rhizoma Atractylodis Macrocephalae), *Chen Pi* (Pericarpium Citri Reticulatae), and *Dang Gui* (Radix Angelicae Sinensis), 10g each, *Sheng Ma* (Rhizoma Cimicifugae), *Chai Hu* (Radix Bupleuri), and mix-fried *Gan Cao* (Radix Glycyrrhizae Uralensis), 6g each. These medicinals were decocted in water and administered in three divided doses. After one packet, the woman had only two bowel movements, the downward falling feeling in her lower abdomen stopped, and her heart palpitations were less. After 24 hours, repeat ECG showed that the atrial fibrillation had disappeared. Thus the woman was prescribed *Bu Zhong Yi Qi Wan* (Supplement the Center & Boost the Qi Pills) to consolidate the treatment results.

From "The Treatment of 654-2-induced Urinary Retention with *Bu Zhong Yi Qi Tang* (Supplement the Center & Boost the Qi Decoction)" by Zhang Jian-jun, *Zhe Jiang Zhong Yi Za Zhi (Zhejiang Journal of Chinese Medicine)*, #6, 2003, p. 239

CASE 40: Medicinally induced urinary retention

The patient was a 72 year-old female who was first seen by Dr. Zhang on Sept. 25, 1999. Seven days earlier the woman had had abdominal pain and diarrhea for two days. When the pain got very bad for over an hour, the woman was hospitalized and diagnosed with acute gastroenteritis and treated with 654-2 (anisodamine) via intravenous drip. This resulted in the woman having difficulty expelling urine. Therefore, she was also treated with 2.5mg of an unidentifiable Western drug (*Lan Di Min*). The next day, the abdominal pain and diarrhea had stopped, but the woman's urination only dribbled and dripped. Warm compresses were used over her lower abdomen and acupuncture was performed, but the treatment effects were not good. Five days previously, the urinary retention had gotten even worse. Ultrasonography was performed and this showed that urinary retention was accompanied by a slight degree of accumulation of water in both kidneys with distention of her ureters. Therefore, the woman was catheterized. Two days previous the woman's urination was still not freely flowing and she had to be catheterized a second time. It was at this point that the patient was referred to Dr. Zhang of the Henan University Huai He Hospital.

When seen by Dr. Zhang, the woman had no thought for eating or drinking. Her facial complexion was a somber white. She had scanty qi and a disinclination to speak and/or a weak, faint voice. Her limbs were fatigued and lacked strength. She was dizzy and had heart palpitations and loose stools. Her tongue was pale, fat, and enlarged with teeth-marks on its edges and thin, white, slimy fur. Her pulse was fine and forceless. She reported that she was habitually vacuous and weak. Based on the foregoing, Dr. Zhang diagnosed her condition as dribbling urinary block due to a combination of senility, unregulated diet, and detriment damage to the spleen and stomach resulting in source qi insufficiency. Hence the clear was not able to be upborne and the turbid was not being downborne. Thus Dr. Zhang prescribed *Bu Zhong Yi Qi Tang* with added flavors: *Dang Shen* (Radix Codonopsitis Pilosulae), *Chen Pi* (Pericarpium Citri Reticulatae), *Dang Gui* (Radix Angelicae Sinensis), and *Zhi Ke* (Fructus Citri Aurantii), 10g each, *Huang Qi* (Radix Astragali Membranacei), 30g, *Bai Zhu* (Rhizoma Atractylodis Macrocephalae), *Sheng Ma* (Rhizoma Cimicifugae), *Chai Hu* (Radix Bupleuri), and *Gan Cao* (Radix Glycyrrhizae Uralensis), 6g each, *Fu Ling* (Sclerotium Poriae Cocos) and *Shan Yao* (Radix Dioscoreae Oppositae), 15g each, *Da Zao* (Fructus Zizyphi Jujubae), 5 pieces, and *Cong Bai* (Bulbus Allii Fistulosi), 3 stalks. These medicinals were decocted in water and administered orally. After taking three packets of these medicinals, the woman was able to urinate freely and her urinary retention disappeared. Therefore, she was administered another three packets of the original formula in order to secure and consolidate the therapeutic results.

From "New Uses of *Sheng Yang Yi Wei Tang* (Upbear Yang & Boost the Stomach Decoction)" by Chen Hai-zhao *et al.*, *Xin Zhong Yi (New Chinese Medicine)*, #1, 2004, p. 187-190

CASE 41: Oligospermia

The patient was a 28 year-old male cadre who had been married for four years without fathering a child. His wife's condition was normal. Examination of the man's reproductive organs was normal. Examination of his seminal fluid showed sperm at 20×10^9/L with poor motility. There were no red or white blood cells in the fluid. The patient had already been treated with chorionic gonadotropin for two years with no effect. The man's signs and symptoms included a thin, weak body, lassitude of the spirit, lack of strength, occasional abdominal distention, a pale red tongue with thin, white fur, and a deep, weak pulse. Therefore, the patient was prescribed *Bu Zhong Yi Qi Tang* with added flavors: *Huang Qi* (Radix Astragali Membranacei), 30g, stir-fried *Bai Zhu* (Rhizoma Atractylodis Macrocephalae) and *Dang Gui* (Radix Angelicae Sinensis), 12g each, *Chen Pi* (Pericarpium Citri Reticulate), 9g, *Sheng Ma* (Rhizoma Cimicifugae) and *Chai Hu* (Radix Bupleuri), 6g each, and *Dang Shen* (Radix Codonopsitis Pilosulae), *Tu Si Zi* (Semen Cuscutae Chinensis), and *Gou Qi Zi* (Fructus Lycii Chinensis), 15g each. One packet of these medicinals was decocted in water and administered per day. After taking 60 packets of this formula, repeat seminal examination showed that the number of sperm had increased as well as their motility. Three grams of *Rou Gui* (Cortex Cinnamomi Cassiae) was added to the above formula and, after taking yet another 60 packets, the man's sperm count was 65 x 10^9/L and their motility was normal. Three months later, the patient's wife conceived and the next year gave birth normally to a healthy daughter.

CASE 42: Postsurgical gastrointestinal dysfunction

The patient was a 58 year-old female who had had a total hysterectomy eight days before. The patient still did not have the strength to stand up. In addition, there was lassitude of the spirit, lack of strength, disinclination to speak and a faint, weak voice, nausea, clamoring stomach, abdominal distention, and lack of power to defecate but loose stools. Her tongue was pale with thin, white fur, and her pulse was vacuous and rapid. Therefore, she was prescribed *Bu Zhong Yi Qi Tang*: *Dang Shen* (Radix Codonopsitis Pilosulae) and *Dang Gui* (Radix Angelicae Sinensis), 15g each, *Huang Qi* (Radix Astragali Membranacei), 30g, *Chen Pi* (Pericarpium Citri Reticulatae) and *Sheng Ma* (Rhizoma Cimicifugae), 9g each, and *Chai Hu* (Radix Bupleuri) and stir-fried *Bai Zhu* (Rhizoma Atractylodis Macrocephalae), 12g each. After taking a single packet of these medicinals, all the patient's symptoms were decreased. After two more packets, the woman was considered cured.

CASE 43: Threatened miscarriage

The patient was a 27 year-old female who had been married for three years and had had four miscarriages. Now she was pregnant again and the day before had shown signs of another miscarriage. The woman had been given progesterone but without effect. There was fetal leakage precipitation of blood. In addition, there was a sallow yellow facial complexion, a thin, weak body, lassitude of the spirit, exhaustion, lack of strength, fatigued limbs, a faint, weak voice, heart palpitations, shortness of breath, stomach duct discomfort, occasional abdominal distention, and no flavor for food taken in. However, the woman's two excretions were normal. Her tongue was pale with thin, white fur, and her pulse was fine and slippery. Therefore, she was treated with *Bu Zhong Yi Qi Tang* with added flavors: *Dang Shen* (Radix Codonopsitis Pilosulae) and *Huang Qi* (Radix Astragali Membranacei), 15g each, stir-fried *Bai Zhu* (Rhizoma Atractylodis Macrocephalae), *Chai Hu* (Radix Bupleuri), *Dang Gui* (Radix Angelicae Sinensis), and *Chen Pi* (Pericarpium Citri Reticulatae), 10g each, *Sheng Ma* (Rhizoma Cimicifugae) and mix-fried *Gan Cao* (Radix Glycyrrhizae Uralensis), 6g each, *E Jiao* (Gelatinum Corii Asini), 12g, stir-fried *Mai Ya* (Fructus Germinatus Hordei Vulgaris) and *Xian He Cao* (Herba Agrimoniae Pilosae), 20g each, *Da Zao* (Fructus Zizyphi Jujubae), 5 pieces, and *Sheng Jiang* (uncooked Rhizoma Zingiberis Officinalis), 3 slices. After taking five packets of these medicinals, the woman's condition had greatly improved. After another 10 packets, her symptoms had completely disappeared and she was cured. After sufficient months, the patient gave birth to a baby girl. Mother and daughter were both healthy.

CASE 44: Galactorrhea resulting in insufficient lactation

The patient was a 21 year-old female peasant who had given birth a half month before. At times, her breast milk leaked making the inside of her clothes damp. Eventually this leakage resulted in insufficient lactation for her child. Other signs and symptoms included dizziness, shortness of breath, lowered appetite and torpid intake, perspiration on movement, fatigue, lack of strength, a pale tongue with thin, white fur, and a deep, fine pulse. Therefore, she was administered *Bu Zhong Yi Qi Tang* with added flavors: mix-fried *Huang Qi* (Radix Astragali Membranacei), 30g, *Dang Shen* (Radix Codonopsitis Pilosulae), stir-fried *Bai Shao* (Radix Albus Paeoniae Lactiflorae), and *Lu Jiao Shuang* (Cornu Degelatinum Cervi), 12g each, stir-fried *Bai Zhu* (Rhizoma Atractylodis Macrocephalae), *Chen Pi* (Pericarpium Citri Reticulatae), *Sheng Ma* (Rhizoma Cimicifugae), and *Chai Hu* (Radix Bupleuri), 9g each, *Dang Gui* (Radix Angelicae Sinensis), *Mai Men Dong* (Tuber Ophiopogonis Japonici), *Wu Wei Zi* (Fructus Schisandrae Chinensis), and mix-fried *Gan Cao* (Radix Glycyrrhizae Uralensis), 10g each, *Sheng Jiang* (uncooked Rhizoma Zingiberis Officinalis), 6g, and *Da Zao* (Fructus Zizyphi Jujubae), 4 pieces. After taking eight packets of these medicinals, the galactorrhea had ceased and her other symptoms had disappeared, the woman's breast milk had increased and she was judged cured.

CASE 45: Postpartum urinary retention

The patient was a 28 year-old female peasant. Due to a difficult delivery, the woman had had to have a C-section. One week after this surgery, she was still having problems with urinary retention. Urination was difficult and dribbled and dripped but did not flow freely. Therefore, she had to be catheterized. This woman's signs and symptoms included a sallow yellow facial complexion, heart palpitations, shortness of breath, incessant spontaneous perspiration, fatigue, somnolence, disinclination to speak and a faint, weak voice, a pale tongue with thin, white fur, and a fine, forceless pulse. Urine examination was one plus positive for white blood cells. The patient was given *Bu Zhong Yi Qi Tang* with added flavors: uncooked *Huang Qi* (Radix Astragali Membranacei), 30g, *Dang Shen* (Radix Codonopsitis Pilosulae), 12g, *Hua Shi* (Talcum), 15g, stir-fried *Bai Zhu* (Rhizoma Atractylodis Macrocephalae), *Sheng Ma* (Rhizoma Cimicifugae), *Chai Hu* (Radix Bupleuri), *Dang Gui* (Radix Angelicae Sinensis), *Gui Zhi* (Ramulus Cinnamomi Cassiae), *Che Qian Zi* (Semen Plantaginis), *Mu Tong* (Caulis Akebiae), and mix-fried *Gan Cao* (Radix Glycyrrhizae Uralensis), 10g each, *Sheng Jiang* (uncooked Rhizoma Zingiberis Officinalis), 6g, and *Da Zao* (Fructus Zizyphi Jujubae), 3 pieces. After taking three packets of these medicinals, the patient was able to urinate on her own. However, her urination was still a little uneasy. Therefore, she was given three more packets, after which her urination was freely flowing and smooth. All her other symptoms were eliminated, and the woman was cured.

CASE 46: Vaginal flatulence

The patient was a 25 year-old female who had given birth 55 days before. For the last half month, this woman experienced vaginal flatulence 10 times per night. This was accompanied by dizziness, bodily fatigue, and lack of strength. She could not eat sweet things, and oily, greasy foods gave her indigestion. There was abdominal fullness and borborygmus, diarrhea, and her lochia had not finished. The patient's tongue was pale and white, and her pulse was choppy. Therefore, she was prescribed *Bu Zhong Yi Qi Tang* plus *Hou Po* (Cortex Magnoliae Officinalis) and *Chen Pi* (Pericarpium Citri Reticulatae). After taking three packets of these medicinals, all the woman's symptoms had decreased. After another 15 packets, she was cured.

From *Qian Jia Miao Fang (Ten Thousand Masters' Miraculous Formulas)* by Li Wen-liang, [People's] Liberation Army Press, Beijing, 1985, Vol. 1, p. 367-368

CASE 47: Urinary incontinence

The patient was a 30 year-old female who was initially seen on Dec. 20, 1971 for urinary incontinence. The woman had a somber white facial complexion and was not able to control her urination. Her tongue had thin fur and her pulse was weak. Therefore, she was treated with *Bu Zhong Yi Qi Tang* with added flavors: *Huang Qi* (Radix Astragali Membranacei), 12g, *Yi Zhi Ren* (Fructus

Alpiniae Oxyphyllae), 9g, *Chai Hu* (Radix Bupleuri), 4.5g, *Dang Shen* (Radix Codonopsitis Pilosulae), 12g, *Sang Piao Xiao* (Ootheca Mantidis), 9g, *Chen Pi* (Pericarpium Citri Reticulatae), 4.5g, *Gan Cao* (Radix Glycyrrhizae Uralensis), 6g, *Fu Pen Zi* (Fructus Rubi Chingii), 12g, *Sheng Ma* (Rhizoma Cimicifugae), 4.5g, *Dang Gui* (Radix Angelicae Sinensis), 9g, and *Bai Zhu* (Rhizoma Atractylodis Macrocephalae), 9g. One packet of these medicinals was decocted in water and administered per day. After taking five packets, the woman's facial complexion had turned normal and all her other symptoms were cured. However, her pulse was still weak and her tongue fur was still thin. Therefore, she was prescribed five more packets in order to secure and consolidate the therapeutic effects.

From *Qian Jia Miao Fang (Ten Thousand Masters' Miraculous Formulas)*, Vol. 2, p. 246-247

CASE 48: Postpartum urinary retention

The patient was a 26 year-old female who was five days postpartum and whose urination was not freely flowing. Delivery had occurred at full term, and, because the child was relatively large, she had had to have a C-section. During this, she lost a lot of blood. In the afternoon, she desired to urinate, but her urine only dribbled and dripped and would not come out. This was accompanied by lower abdominal distention and pain. She had been catheterized, had taken anti-inflammatory and urination-disinhibiting medicinals, and had undergone acupuncture and cupping, all without effect. At the time of her present diagnosis, her facial complexion was pale and white and there was fatigue, lack of strength, occasional spontaneous perspiration, heart palpitations, occasional low back soreness, a profuse lochia, a pale, whitish tongue, and a vacuous, fine pulse. Based on these signs and symptoms, the patient's pattern was categorized as postpartum kidney qi damage and detriment, central qi falling downward, and inhibition of the urinary bladder's qi transformation. Therefore, the woman was prescribed *Bu Zhong Yi Qi Tang* plus *Wu Ling San* (Five [Ingredients] Poria Powder) with additions and subtractions: *Huang Qi* (Radix Astragali Membranacei), 20g, *Dang Shen* (Radix Codonopsitis Pilosulae), 15g, *Bai Zhu* (Rhizoma Atractylodis Macrocephalae), 12g, mix-fried *Sheng Ma* (Rhizoma Cimicifugae), 6g, *Fu Ling* (Sclerotium Poriae Cocos), 10g, *Zhu Ling* (Sclerotium Polypori Umbellati), 10g, *Ze Xie* (Rhizoma Alismatis Orientalis), 10g, *Che Qian Zi* (Semen Plantaginis), 10g, *Chai Hu* (Radix Bupleuri), 10g, *Gui Zhi* (Ramulus Cinnamomi Cassiae), 10g, and *Gan Cao* (Radix Glycyrrhizae Uralensis), 3g. One packet of these medicinals was decocted in water and administered per day. After taking six packets, the patient's urination was smoothly and freely flowing.

CASE 49: Postpartum urinary retention

The patient was a 25 year-old female who was first seen on Feb. 25, 1980. After delivering, the woman had developed uirnary retention. For the last four days, her urine had only dribbled and dripped and not truly flowed. There was also lower abdominal drum distention, a sallow yellow facial complexion, lassitude of the spirit, lack of strength, profuse sweating, decreased appetite, a low, faint voice and disinclination to speak, a pale tongue with thin fur, and a fine, weak pulse. The patient's pattern was categorized as central qi insufficiency and thus was prescribed modified *Bu Zhong Yi Qi Tang*: *Dang Shen* (Radix Codonopsitis Pilosulae), 12g, mix-fried *Huang Qi* (Radix Astragali Membranacei), 9g, *Bai Zhu* (Rhizoma Atractylodis Macrocephalae), 9g, vinegar stir-fried *Chai Hu* (Radix Bupleuri), 4.5g, mix-fried *Sheng Ma* (Rhizoma Cimicifugae), 3g, *Dang Gui* (Radix Angelicae Sinensis), 9g, *Chen Pi* (Pericarpium Citri Reticulatae), 9g, *Gan Cao* (Radix Glycyrrhizae Uralensis), 3g, *Guan Gui* (Cortex Tubiformis Cinnamomi Cassiae), 2g, and *Jie Geng* (Radix Platycodi Grandiflori), 9g. One packet of these medicinals was decocted in water and administered per day. The next morning the patient reported that she had urinated six times the night before. She was prescribed one more packet of the above medicinals and was cured.

From *Qian Jia Miao Fang (Ten Thousand Masters' Miraculous Formulas)*, Vol. 2, p. 252-254

CASE 50: Uterine prolapse

The patient was a 42 year-old female who had suffered from uterine prolapse for nine years. This was usually accompanied by low back and lower abdominal pain and a feeling of oppression and sagging in the perineal area. Other symptoms included discomfort when defecating and urinary incontinence. Gynecological examination revealed that the woman's uterus had completely prolapsed into her vaginal tract and was pressing against her intestines and bladder. The patient's tongue was pale with thin, white fur, and her pulse was fine. Her Western medical diagnosis was third degree uterine prolapse, and she was prescribed *Bu Zhong Yi Qi Tang* with added flavors: *Huang Qi* (Radix Astragali Membranacei), 30g, mix-fried *Gan Cao* (Radix Glycyrrhizae Uralensis), 4.5g, *Ren Shen* (Radix Panacis Ginseng), 4.5g, *Bai Zhu* (Rhizoma Atractylodis Macrocephalae), 15g, *Dang Gui* (Radix Angelicae Sinensis), 15g, *Shu Di* (cooked Radix Rehmanniae Glutinosae), 15g, *Jin Ying Zi* (Fructus Rosae Laevigatae), 18g, *Tu Si Zi* (Semen Cuscutae Chinensis), 18g, *Ge Gen* (Radix Puerariae), 9g, *Wu Wei Zi* (Fructus Schisandrae Chinensis), 9g, *Sheng Ma* (Rhizoma Cimicifugae), 6g, and *Chai Hu* (Radix Bupleuri), 6g. One packet of these medicinals was decocted in water and administered per day. In addition, the woman bathed each day in a sitz bath made from 120 grams of *Zhi Ke* (Fructus Citri Aurantii) and 15 grams of *Sheng Ma* (Rhizoma Cimicifugae). After taking six packets of medicinals, her uterus was markedly shrunken. Therefore, the same formula was prescribed again with the addition of *Yi Zhi Ren* (Fructus Alpiniae Oxyphyllae), *Xu Duan* (Radix Dipsaci), and *Zhi Ke* (Fructus Citri Aurantii). After taking another five packets of medicinals, the woman's uterus had returned to normal and all her symptoms had disappeared. On follow-up (after an undisclosed amount of time), there had been no recurrence. Some time later, the woman conceived and gave birth to a son.

CASE 51: Uterine prolapse

The patient was a 41 year-old female who was initially seen in February of 1979. After her second child's birth, the woman had not been able to get adequate rest or nourishment and, not long after, had experienced uterine prolapse for which she had been treated. Sometimes this prolapse was good and sometimes it was not. This had gone on for 10 years. Two years before, the prolapse had gotten worse and the uterus would emerge from the vaginal meatus. The pain and suffering were difficult for the patient to bear. She was diagnosed at her local hospital as suffering from a third degree uterine prolapse and was urged to undergo a complete hysterectomy. The patient decided to seek a second opinion before undergoing this treatment. When examined, the woman's nourishment was poor and there was profuse leukorrhea. Because of enduring disease and qi vacuity, it was decided to treat the woman with modified *Bu Zhong Yi Qi Tang*: *Huang Qi* (Radix Astragali Membranacei), 15g, *Dang Shen* (Radix Codonopsitis Pilosulae), 15g, uncooked *Gan Cao* (Radix Glycyrrhizae Uralensis), 6g, *Cang Zhu* (Rhizoma Atractylodis), 9g, *Bai Zhu* (Rhizoma Atractylodis Macrocephalae), 9g, *Bi Xie* (Rhizoma Dioscoreae Hypoglaucae), 9g, *Chun Gen Pi* (Cortex Cedrelae), 9g, *Chen Pi* (Pericarpium Citri Reticulatae), 9g, *Dang Gui* (Radix Angelicae Sinensis), 12g, *Sheng Ma* (Rhizoma Cimicifugae), 15g, *Chai Hu* (Radix Bupleuri), 9g, and *Da Zao* (Fructus Zizyphi Jujubae), 5 pieces. One packet of these medicinals was decocted in water and administered per day. One week later, the woman reported that her bodily strength had gradually returned, her leukorrhea had decreased, and her uterine prolapse had also improved. Therefore, she was told to continue taking the same formula combined with a daily wash and external application. After a half month more of treatment, the leukorrhea was cured and the woman's facial complexion was red and lustrous. Her strength had increased yet again and now there was only slight prolapse in the afternoon. Hence *Cang Zhu*, *Bi Xie*, and *Chun Gen Pi* were removed from the original formula. The woman was also told to continue the external applications and wash, to increase her nutrition, and to stay away from acrid, hot, fire-stirring drinks and foods. On her fourth visit, the woman reported that she had gone 20 days without any uterine prolapse and that her menstruation had become more normal than before. In order to keep this patient moving in the right direction, she was prescribed 500 pills of *Shi Quan Da Bu Wan* (Ten [Ingredients] Completely & Greatly Supplementing Pills). She was told to take 15 grams of these pills each time, morning and evening. On follow-up after one years, there had been no recurrence and the patient's health was sound and normal.

From *Qian Jia Miao Fang (Ten Thousand Masters' Miraculous Formulas)*, Vol. 2, p. 246-247

CASE 52: Drooping eyelid (associated with myasthenia gravis)

The patient was a 12 year-old boy student in Tianjin whose right lower eyelid had been drooping for the last three months. His Western medical diagnosis was myasthenia gravis, for which he had been given medicines which had been ineffective. Therefore, his parents brought him to a Chinese doctor. At the time of examination, the child could not open his eyelids. In addition, there was lassitude of the spirit, lack of strength, decreased appetite, disinclination to speak, excessive daytime somnolence, no thought for activity, no thirst, a pale red, moist tongue, and a moderate (*i.e.*, slightly slow), weak, forceless pulse. Based on these findings, it was determined that the child suffered from spleen vacuity with dampness. Therefore, he was prescribed *Bu Zhong Yi Qi Tang* with additions and subtractions: *Dang Shen* (Radix Codonopsitis Pilosulae), 12g, *Bai Zhu* (Rhizoma Atractylodis Macrocephalae), 10g, *Fu Ling* (Sclerotium Poriae Cocos), 10g, mix-fried *Gan Cao* (Radix Glycyrrhizae Uralensis), 6g, *Huang Qi* (Radix Astragali Membranacei), 10g, *Dang Gui* (Radix Angelicae Sinensis), 10g, *Chen Pi* (Pericarpium Citri Reticulatae), 3g, *Sheng Ma* (Rhizoma Cimicifugae), 3g, *Jie Geng* (Radix Platycodi Grandiflori), 3g, *Cang Zhu* (Rhizoma Atractylodis), 5g, and *Wan Can Sha* (Excrementum Bombycis Mori), 10g. One packet of these medicinals was decocted in water and administered per day. After taking 30 packets of this formula, the patient's appetite had gradually increased, his affect had become more animated, and he was able to open his eye halfway. However, his vision was still weak. Therefore, *Jie Geng* was removed from the original formula and 10 grams each of *Gou Qi Zi* (Fructus Lycii Chinensis), *Tu Si Zi* (Semen Cuscutae Chinensis), and *Sang Ye* (Folium Mori Albi) were added. The boy continued taking another 20 packets of these medicinals, at which time he was able to open his right eye just as wide as his left. He continued with this treatment for an unspecified period of time. Six years later, he entered university and his treatment was considered secure.

From *Qian Jia Miao Fang (Ten Thousand Masters' Miraculous Formulas)*, Vol. 2, p. 428-429

CASE 53: Thickened vocal cords

The patient was a 26 year-old male worker from Gansu who was initially seen on Jan. 15, 1980. Five months before, the man had lost his voice. He was treated at his local hospital but without success. So he came to Shanghai where he was diagnosed in an ENT department with thickening of his vocal cords. The man was given Western medicines for many days but also without result. Hence he decided to try Chinese medicine. At the time of examination, there was decreased facial luster, aphonia, occasional itchy throat, slight cough, heart fluster, dizziness, decreased appetite, and lack of strength. The man's two excretions were ok. His tongue was pale with thin fur and teeth-marks on its edges. His pulse was soggy and fine. Therefore, his pattern was categorized as central qi insufficiency with lungs loss of moistening and nourishment. The patient was prescribed *Bu Zhong Yi Qi Tang* with additions and subtractions: *Dang Shen* (Radix Codonopsitis Pilosulae), 12g, *Dang Gui* (Radix Angelicae Sinensis), 9g, *Jie Geng* (Radix Platycodi Grandiflori), 6g, uncooked *Huang Qi* (Radix Astragali Membranacei), 12g, mix-fried *Sheng Ma* (Rhizoma Cimicifugae), 6g, *Xiao Mai* (Fructus Tritici Aestivi), 30g, uncooked *Bai Zhu* (Rhizoma Atractylodis Macrocephalae), 9g, *Gan Cao* (Radix Glycyrrhizae Uralensis), 4.5g, *Mu Hu Die* (Semen Oroxyli Indici), 15g, *Pang Da Hai* (Fructus Sterculiae Scaphageriae), 9g, and *Feng Huang Yi* (the white membrane within chicken eggs), 3g. One packet of these medicinals was decocted in water and administered per day for seven days. At that time, the patient communicated that his throat felt more comfortable than before. However, his pulse and tongue were the same as before. So 12 grams each of *Sha Shen* (Radix Glehniae Littoralis) and *Tian Men Dong* (Tuber Asparagi Cochinensis) were added to the original formula and another seven packets were prescribed. On the patient's third visit, he was able to talk normally and was exceedingly happy. Several more packets of the same formula were prescribed to secure and consolidate the therapeutic results.

From "Lifting the Borders of the Use of *Bu Zhong Yi Qi Tang* in External Medicine" by Tan Cheng-bang & Tan Xin-le, *Hu Nan Zhong Yi Za Zhi (Hunan Journal of Chinese Medicine)*, #2, 2004, p. 14

CASE 54: Sub-occipital abscess

The patient was a 72 year-old female who had developed a sub-occipital abscess within the last month. She had already been treated by several different doctors in the internal and external medicine departments, but the lesion would not heal. At the time of examination, the surface of the lesion was ulcerated and exuded pussy water. There was some necrosis, and granulation was retarded. Accompanying signs and symptoms included torpid intake, disinclination to speak, shortness of breath, a lusterless facial complexion, lack of strength, a pale, white tongue, and a vacuous, forceless pulse. Therefore, she was diagnosed as suffering the latter stages of a "brain flat abscess," and her Chinese medical pattern was categorized as spleen- stomach vacuity weakness with qi and blood dual vacuity. The formula used to treat this was *Bu Zhong Yi Qi Tang*: *Huang Qi* (Radix Astragali Membranacei), 30g, *Dang Shen* (Radix Codonopsitis Pilosulae), 20g, *Bai Zhu* (Rhizoma Atractylodis Macrocephalae), *Chen Pi* (Pericarpium Citri Reticulatae), *Dang Gui* (Radix Angelicae Sinensis), and *Chai Hu* (Radix Bupleuri), 10g each, mix-fried *Gan Cao* (Radix Glycyrrhizae Uralensis), 5g, and *Sheng Ma* (Rhizoma Cimicifugae), 6g. After taking 15 packets of these medicinals as well as applying *Jiu Yi Dan* (Nine [to] One Elixir) externally to the affected region, the woman's appetite was better, her central qi was sufficient, her four limbs had strength, all her other symptoms had disappeared, and the abscess had completely healed.

CASE 55: Internal bleeding hemorrhoids

The patient was a 50 year-old male who had had hemafecia for one week. The patient had already been diagnosed with internal hemorrhoids and had been treated with medicinal injection therapy. However, the hemafecia was the same as before. At the time of examination, accompanying signs and symptoms included poor appetite, lassitude of the spirit, lack of strength, dizziness, vertigo, a somber white facial complexion, heart palpitations, shortness of breath, white lips and a pale tongue, and a fine, forceless pulse. Based on the foregoing, the man was diagnosed with internal hemorrhoidal hemafecia with detriment and damage to the middle burner-spleen earth which was failing to do its duty of gathering and containing. Therefore, the formula used was *Bu Zhong Yi Qi Tang* with additions and subtractions: *Huang Qi* (Radix Astragali Membranacei), 50g, *Dang Shen* (Radix Codonopsitis Pilosulae), 15g, mix-fried *Gan Cao* (Radix Glycyrrhizae Uralensis), stir-fried *Dang Gui* (Radix Angelicae Sinensis), and *Chen Pi* (Pericarpium Citri Reticulatae), 6g each, stir-fried *Bai Zhu* (Rhizoma Atractylodis Macrocephalae) and *Chai Hu* (Radix Bupleuri), 10g each, carbonized *Di Yu* (Radix Sanguisorbae) and carbonized *Sheng Di* (uncooked Radix Rehmanniae Glutinosae), 12g each, and *Bai Ji* (Radix Bletillae Striatae), 20g. After taking two packets of these medicinals, the hemafecia had stopped and all the other symptoms were greatly reduced. The man continued on this prescription for another two weeks in order to consolidate and secure the therapeutic effects.

CASE 56: Urticaria

The patient was a four year-old little boy who had had urticaria for one year without cure. Recently the hives had gotten worse. Each time the child sweat, he would develop these hives which were accompanied by incessant itching. Other signs and symptoms included devitalized eating and drinking, lassitude of the spirit, fatigue, an ashen white facial complexion, a pale tongue with thin fur, and a moderate, *i.e.*, slightly slow, pulse. Based on these signs and symptoms, the boy's Chinese medical pattern was categorized as spleen-stomach vacuity weakness with insecurity of the defensive exterior. Therefore, he was prescribed *Bu Zhong Yi Qi Tang* with added flavors: *Dang Shen* (Radix Codonopsitis Pilosulae) and *Bai Zhu* (Rhizoma Atractylodis Macrocephalae), 6g each, *Huang Qi* (Radix Astragali Membranacei), 10g, *Chen Pi* (Pericarpium Citri Reticulatae), *Dang Gui* (Radix Angelicae Sinensis), and *Chai Hu* (Radix Bupleuri), 5g each, and *Sheng Ma* (Rhizoma Cimicifugae), mix-fried *Gan Cao* (Radix Glycyrrhizae Uralensis), and *Fang Feng* (Radix Ledebouriellae Divaricatae), 3g each. After taking three packets of these medicinals, the child's spleen and stomach were healthy, all his symptoms disappeared, and the rash receded. Another two packets worth of the same medicinals were prescribed in order to make the child even stronger. On follow-up after three months there had been no recurrence.

From "Lifting the Borders of the Clinical Use of *Bu Zhong Yi Qi Tang*" by Xu Yu-feng, *Shan Dong Zhong Yi (Shandong Chinese Medicine)*, #2, 2004, p. 36

CASE 57: Intestinal adhesions

The patient was a 46 year-old male who was initially seen on Oct. 8, 2000. Due to liver cirrhosis and portal hypertension, the man had had a splenectomy in September 1999. The previous week, the man had been diagnosed with intestinal obstruction and had come in for surgery. After surgery, his defecation was still not normal. Therefore, another doctor prescribed a *Cheng Qi* (Order the Qi) type formula, but no improvement in the man's condition was seen. Instead, the patient's respiration became faint and weak. When examined by Dr. Xu, the patient had a somber yellow facial complexion, difficulty speaking for any length of time, slight abdominal distention and fullness which got slightly worse with defecation, some abdominal pain, uneasy passage of gas, no desire to eat, a pale, fat tongue with thin, white, slightly slimy fur, and a deep, fine, weak pulse. Based on these signs and symptoms, the man's pattern was categorized as central qi insufficiency and he was, thus, prescribed: *Huang Qi* (Radix Astragali Membranacei), 30g, *Dang Shen* (Radix Codonopsitis Pilosulae), 20g, *Bai Zhu* (Rhizoma Atractylodis Macrocephalae), *Chen Pi* (Pericarpium Citri Reticulatae), mix-fried *Gan Cao* (Radix Glycyrrhizae

Uralensis), *Dang Gui* (Radix Angelicae Sinensis), and *Bai Shao* (Radix Albus Paeoniae Lactiflorae), 15g each, *Chai Hu* (Radix Bupleuri), *Tao Ren* (Semen Pruni Persicae), *Hong Hua* (Flos Carthami Tinctorii), and *Sha Ren* (Fructus Amomi), 10g each, *Sheng Ma* (Rhizoma Cimicifugae), 5g, *Sheng Jiang* (uncooked Rhizoma Zingiberis Officinalis), 3 slices, and *Da Zao* (Fructus Zizyphi Jujubae), 4 pieces. Two packets were prescribed, and, after taking one packet of these medicinals, the man felt his abdomen become warm inside and, after passing gas, felt comfortable and easy. He was then able to eat some thin porridge and his mood improved. Therefore, Dr. Xu prescribed two more packets of the original formula and discharged the man from the hospital. The patient continued taking this formula for a few days as an outpatient. On follow-up after two years, there had been no recurrence and the man was able to perform his usual activities.

CASE 58: Recalcitrant headache

The patient was a 28 year-old female who was first seen on Nov. 18, 1997. The patient had had intermittent headaches for more than five years. However, in the last half year, the headaches had become more frequent and the symptoms had gradually gotten worse. Each month, the woman would have 5-6 attacks. The main symptoms were pain at the vertex or forehead region accompanied by dizziness and insomnia. The patient had had a CT scan at her local hospital as well as an EEG, but no abnormalities were found. She also had tried several Western and Chinese medical prescriptions, but without much effect. At the time of Dr. Xu's examination, besides the foregoing signs and symptoms, there were profuse dreams, lassitude of the spirit, bodily fatigue, lack of strength, a cold body and chilled limbs, and devitalized eating and drinking. Taxation made all these symptoms worse and provoked an attack of headache. Her stools were unformed, but her urination was ok. Her tongue was pale with white fur, and her pulse was deep, fine, and weak. Therefore, the pattern was categorized as qi vacuity headache and she was prescribed *Bu Zhong Yi Qi Tang* with added flavors: *Huang Qi* (Radix Astragali Membranacei), 30g, *Dang Shen* (Radix Codonopsitis Pilosulae), *Shu Di* (cooked Radix Rehmanniae Glutinosae), *Chuan Xiong* (Radix Ligustici Wallichii), and stir-fried *Suan Zao Ren* (Semen Zizyphi Spinosae), 20g each, *Bai Zhu* (Rhizoma Atractylodis Macrocephalae) and *Gao Ben* (Radix Et Rhizoma Ligustici Chinensis), 15g each, *Chen Pi* (Pericarpium Citri Reticulatae), *Sheng Ma* (Rhizoma Cimicifugae), *Bai Zhi* (Radix Angelicae Dahuricae), and *Yuan Zhi* (Radix Polygalae Tenuifoliae), 10g each. After taking four packets of these medicinals, the headaches seemed less. So four more of the same prescription were administered and the woman's symptoms decreased greatly. However, during this time, she did still have one slight headache. Yet another six packets of the same formula were given due to the chronic, enduring nature of her disease. At the end of this time, the woman was considered cured. On follow-up after one year, there had not been a single attack of headache.

From "Experience in the Treatment of Ear, Nose & Throat Diseases with Dong-yuan's Spleen-stomach Theory" by Ren Wei, *Shang Hai Zhong Yi Yao Za Zhi (Shanghai Journal of Chinese Medicine & Medicinals),* #6, 2004, p. 39-40

CASE 59: Chronic otitis media

The patient was a 56 year-old male cadre who was first seen on Mar. 7, 2003. This man had had continuous suppuration from his right ear for several years. During the last half year, the pus was white, clear, and thin. The patient had previously been treated with various types of eardrops at a university ENT department but without effect. The pussy discharge had still not stopped. When examined, there was no abnormality of the man's outer ear. However, his right tympanic membrane had a hole 4 x 4mm in size through which the pus was flowing and the entire membrane was pale red in color and edematous. The patient's tongue was pale and slightly enlarged or fat with slightly slimy, white fur. His pulse was deep and fine. Based on the foregoing signs and symptoms, the man's pattern was categorized as righteous qi vacuity detriment with evils stagnating in the orifice of the ear. Therefore, the treatment principles were to boost the qi and engender the clear, downbear the turbid and open the orifices. The formula used was a modification of *Bu Zhong Yi Qi Tang* which consisted of: *Huang Qi* (Radix Astragali Membranacei), 30g, *Dang Shen* (Radix Codonopsitis Pilosulae), 15g, *Bai Zhu* (Rhizoma Atractylodis Macrocephalae), 15g, *Fu Ling* (Sclerotium Poriae Cocos), 20g, *Yi Yi Ren* (Semen Coicis Lachryma-jobi), 30g, *Sheng Ma* (Rhizoma Cimicifugae), 6g, *Chai Hu* (Radix Bupleuri), 6g, *Bai Jiang Cao* (Herba Patriniae Heterophyllae), 30g, *Bai Hua She She Cao* (Herba Oldenlandiae Diffusae Cum Radice), 30g, *Zao Jiao Ci* (Spina Gleditschiae Chinensis), 12g, and *Shi Chang Pu* (Rhizoma Acori Graminei), 10g. The cadre was given seven packets of these medicinals plus another Western medical eardrop for his right ear and told to come back in half a month. When the patient returned, he said that, after taking the seven packets of herbs, the pussy discharge had stopped. The pale red color and edema of the tympanic membrane had disappeared. Now it was only slightly moist. The man was given another seven packets of the same formula, after which he was cured.

CASE 60: Chronic rhinitis

The patient was a 30 year-old female teacher who was first seen on Jan. 13, 2002. The patient said that she had recurrent nasal congestion with scanty white, sticky snivel. She had used several over-the-counter remedies and had taken antibiotics but with no effect. Sometimes her condition was worse and sometimes it was better. However, typically, she feared cold and her four limbs were not warm. After catching a chill, her condition was worse. When examined, the woman's nasal mucosa were pale but dark. Both lower conchae were enlarged, but neither middle conchae were enlarged. The patient's tongue was pale and slightly enlarged or fat with teeth-marks on its edges and thin, slimy, glossy fur. Her pulse was deep and fine. Based on these signs and symptoms, the patient's Chinese medical pattern was categorized as lung-spleen qi vacuity, and the treatment principles were to fortify the spleen and boost the qi, upbear the clear and downbear the turbid. Therefore, she was given: *Huang Qi* (Radix Astragali Membranacei), 30g, *Dang Shen* (Radix Codonopsitis Pilosulae), 15g, *Bai Zhu* (Rhizoma Atractylodis Macrocephalae), 15g, *Fu Ling* (Sclerotium Poriae Cocos), 20g, *Chen Pi* (Pericarpium Citri Reticulatae), 12g, *Dang Gui* (Radix Angelicae Sinensis), 15g, *Chai Hu* (Radix Bupleuri), 6g, *Sheng Ma* (Rhizoma Cimicifugae), 6g, *Cang Er Zi* (Fructus Xanthii Sibirici), 9g, *Xin Yi Hua* (Flos Magnoliae Liliflorae), 9g, *Bai Zhi* (Radix Angelicae Dahuricae), 9g, *Gui Zhi* (Ramulus Cinnamomi Cassiae), 6g, and *Gan Cao* (Radix Glycyrrhizae Uralensis), 3g. After taking six packets of these medicinals, the woman was examined again and all her symptoms were greatly diminished. After taking another 10 packets of the same formula, she was judged cured. The patient was then prescribed *Bu Zhong Yi Qi Wan* (Supplement the Center & Boost the Qi Pills) to take on a continuous or regular basis in order to continue regulating and nourishing her condition.

CASE 61: Chronic sinusitis

The patient was a 13 year-old male student who was first seen on Jan. 29, 2003. The patient reported that he had had nasal congestion and yellow, pussy nasal snivel for three years. Sometimes this was mild and sometimes it was heavy. In that case, it was accompanied by headache. For the last three months it had been serious. Originally, this condition had been precipitated by catching cold, and it had been diagnosed as chronic sinusitis. The young man had been prescribed antibiotics and nose drops, after which his condition was somewhat less. However, after catching cold again, it was as bad as originally. The nasal mucosa were hyperemic and both the inferior and middle conchae were enlarged. The patient's tongue was pale with slightly thick, white fur, and his pulse was deep. Therefore, his pattern was categorized as a righteous vacuity with evil repletion, and the treatment principles were to support the righteous and dispel evils, open the orifices and expel pus, for which he was prescribed: *Huang Qi* (Radix Astragali Membranacei), 9g, *Dang Shen* (Radix Codonopsitis Pilosulae), 9g, *Bai Zhu* (Rhizoma Atractylodis

Macrocephalae), 9g, *Fu Ling* (Sclerotium Poriae Cocos), 10g, *Yi Yi Ren* (Semen Coicis Lachryma-jobi), 20g, *Bai Jiang Cao* (Herba Patriniae Heterophyllae), 15g, *Bai Hua She She Cao* (Herba Oldenlandiae Diffusae Cum Radice), 15g, *Yu Xing Cao* (Herba Houttuyniae Cordatae Cum Radice), 15g, *Bai Zhi* (Radix Angelicae Dahuricae), 8g, *Chuan Xiong* (Radix Ligustici Wallichii), 6g, *Ju Hua* (Flos Chrysanthemi Morifolii), 6g, *Sheng Ma* (Rhizoma Cimicifugae), 3g, and *Chai Hu* (Radix Bupleuri), 3g. After taking seven packets of these medicinals, the nasal discharge was greatly reduced and his nasal passageways were more freely flowing. In addition, his headache was less, and intranasal examination showed that his mucosal membranes were only slightly hyperemic. Both inferior conchae were only slightly enlarged, while the middle conchae were still enlarged. Thus the same formula with additions and subtractions was continued for another two months, after which the nasal discharge had completely disappeared and his breathing through his nose was no longer obstructed. However, when the patient attempted to stop treatment, his condition recurred. Therefore, he was prescribed the above formula plus 10 grams of *Gong Cheng Wan* (Work-accomplishing Pills, an unidentified Chinese ready-made medicine) three times per day for another month. At this point, the patient's condition had returned to normal and he was judged cured.

CASE 62: Chronic laryngitis

The patient was a 35 year-old male peasant who was first seen on Jul. 4, 2002. The man said that his throat had been dry and he had been thirsty for one whole year. This had been accompanied by fatigue, lack of strength, torpid intake, and sometimes clamoring stomach and discomfort or even pain. In May 2001, the man's stomach lining had been examined and he had been diagnosed with gastritis and duodenitis for which he had been prescribed various Western medicines. Most medicines for gastritis are cool or cold in nature. Therefore, these medicines had caused vacuity cold to be engendered internally. Because the man still had discomfort whenever he ate or drank anything, he had continued to take these anti-inflammatory stomach medicines on a regular basis. Gradually, this had come to involve throat dryness and thirst in the last year. When the patient's throat was examined, the mucus membranes were pale red and slightly dry, but, otherwise, the throat was normal. The man's tongue was pale and slightly enlarged with thin, white fur, and his pulse was deep, fine, and forceless. Therefore, his disease diagnosis was categorized as chronic laryngitis, his pattern was categorized as spleen vacuity failing to transport fluids upward, the treatment principles were to fortify the spleen, boost the qi, and engender fluids, and the man was prescribed: *Huang Qi* (Radix Astragali Membranacei), 20g, *Dang Shen* (Radix Codonopsitis Piliosulae), 15g, *Bai Zhu* (Rhizoma Atractylodis Macrocephalae), 15g, *Fu Ling* (Sclerotium Poriae Cocos), 20g, *Shan Yao* (Radix

Dioscoreae Oppositae), 15g, *Sheng Ma* (Rhizoma Cimcifugae), 6g, *Chai Hu* (Radix Bupleuri), 6g, mix-fried *Pi Pa Ye* (Folium Eriobotryae Japonicae), 15g, *Sha Shen* (Radix Glehniae Littoralis), 15g, and *Zhu Ru* (Caulis Bambusae In Taeniis), 15g. After taking nine packets of these medicinals, the dry throat was greatly diminished. After taking various additions and subtractions of this formula for an unspecified period of time, the condition was cured.

REPRESENTATIVE CLINICAL TRIALS:

Below are only a tiny selection of representative clinical trials published in the Chinese medical journal literature which use *Bu Zhong Yi Qi Tang* as the main treatment protocol. All demonstrate the clinical efficacy of this remarkable formula.

CLINICAL TRIAL 1: Altitude-induced low blood pressure

From "Observations on the Therapeutic Effect of Treating 24 Cases of High Altitude Low Blood Pressure with *Bu Zhong Yi Qi Tang Jia Wei* (Supplement the Center & Boost the Qi Decoction with Added Flavors)," Yao Yun-qing, *Yun Nan Zhong Yi Zhong Yao Za Zhi (Yunnan Journal of Chinese Medicine & Chinese Medicinals)*, #5, 2003, p. 17

Cohort description:

All the patients in this study had moved from sea level to high altitude areas. The course of their disease ranged from 10 days to 1.5 years. There were nine males and 15 females 17-52 years of age. Twelve cases had headaches and dizziness as their main complaint, six were fatigued and had decreased appetites, two experienced mainly chest oppression and numbness of their limbs, and the other four complained of fatigue, insomnia, and a clear decrease in memory. All patients had their blood arterial blood pressure measured on their upper arms three times, and their blood pressure was as low as 12.0/8.0kPa.

Treatment method:

The basic formula consisted of: *Dang Shen* (Radix Codonopsitis Pilosulae), 30-50g, *Huang Qi* (Radix Astragali Membranacei), 30-50g, mix-fried *Gan Cao* (Radix Glycyrrhizae Uralensis), 10-20g, *Dang Gui* (Radix Angelicae Sinensis), 10-20g, *Chen Pi* (Pericarpium Citri Reticulatae), 6-10g, *Sheng Ma* (Rhizoma Cimicifugae), 10-15g, *Chai Hu* (Radix Bupleuri), 10-15g, uncooked *Bai Zhu* (Rhizoma Atractylodes Macrocephalae), 10-15g, and *Xian Ling Pi* (Herba Epimedii), 10-15g. If there was abdominal distention and torpid intake, *Sha Ren* (Fructus Amomi), *Rou Dou Kou* (Semen Myristicae Fragrantis), and *Zhi Ke* (Fructus Citri Aurantii) were added. If there was insomnia, *Fu Shen* (Sclerotium Pararadicis Poriae Cocos), *Lian Zi* (Semen Nelumbinis Nuciferae), and *Suan*

Zao Ren (Semen Zizyphi Spinosae) were added. If there was numbness of the limbs, *Gui Zhi* (Ramulus Cinnamomi Cassiae) and *Rou Gui* (Cortex Cinnamomi Cassiae) were added. If there was easy contraction of common colds, *Fang Feng* (Radix Ledebouriellae Divaricatae) was added and the amount of *Huang Qi* increased. If there was headache, *Xi Xin* (Herba Asari Cum Radice) and *Qiang Huo* (Radix Et Rhizoma Notopterygii) were added. One packet of these medicinals was decocted in water and administered per day, with 10 days equaling one course of treatment.

Study outcomes:

Cure was defined as normalization of blood pressure, disappearance of clinical symptoms, and no recurrence on follow-up after half a year. Improvement was defined as normalization of clinical symptoms and blood pressure. However, within one month of stopping the above medicinals, the condition returned. No effect meant that there was no obvious improvement in either the blood pressure or clinical symptoms. Based on these criteria, 16 cases were judged cured, six improved, and two got no effect, for a total effectiveness rate of 91.7%.

CLINICAL TRIAL 2: Systolic hypertension

From "The Treatment of Systolic Hypertension with *Bu Zhong Yi Qi Tang* (Supplement the Center & Boost the Qi Decoction)" by Wang Shao-qing, *Bei Jing Zhong Yi (Beijing Chinese Medicine)*, #5, 2003, p. 40-41

Cohort description:

There were 37 outpatients included in this study which was conducted in the Chinese medical department of the Public Security Hospital in Beijing. Systolic hypertension is defined as a systolic blood pressure of more than 160mmHg and a diastolic blood pressure of less than 90mmHg. Among these 37 patients, there were 22 males and 15 females aged 56-78 years, with an average age of 67 years. The shortest course of disease was seven months and the longest was five years. Three cases had had systolic hypertension for one year or less, 11 had had it for two years, seven for three years, 10 for four years, and six for five or more years. Among these 37 patients, four cases had a systolic blood pressure of 200-190mmHg, seven had 190-180mmHg, 17 had 180-170mmHg, and nine had a systolic blood pressure of 170-160mmHg. In eight cases, there had been no obvious decrease in systolic pressure after taking Western drugs. In 29 cases, the systolic pressure had been reduced, at least sometimes, by Western drugs, but these drugs also reduced their diastolic pressure, sometimes as low as 35mmHg. These patients complained of headache, dizziness, nausea, and even episodic angina pectoris. Therefore, they were forced to stop taking the Western medicines. Based on presenting signs and symptoms of dizziness, tinnitus, a desire to lie down, fatigue, disinclination to speak and/or low, weak voice, shortness of breath, lack of strength, decreased intake of food, loose stools, a pale tongue with white fur, and a vacuous, weak or floating, large pulse, these patients' Chinese medical pattern was categorized as spleen vacuity and qi depletion with non-upbearing of the clear yang.

Treatment method:

All 37 patients were orally administered *Bu Zhong Yi Qi Tang* (Supplement the Center & Boost the Qi Decoction) at a rate of one packet per day. Exact dosages of the ingredients of this standard formula were not given. If dampness was exuberant, *Ban Xia* (Rhizoma Pinelliae Ternatae) was added. If kidney vacuity was marked, *He Shou Wu* (Radix Polygoni Multiflori) and *Gou Qi Zi* (Fructus Lycii Chinensis) were added. Fourteen days equaled one course of treatment, and treatment outcomes were assessed after two consecutive courses. During this time of treatment, patients did not take any other medications besides these Chinese medicinals.

Study outcomes:

Cure was defined as disappearance of symptoms, a systolic blood pressure of 140-120mmHg, and a diastolic pressure of 60-85mmHg. Some effect was defined as improvement in symptoms, a decrease of 10mmHg in systolic blood pressure, and a diastolic pressure of 60-85mmHg. No effect meant that there was no improvement in symptoms. Based on these criteria, 13 patients (35.1%) were cured after two courses of treatment, 18 got some effect, and six got no effect. Thus the total effectiveness rate was reported as 83.7%.

CLINICAL TRIAL 3:
Late stage lower extremity fracture swelling & distention

From "The Treatment of 48 Cases of Late Stage Lower Extremity Fracture Swelling & Distention with *Bu Zhong Yi Qi Tang Jia Wei* (Supplement the Center & Boost the Qi Decoction with Added Flavors)" by Zhang Xing-jun, *Zhe Jiang Zhong Yi Za Zhi (Zhejiang Journal of Chinese Medicine)*, #6, 2003, p. 236

Cohort description:

Of the 48 patients enrolled in this study, 32 were male and 16 were female. These patients ranged in age from 14-62 years, with an average age of 32. The shortest course of disease was 45 days and the longest was eight months. The clinical manifestations were late stage lower extremity fracture swelling and distention and disturbance in joint movement. Twelve cases had broken their femur, 15 had broken their tibia, and 21 had broken their anklebone. Twenty-eight cases had had surgery to fix the break, while the other 20 had only had external manual reduction and stabilization.

Treatment method:

The basic formula consisted of: *Huang Qi* (Radix Astragali Membranacei), *Dang Shen* (Radix Codonopsitis Pilosulae), and *Dan Shen* (Radix Salviae Miltiorrhizae), 30g each, *Bai Zhu* (Rhizoma Atractylodis Macrocephalae), *Chai Hu* (Radix Bupleuri), *Sheng Ma* (Rhizoma Cimicifugae), *Dang Gui* (Radix Angelicae Sinensis), *Chen Pi* (Pericarpium Citri Reticulatae), *Gui Zhi* (Ramulus Cinnamomi Cassiae), *Bi Xie* (Rhizoma Dioscoreae Hypoglaucae), and *Fang Ji* (Radix Stephaniae Tetrandrae), 10g each, *Yi Yi Ren* (Semen Coicis Lachryma-jobi), 20g, and *Gan Cao* (Radix Glycyrrhizae Uralensis), 6g. One packet of these medicinals was decocted in water two times and administered orally in two divided doses, morning and evening. In addition, at night, these medicinals were decocted yet again and then used to fumigate and wash the affected area.

Study outcomes:

This protocol proved effective for all 48 patients. Therefore, the total effectiveness rate was 100%. In all cases, the lower extremity swelling and distention disappeared and function of the affected limb returned to normal. The shortest course of treatment with this regime was 10 days and the longest was 45 days, with an average duration of treatment of 20 days.

CLINICAL TRIAL 4: Hypotension

From "*Jia Wei Bu Zhong Yi Qi Tang* (Added Flavors Supplement the Center & Boost the Qi Decoction) in the Treatment of Primary Hypotension" by Lin Lu-dong, *Si Chuan Zhong Yi (Sichuan Journal of Chinese Medicine)*, #2, 1999, p. 20-21

Cohort description:

This study included 39 cases, 14 of whom were male and 25 of whom were female. These patients ranged in age from 15-67 years, with an average age of 31.4 years. In all cases, the blood pressure was below 90/60mmHg. The presenting signs were as follows: 100% suffered from lack of strength, 87.2% suffered from dizziness, 51.2% suffered from reduced intake, 38.5% suffered from a lusterless facial complexion, 38.5% suffered from shortness of breath, 23% suffered from loose stools, 23% suffered from spontaneous perspiration, 17.9% had a desire to lie down, 17.9% had heart palpitations, and 2.6% suffered from syncope. The tongue was pale or pale red in 94.8%, with thin or thin white fur in 87.1%. The pulse was soggy in 35.9%.

Treatment method:

The basic treatment formula was *Bu Zhong Yi Qi Tang* (Supplement the Center & Boost the Qi Decoction): *Huang Qi* (Radix Astragali Membranancei), 30-60g, *Ren Shen* (Radix Panacis Ginseng), 3-5g, *Bai Zhu* (Rhizoma Atractylodis

Macrocephalae) and mix-fried *Gan Cao* (Radix Glycyrrhizae Uralensis), 10g each, *Sheng Ma* (Radix Cimicifugae) and *Chai Hu* (Radix Bupleuri), 6-10g each, *Dang Gui* (Radix Angelicae Sinensis), 10-15g, and *Chen Pi* (Pericarpium Citri Reticulatae), 6g. Depending on the patient's individual symptoms, the following additions were considered: *Shu Di* (cooked Radix Rehmanniae Glutinosae) and *He Shou Wu* (Radix Polygoni Multiflori), 15g each, and *E Jiao* (Gelatinum Corii Asini) and *Gui Zhi* (Ramulus Cinnamomi Cassiae), 10g each.

Study outcomes:

Out of the 39 cases, 27 (69.2%) improved markedly. This meant that their blood pressure was at or above 90/60mmHg and all symptoms had markedly improved. Eleven cases (28.2%) experienced some effect. This meant that even though the blood pressure did not normalize, all other symptoms markedly improved. One case (2.6%) did not experience any effect. The length of treatment varied. The shortest period after which an effect was seen was five days, while the longest was 20 days. The average length of treatment was 10 days.

CLINICAL TRIAL 5: Cancer anorexia-cachexia syndrome (CACS)

From "A Clinical Audit of the Treatment of 30 Cases of Cancer Anorexia-cachexia Syndrome with *Bu Zhong Yi Qi Tang*" by Cai Hong-bing *et al., Xin Zhong Yi (New Chinese Medicine)*, #3, 2003, p. 25-26

Cohort description:

All the patients in this study were diagnosed with incurable malignant tumors but had a life expectancy of more than one month. Altogether, there were 90 patients who were randomly divided into three groups for comparison. Among these 90, there were 52 males and 38 females 36-72 years of age, with an average age of 46 years. Thirty-four cases had nasopharyngeal cancer, 18 had lung cancer, 13 had breast cancer, six had lymphoma cancer, six had esophageal cancer, and 13 had colon cancer. The treatment group consisted of 30 patients, the comparison group consisted of 34 patients, and blank group consisted of 26 patients. In terms of sex, age, clinical staging, and type of cancer, these groups were all comparable.

Treatment method:

Members of the treatment group received the following version of modified *Bu Zhong Yi Qi Tang* (Supplement the Center & Boost the Qi Decoction): *Dang Shen* (Radix Codonopsitis Pilosulae), *Fu Ling* (Sclerotium Poriae Cocos), *Bai Zhu* (Rhizoma Atractylodis Macrocephalae), *Dang Gui* (Radix Angelicae Sinensis), stir-fried *Gu Ya* (Fructus Germinatus Oryzae Sativae), and stir-fried *Mai Ya* (Fructus Germinatus Hordei Vulgaris), 15g each, *Huang Qi* (Radix Astragali

Membranacei), 30g, *Sheng Ma* (Rhizoma Cimicifugae) and *Chai Hu* (Radix Bupleuri), 9g each, and *Sha Ren* (Fructus Amomi) and *Gan Cao* (Radix Glycyrrhizae Uralensis), 6g each. This basic formula was modified depending on each patient's personal presenting signs and symptoms. One packet of these medicinals was decocted in water and administered orally per day. The comparison group received 600mg one time per day of medroxyproges-terone (Provera), while the blank group was not given any medicine for their CACS. Four weeks equaled one course of treatment.

Study outcomes:

Marked effect was defined as an increase of 100g or more of food per day over the amount eaten before undergoing treatment for CACS or an increase in body weight of 0.5kg or more. No change meant that there was no marked change in either the patient's intake or weight, and no effect meant that the patient's food intake went down approximately 100g per day or that they lost more than 0.5kg of weight. Based on these criteria, in the treatment group, 66.7% of cases got a marked effect in terms of increased food intake, 20% saw no change in their food intake, and 13.3% got no effect. In the comparison group, 76.5% got a marked effect in terms of food intake, 11.8% had no change, and 11.8% got no effect. In the blank group, 19.2% got a marked effect, 26.9% saw no change, and 53.8% got no effect. In terms of body weight, in the treatment group, 63.3% got a marked effect, 16.7% saw no change, and 20% got no effect. In the comparison group, 79.4% got a marked effect, 8.8% saw no change, and 11.8% got no effect, and in the blank group, 23.1% got a marked effect, 30.8% saw no change, and 46.2% got no effect. Although treatment with Provera was more effective than treat-ment with *Bu Zhong Yi Qi Tang* both for increasing appetite and body weight, some of the patients in the comparison group experienced such side effects as pedal edema, vaginal bleeding, and hypertension. In fact, one patient had to stop taking the medication because of vaginal bleeding and hypertension. In the treatment group, there were no side effects. Further, although the food intake and increase in body weight was slightly lower in the treatment group than in the comparison group, it was markedly higher than those two param-eters in the blank group. Therefore, it was concluded that *Bu Zhong Yi Qi Tang* is capable of improving appetite, increasing body weight, and improving quality of life in those with CACS.

CLINICAL TRIAL 6: Outlet obstruction constipation[6]

From "The Treatment of 96 Cases of Outlet Obstruction Constipation with *Bu Zhong Yi Qi Tang* with Additions & Subtractions" by Gao Feng *et al.*, *Fu Jian Zhong Yi Yao (Fujian Chinese Medicine & Medicinals)*, #2, 2004, p. 30

Cohort description:

There were 146 patients altogether enrolled in this two-wing comparison study. In the treatment group there were 96: 19 males and 77 females 21-86 years old, with an average age of 42.8 years and a disease duration from one week to 32 years. In the comparison group there were 50 patients: 11 males and 39 females 20-84 years of age, with an average age of 41.3 years and a disease duration of one week to 30 years.

Treatment method:

All the members of the treatment group were orally administered the following version of *Bu Zhong Yi Qi Tang*: *Huang Qi* (Radix Astragali Membranacei), 30g, *Dang Shen* (Radix Codonopsitis Pilosulae), 30g, *Bai Zhu* (Rhizoma Atractylodis Macrocephalae), 40g, *Chai Hu* (Radix Bupleuri), 9g, *Sheng Ma* (Rhizoma Cimicifugae), 9g, *Dang Gui* (Radix Angelicae Sinensis), 9g, *Chen Pi* (Pericarpium Citri Reticulatae), 6g, *Rou Cong Rong* (Herba Cistanchis Deserticolae), 15g, and *Gan Cao* (Radix Glycyrrhizae Uralensis), 3g. If the patient was elderly and weak, 15 grams each of *He Shou Wu* (Radix Polygoni Multiflori) and *Sang Shen* (Fructus Mori Albi) were added. If the main symptoms was that the sensation of the expulsion of feces was slow, *Rou Cong Rong* was removed and more *Bai Zhu* was added. If there was hemafecia, 15 grams each of *Di Yu* (Radix Sanguisorbae Officinalis) and *Qian Cao Gen* (Radix Rubiae Cordifoliae) were added. If there was perianal aching and pain, 15 grams of *Bai Shao* (Radix Albus Paeoniae Lactiflorae) were added. If dry mouth was marked, *Huang Qi* and *Dang Shen* were both reduced to 15 grams each and 15 grams each of *Sha Shen* (Radix Glehniae Littoralis) and *Mai Men Dong* (Tuber Ophiopogoni Japonici) were added. One packet of these medicinals was decocted in water and administered per day in two divided doses. Members of the comparison group were orally administered 15 grams of *Ma Ren Wan* (Cannabis Pills) once per day. Three days equaled one course of treatment for both groups. During the administration of these medicinals, acrid, peppery, fatty, sweet, thick-flavored, and fried foods were prohibited.

Study outcomes:

Marked effect was defined as complete disappearance of clinical symptoms after one course of treatment. Some effect was defined as reduction of symptoms after one course and complete disappearance after two courses. No effect meant that, after two courses of treatment, there was no improvement. Based on these criteria, in the treatment group, 39 cases got a marked effect, 55 got some effect, and only two got no effect, for a total effectiveness rate of 97.9%. In the comparison group, seven cases got a marked effect, 16 got some effect, and 27 got no effect, for a total effectiveness rate of only 46%.

CLINICAL TRIAL 7: Liver cirrhosis hypoproteinemia

From "The Treatment of 62 Cases of Liver Cirrhosis Hypoproteinemia with *Bu Zhong Yi Qi Tang* Combined with Western Medicine" by Fang Wen-jia, *Shang Hai Zhong Yi Yao Za Zhi (Shanghai Journal of Chinese Medicine & Medicinals)*, #5, 2004, p. 33-34

Cohort description:

All 100 patients enrolled in this two-wing comparison study met the diagnostic criteria for liver cirrhosis set forth in the Fifth National Symposium on Infectious & Parasitic Diseases and all had hypoproteinemia. For instance, serum albumin was as low as 35g/L. These 100 patients were randomly divided into two groups, a treatment group and a comparison group. There were 62 patients in the treatment group, 46 males and 16 females 34-68 years of age, with an average age of 51.3 years. These patients' disease course had lasted from 0.5-12.5 years, with an average duration of 3.5 years. There were 38 patients in the comparison group, 25 males and 13 females 31-69 years of age, with an average age of 53.2 years. These patients' disease course had lasted from 0.8-13 years, with an average duration of four years. Therefore, in terms of sex, age, and disease duration, there was no significant statistical differences between these two groups.

Treatment method:

All members of both groups received standard Western medical care for liver cirrhosis, such as liver-protecting and urine-disinhibiting medicinals as well as supplemental albumin and other supporting medications. In addition to this basis, the members of the treatment group also received the following version of *Bu Zhong Yi Qi Tang*: *Huang Qi* (Radix Astragali Membranacei), 30g, *Dang Shen* (Radix Codonopsitis Pilosulae), 15g, *Bai Zhu* (Rhizoma Atractylodis Macrocephalae), 30g, *Dang Gui* (Radix Angelicae Sinensis), 15g, *Chen Pi* (Pericarpium Citri Reticulatae), 9g, *Chai Hu* (Radix Bupleuri), 6g, *Sheng Ma* (Rhizoma Cimicifugae), 9g, and *Gan Cao* (Radix Glycyrrhizae Uralensis), 6g. If torpid intake was pronounced, 12 grams of processed *Hou Po* (Cortex Magnoliae Officinalis), 30 grams of scorched *Shen Qu* (Massa Medica Fermentata), 15 grams of scorched *Mai Ya* (Fructus Germinatus Hordei Vulgaris), and nine grams of stir-fried *Ji Nei Jin* (Endothelium Corneum Gigeriae Galli) were added. If abdominal distention was marked and urination was scanty, 30 grams of *Fu Ling* (Sclerotium Poriae Cocos), 12 grams of *Da Fu Pi* (Pericarpium Arecae Catechu), and four grams of uncooked *Jiang Pi* (Cortex Rhizomatis Zingiberis Officinalis) were added. These medicinals were cooked as a standard decoction. Six weeks equaled one course of treatment for both groups, and total serum protein (TP), albumin (ALB), globulin (GLB), and the albumin to globulin ratio (A/G) were measured before and after treatment.

Study outcomes:

Marked effect was defined as complete disappearance of clinical symptoms, such as ascites, lower extremity edema, generalized edema, and torpid intake, a stable reduction in size of the liver and spleen, and normalization of ALB, GLB, and A/G. Some effect was defined as disappearance of symptoms or marked improvement, no change in hepato- and/or splenomegaly, and an increase in serum protein by 50% or more. No effect meant that none of these criteria were met. Based on these criteria, in the treatment group, 31 patients got a marked effect, 23 improved, and eight got no effect, for a total effectiveness rate of 87.25%. In the comparison group, 13 got a marked effect, 11 improved, and 14 got no effect, for a total effectiveness rate of 63.16%. Therefore, it was concluded that the combined Chinese-Western protocol was more effective than the simple Western medical protocol. Further, the mean ALB and A/G increased significantly and the GLB dropped strikingly after treatment, while, in the comparison group, the ALB changed little after treatment. And finally, the recurrence rate was lower in the treatment group than in the comparison group.

From 1999-2003, 44 articles were published in Chinese medical journals in the People's Republic of China on *Bu Zhong Yi Qi Tang*.[7] A large number of these were accounts of clinical trials. Based on those reports, some of the diseases that this formula has been able to successfully treat include digestive ulcers, chronic hepatitis B, irritable bowel syndrome (IBS), biliary duct stones, recalcitrant constipation, chronic obstructive pulmonary disease (COPD), recurrent respiratory tract infections, low blood pressure, unstable angina, diabetic constipation, diabetic neurogenic bladder, myasthenia gravis, Meniere's syndrome, low intracranial pressure, recalcitrant headache, insomnia, chronic glomerulonephritis, allergic purpura, menometrorrhagia, adolescent menorrhagia, abdominal pain accompanying menstruation, chronic pelvic inflammatory disease (PID), decreased female libido, retroversion of the uterus, menopausal syndrome, pediatric enuresis, pediatric polyuria, pediatric hyperactivity, opthalmological bleeding, chronic otitis media, tinnitus, allergic rhinitis, sinusitis, epistaxis, recurrent oral apthae, halitosis, and seminal emission. Clearly, this formula has one of the widest scopes of indication of any Chinese medicinal formula.

Endnotes

[1] A long lost, ancient medical work supposed to be written by the Yellow Emperor.

[2] *Su Wen*, Ch. 74. A later editor says boosted for the second warmed, but the present translator believes Li specifically meant warmed for boosted.

[3] This formula is composed of: *Qiang Huo* (Radix Et Rhizoma Notopterygii), *Huang Qin* (Radix Scutellariae Baicalensis), *Huang Lian* (Rhizoma Coptidis Chinensis), *Fang Feng* (Radix

Ledebouriellae Divaricatae), *Chai Hu* (Radix Bupleuri), *Chuan Xiong* (Radix Ligustici Wallichii), and *Gan Cao* (Radix Glycyrrhizae Uralensis) ground and made into a paste with a little tea water. Dosage: 2-5 *qian*.

4 The composition of both the *tang* (decoction) and the *wan* (pill) are the same: *Shui Zhi* (Hirudo Seu Whitmania), *Meng Chong* (Tabanus), *Tao Ren* (Semen Pruni Persicae), and *Da Huang* (Radix Et Rhizoma Rhei).

5 *Ling Shu*, Vol. 1, Ch. 4

6 *I.e.*, constipation secondary to outlet obstruction due to pelvic floor dysenergia, intussusception, or a non-emptying rectocele

7 Mao Zhi & Wei Ke-feng, "A Survey of the Clinical Uses of *Bu Zhong Yi Qi Tang*," *Jiang Su Zhong Yi Yao (Jiangsu Chinese Medicine & Medicinals)*, #3, 2004, p. 56-58

3

Diseases in the Different Seasons Due to Spleen & Stomach Vacuity Weakness and Formula Composing According to Different Diseases

When the spleen and stomach are vacuous and weak, the qi of the upper burner is insufficient. It is extremely important in clinical practice to keep in mind that the qi of both the heart and lungs is mainly derived from the spleen. In summer, the original qi is damaged by intense heat, [giving rise to] fatigue, somnolence, debilitated limbs, insufficient essence spirit, wilting flaccidity of the legs, cold reversal in the mornings and evenings, and fire-like heat coming back with the yang qi becoming effulgent when the sun is hanging high. Summer is a time of intense heat, and fire or intense heat eats qi. That means that the spleen-stomach may be damaged by intense heat. Since both yin and yang, qi and blood are insufficient, there occurs heat reversal with yin vacuity or cold reversal with qi vacuity [with] inability to taste food, fire sparks emitted in the eyes, blurred vision, frequent urination, difficult voiding of bound stools, ductal pain in the cardiac region, rib-side pain or acute spasm, tightening below the umbilicus as if bound by rope or, in the extreme, stabbing [lower abdominal] pain, difficulty relaxing the abdomen, obstruction in the chest, frequent retching or dry retching or coughing with phlegm, foaming at the mouth, rigidity of the tongue, pain in the upper and lower back, scapulae, and eyes, frequent headache, inability to take in food or [too easily] feeling satiated on eating, no desire to eat, particularly severe spontaneous perspiration, and [a feeling of] yin qi shrouding the skin and hair [*i.e.*, chills or a feeling of cold]. It is hot weather that exacerbates this disease. All this is brought about by *geng*, the large intestine and *xin*, lung metal, which are overwhelmed by heat. [In this case,] one must first assist the original qi and regulate the insufficient *geng* and *xin*. [For this,] *Huang Qi Ren Shen [Tang]* (Astragalus & Ginseng Decoction) is indicated.

Huang Qi Ren Shen Tang (Astragalus & Ginseng Decoction)

Huang Qi (Radix Astragali Membranacei), 1 *qian*; add 1 *qian* in case of excessive spontaneous sweating

Sheng Ma (Rhizoma Cimicifugae), 6 *fen*
Ren Shen (Radix Panacis Ginseng), stemmed
Chen Pi (Pericarpium Citri Reticulatae), with the white inner skin preserved
Mai Men Dong (Tuber Ophiopogonis Japonici), cored
Cang Zhu (Rhizoma Atractylodis), increase by 5 *fen* in the absence of sweating
Bai Zhu (Rhizoma Atractylodis Macrocephalae), 5 *fen* for each of the above
Huang Bai (Cortex Phellodendri), washed with wine to rescue the
    origin of water
Shen Qu (Massa Medica Fermentata), stir-fried, 3 *fen* [for each of] the above
Dang Gui (Radix Angelicae Sinensis), washed with wine
mix-fried *Gan Cao* (Radix Glycyrrhizae Uralensis), 2 *fen* [for each of]
    the above
Wu Wei Zi (Fructus Schisandrae Chinensis), 9 pieces

Slice the above ingredients [and take] as one dose, boiled in two cups of water down to one cupful and taken moderately hot between meals or on an empty stomach after removing the dregs. Refrain from wine, sodden wheat food, spices, and eating too much cold food.

During the heat of summer, the spleen is also commonly damaged by over-drinking chilled liquids and eating chilled foods, and eating too many uncooked, raw fruits and vegetables. Not only does this cause the spleen to be vacuous and weak, but it also causes the internal engenderment of dampness. It is said in Chinese medicine, the spleen is the root of phlegm engenderment, [but] the lungs are the place where phlegm is stored. Therefore, if dampness congeals into phlegm, this phlegm may be stored in the lungs where it hides or lies deeply until something else provokes its spilling over. In addition, a vacuous, weak spleen leading to lung qi vacuity leads to defensive qi vacuity and insecurity. Thus the person is easily invaded by wind evils (*i.e.*, unseen airborne pathogens). This helps explain a prevalence to allergic rhinitis in the fall, and it is my experience that this formula can be used to prevent just that. In this case, it should be taken during the heat of summer, 6-8 weeks before the expected seasonal onset of hayfever. Along with this formula, the patient should also strive to eat a clear, bland diet and avoid overeating chilled, uncooked foods as well as too many sugars and sweets.

In case of glomus and oppression below the heart, add *Huang Lian* (Rhizoma Coptidis Chinensis), 2-3 *fen*. Glomus below the heart suggests that there is more severe food stagnation due to spleen vacuity not moving and transforming water grains. Because food stagnation depresses the free flow of yang qi, this may give rise to concomitant depressive or transformative heat. Thus the addition of bitter, cold *Huang Lian*. In case of stomach ductal pain in the cardiac region, reduce the intensely cold medicinals and add *Cao Dou Kou* (Semen Alpiniae Katsumadai), five *fen*. In case of rib-side pain or spasm and tightness, add *Chai Hu* (Radix Bupleuri), 2-3 *fen*. In case of headache and fire sparks emitting in the eyes, add *Huang Lian* (Rhizoma Coptidis Chinensis), 2-3 *fen*, and *Chuan Xiong* (Radix Ligustici Wallichii), three *fen*. The *Huang Lian* is to clear heat, while the *Chuan Xiong* is to guide the effect of these medicinals upward to the region of the head and eyes. In case of headache and unclear vision [which is due to] congested heat in the upper, add *Man Jing Zi* (Fructus Viticis) and *Chuan Xiong* (Radix Ligustici Wallichii), both three *fen*, *Gao Ben* (Radix Et Rhizoma Ligustici Sinensis) and *Sheng Di* (uncooked Radix Rehmanniae Glutinosae), both two *fen*, and *Xi Xin* (Herba Asari Cum Radice), one *fen*. In case of shortness of breath, [clouding of] essence spirit as if vacillating on the border of sleeping and waking, drowsiness, and weakness, add *Wu Wei Zi* (Fructus Schisandrae Chinensis), nine pieces.

If astringent, stagnant defecation with no movement for one or two days running results in low food intake or inability to take in food, [this is due to] scanty blood with fire hidden within it and [which] is not moistened. [In this case,] add *Dang Gui* (Radix Angelicae Sinensis), *Sheng Di* (uncooked Radix Rehmanniae Glutinosae), and ground *Huo Ma Ren* (Semen Cannabis Sativae), five *fen* for the above, and *Tao Ren* (Semen Pruni Persicae), three pieces, soaked in boiled water, skinned, tipped, and ground separately. When the stools move freely [again], do not administer the added medicinals any longer. Thus it is entirely possible to have a damp, vacuous spleen at the same time as having dry, bound stools in the large intestine.

If defecation is still not disinhibited, do not introduce any other medicinals but add a small amount of *Da Huang* (Radix Et Rhizoma Rhei), five *fen*, simmered. If [even yet] defecation is not disinhibited, [this] is not [due to] blood binding but blood blockage that causes [the stools] to be non-freely flowing. Binding means dryness and blockage means stagnation and discontinuation of circulation. This is heat leading to the engenderment of wind, and, therefore, the patient must [manifest] a wind pattern. [In this case,] it is not ok to only add more blood medicinals and to stop regularly administering *Huang Qi Ren Shen Tang* (Astragalus & Ginseng Decoction). As for the medicinals, only *Qiang Huo* (Radix Et Rhizoma Notoptergyii) and *Fang Feng* (Radix Ledebouriellae Divaricatae), five *qian* each, should be used. Slice and boil these in four cups of water down to one cupful. Remove the dregs and take the decoction on an empty stomach. Then the stool will for sure be loosened and one dose is sufficient. In other words, one should continue taking *Huang Qi Ren Shen Tang* plus a single dose of a decoction of *Qiang Huo* and *Fang Feng* to treat the wind engendered by the heat.

In case of stagnant qi in the chest, add *Qing Pi* (Pericarpium Citri Reticulatae Viride), 1-2 *fen*, and double the amount of *Chen Pi* with the white inner skin removed in order to eliminate evil qi. This disease is due to insufficient original qi, and, therefore, it is necessary to supplement rather than drain the original qi. In other words, due to spleen vacuity leading to lung qi vacuity, the lungs are not diffusing and downbearing correctly. Although nondiffused qi may be stagnating in the chest, this is only a tip or branch repletion. The root of this condition is a qi vacuity. In case of severe qi stagnation possibly [due to] excessive supplementing medicinals [with a sensation of] worry, stagnation, depression, and binding below the patient's heart, add *Mu Xiang* (Radix Auklandia Lappae) and *Sha Ren* (Fructus Amomi), 2-3 *fen* for each of the above, and *Bai Dou Kou* (Fructus Cardamomi), two *fen*, to be boiled together with the standard formula [*i.e.*, *Huang Qi Ren Shen Tang*]. In case of abdominal pain without aversion to cold, add *Bai Shao* (Radix Albus Paeoniae Lactiflorae), five *fen*, and *Huang Qin* (Radix Scutellariae Baicalensis), two *fen*, but delete *Wu Wei Zi*.

In the sixth and the seventh months, rivers are flooding, it rains continually, everything gets wet, and clothes are soaked with sweat. If the spleen and stomach are vacuous and weak, generalized heaviness and shortness of breath and, in the extreme, wilting and limpness of the limbs, unsteady steps, feet awry, and liability to collapse with dark eyes are all signs of exhaustion of both kidney water and the urinary bladder. [For such conditions,] it is necessary to apply emergency aids. Lung qi should be enriched to supplement the upper source of water as well as to rid *geng*, the large intestine, of evil heat and check perspiration from exuding profusely. Massive discharge of perspiration means collapse of fluids and, when fluids collapse, the seven spirits have nothing upon which to rely. The seven spirits include the ethereal soul, corporeal soul, essence, spirit, reflection, wisdom, and will. The classic explains, "When fluids and humor are engendered, spirit is engendered by itself."[1] Fluids [and humors] are governed by *geng*, the large intestine. So-called triple hiding means nothing other than *geng* metal in confinement. The triple hiding refers to the three 10 day periods of the hot seasons, the first hiding commencing on the third *geng* day after the summer solstice, the second (middle) hiding on the fourth *geng* day, and the third (last) hiding on the first *geng* day after the beginning of autumn. If fluids and humors collapse with profuse drainage of perspiration and dampness governs in a hyperactive way, dry metal will be still confined and wind wood will go unchecked [even] when the clearing and depurating qi should prevail. This implies that as dampness overwhelms, when autumn (whose qi is clear and depurating) comes, lung metal is affected. As a result, wind and dampness are locked in a struggle, causing distressing pain in the joints and generalized pain. Hyperactivity is harmful, and it should be counteracted by restraint. Sun Si-miao[2] instructed that *Wu*

Wei Zi (Fructus Schisandrae Chinensis) should be administered frequently in the fifth month. [The object] is to drain *bing* fire, to supplement *geng*, the large intestine, and to boost the original qi of the five viscera. *Ren*, the cold water of the urinary bladder, has expired in *si* (S10) and *gui* (S2), kidney water has expired in *wu*. In terms of the earthly branches, the associations of the months and the five viscera are:

Phase	Viscus-bowel	Earthly Branches	Month
Water	Kidney/urinary bladder	*Hai* (B12), *zi* (B1)	10 -11th
Earth	Spleen/stomach	*Chou* (B2)	12th
Wood	Liver/gallbladder	*Yin* (B3), *mou* (S4)	1st, 2nd
Earth	Spleen/stomach	*Chen* (B5)	3rd
Fire	Heart/small intestine	*Si* (B6), *wu* (B7)	4th, 5th
Earth	Spleen/stomach	*Wei* (B8)	6th
Metal	Lung/large intestine	*Shen* (B9), *you* (B10)	7th, 8th
Earth	Spleen/stomach	*Xu* (B11)	9th

This sentence seems to imply that *si* and *wu* are the fire phase which restrain cold water. In other words, the kidneys and urinary bladder may experience detriment in the 4th (*si*) and 5th (*wu*) months.

Now, what is worse, since dampness is effulgent, it conspires with heat, and the clear and cold of the west and north both expire. In terms of five phase theory, north is *ren* and *gui*, i.e., the kidney/urinary bladder, and west is *geng* and *xin*, i.e., the lungs/large intestine. Remember that lung qi is clear and kidney qi is cold. Summer months make supplementation necessary, but what should be supplemented is the true qi of the heavenly origin rather than hot fire. That is, people should be made to take cold food in summer months. This is because the original qi is damaged by heat. True, but cold food should not be eaten to excess even in summer. Administer *Ren Shen* (Radix Panacis Ginseng), *Mai Men Dong* (Tuber Ophiopogonis Japonici), and *Wu Wei Zi* (Fructus Schisandrae Chinensis) to engender the pulse. What is known as the pulse is [actually] the original qi. *Ren Shen* (Radix Panacis Ginseng) supplements the original qi and drains hot fire with its sweetness. *Mai Men Dong* (Tuber Ophiopogonis Japonici) supplements the source of water as well as clears and depurates dry metal with its bitterness (sweetness [later editor]) and cold. *Wu Wei Zi* (Fructus Schisandrae Chinensis) drains fire and supplements *geng*, the large intestine, and lung metal with its sourness.

On occasion, even healthy persons are liable to two pathoconditions. That which arises as a result of enjoying the cool in a spacious court or large building to escape from the summer heat is called summer heat stroke. This disease invariably manifests as headache, aversion to cold, rigidity of the formal body, distressing pain in the joints, heart vexation, intense heat in the skin and flesh, and absence of sweating. [The cause is that] the yang qi around the body is deterred by the yin cold inside the house from diffusing and spreading. For most such cases, physicians prescribe *Da Shun San* (The Great Normalizing Powder).[3] Air-conditioning also can keep the yang qi from naturally diffusing and emitting from the inside of the body via perspiration.

That which occurs to the traveler or farmer toiling in the sun is called heat stroke. This disease invariably manifests as tormenting headache, agitating fever, aversion to heat, and intense heat felt in the skin and flesh when pressed as well as intense thirst, much drinking, massive drainage of perspiration, and qi being too scanty to move [the body]. This is hot weather damaging the lungs from the outside or qi from the external. *Cang Zhu Bai Hu Tang* (Atractylodes White Tiger Decoction)[4] is indicated.

Jie-gu[5] explains, "That which arises on movement is heat stroke, while that which arises at rest is summer heat stroke." Summer heat stroke is a yin pattern. It requires perfusion and dissipation. Heat stroke is a yang pattern. In it, the original qi is damaged by heat, but the formal body remains free from disease.

If, [during] the heaven's summerheat, a person with perduring disease due to spleen-stomach vacuity detriment neglects to nurture and adapt themself, acting counter to the season and attacking transformation, they must be encumbered and fatigued and [experience] loss of strength, disinclination to speak [and/or a faint, weak voice], shortness of breath, qi weakness, distressed rapid breathing, sometimes panting [and sometimes] not panting, fatigued and weak bones, a dreamy, somnolent appearance, clouded vision as if shrouded in clouds of smoke, and lack of consciousness of one's own body. Transformation here means a natural transforming process carried on in the body. [In this case,] one must massively discharge sweat.

If wind invades the sweat eyes [or pores], there must be convulsed [*i.e.*, puckered] skin, [exposure of the prominent] sinews [or veins] in the neck, dry skin, scorched hair, generalized heaviness, and intermittent vexatious pain in the joints of the limbs or pain all over the body, possible thirst or no thirst, and/or yellow, astringent urination. All this demonstrates the mutual struggle between wind and dampness, while headache or heavy-headedness, congested and exuberant heat in the upper, shortness of breath through the mouth or nose, distressed rapid breathing, vexed and agitated body and heart, pessimism, sadness, and despondency demonstrate yin being exuberant [over] yang in the extreme.

[If] this gets worse, the disease will transmit to the kidneys and liver, resulting in wilting and reversal. The limbs [as hot] as if amid a fire [indicate] heat reversal, while cold limbs [indicate] cold reversal. [In the case of] cold reversal, there is cold in the abdomen. [In the case of] heat reversal, there is heat in the abdomen. The reason [for the body pain] is that the limbs are ruled by the spleen. If the muscles become wet, impediment with insensitivity can transmute into the pattern of flesh wilting. This pattern is invariably accompanied by lung disease and physicians must base their medication on this condition.

In clinical practice, it is common to see certain autoimmune diseases, such as multiple sclerosis, get worse in the summer. Multiple sclerosis is mainly categorized as a wilting disease in Chinese medicine. However, any nerve insensitivity in MS may be considered a manifestation of local impediment of the skin and flesh. Such aggravation of autoimmune diseases in the summer is typically due to damage to the spleen due to a combination of external heat and improper diet.

Qi ascent surging into the chest is always a reversal pattern. Wilting is withered flaccidity and limpness of the limbs with incessant vexation and oppression of the heart. Reversal is qi counterflow. In the extreme, it can be a major counterflow and hence is termed reversal counterflow. Reversal and wilting are usually interrelated. [For this,] add to one dose of the above *Huang Qi Ren Shen Wu Wei Zi Mai Men Dong Tang* (Astragalus, Ginseng, Schisandra, & Ophiopogon Decoction),[6] *Fu Ling* (Sclerotium Poriae Cocos), two *fen*, *Ze Xie* (Rhizoma Alismatis Orientalis), four *fen*, and *Zhu Ling* (Sclerotium Polypori Umbellati) and *Bai Zhu* (Rhizoma Atractylodis Macrocephalae), one *fen* each. In case of free, uninhibited voiding of urine other than yellow, merely add *Ze Xie* (Rhizoma Alismatis Orientalis), two *fen*, to separate and disperse dampness in the upper and lower together with the two *Zhu*.[7] Unsteady step, wilting and limpness of the legs and knees, and the feet awry indicate that the wilting evil has already struck [the body]. [In that case,] add wine-washed *Huang Bai* (Cortex Phellodendri) and *Zhi Mu* (Rhizoma Anemarrhenae Aspheloidis), 3-5 *fen*, to enable the feet to issue forth abundant strength. The evil in this case is damp heat with or without concomitant yin vacuity.

If sweat is drained massively, fluids will desert. To quickly stop this, add *Wu Wei Zi* (Fructus Schisandrae Chinensis), six pieces, stir-fried *Huang Bai* (Cortex Phellodendri), five *fen*, and stir-fried *Zhi Mu* (Rhizoma Anemarrhenae Aspheloidis), three *fen*. Careful weighing is demanded so that [these medicinals] not interfere with food, [*i.e.*, eating]. Should they interfere with appetite, stop [administering them] till food intake returns [to normal]. Prick [*Zu*] *San Li* (St 36) and *Qi Jie* (St 30) with a three-edged needle to bleed. Should perspiration not be reduced or checked, prick to bleed the upper ridge three *cun* below *San Li* [*i.e.*, *Shang Ju Xu*, St 37] . Wine and sodden wheat food are prohibited.

Wilting is [due to] damp heat assailing the kidneys and liver. Here again we are talking about such autoimmune diseases as MS. [This damp heat] must be eliminated quickly. If not, the lower burner original qi will be exhausted completely causing limpness and paralysis. [In that case,] there must be inability to move [the parts] below the low back and incessant heart vexation and oppression. If the heaviness of the body has lessened with no shortness of breath and normalized urination, or, if the complicated disease qi has retreated with the retreating of the dampness and heat in the season, do not use *Wu Wei Zi* (Fructus Schisandrae Chinensis), *Ze Xie* (Rhizoma Alismatis Orientalis), *Fu Ling* (Sclerotium Poriae Cocos), *Zhu Ling* (Sclerotium Polypori Umbellati), *Huang Bai* (Cortex Phellodendri), *Zhi Mu* (Rhizoma Anemarrhenae Aspheloidis), *Cang Zhu* (Rhizoma Atractylodis), or *Bai Zhu* (Rhizoma Atractylodis Macrocephalae), but just vary the formula in accordance with the signs of the disease indicated by the formula. Among the commonly administered medicinals, wine[-processed] *Haung Bai* (Cortex Phellodendri) must also be used at 2-3 *fen*. When the season changes and the clear, dry qi moves greatly [or advances in a big way], add acrid, warm [medicinals] to drain [dampness]. If damp qi overwhelms and the wind signs do not recede [with] incessant dizziness and constant numbness, *Chu Feng Shi Qiang Huo Tang* (Eliminate Wind Dampness Notopterygium Decoction) governs this.

Chu Feng Shi Qiang Huo Tang (Eliminate Wind Dampness Notopterygium Decoction)

Qiang Huo (Radix Et Rhizoma Notopterygii), 1 *liang*
Fang Feng (Radix Ledebouriellae Divaricatae), stemmed
Cang Zhu (Rhizoma Atractylodis), soaked with wine, skinned
Huang Qi (Radix Astragali Membranacei), 1 *qian* [for each of] the above
Sheng Ma (Rhizoma Cimicifugae), 7 *fen*
mix-fried *Gan Cao* (Radix Glycyrrhizae Uralensis)
Du Huo (Radix Angelicae Pubescentis)
Chai Hu (Radix Bupleuri), 5 *fen* [for each of] the above
Chuan Xiong (Radix Ligustici Wallichii), to relieve headache
Huang Bai (Cortex Phellodendri)
Chen Pi (Pericarpium Citri Reticulatae)
Gao Ben (Radix Et Rhizoma Ligustici Sinensis), 3 *fen* [for each of]
    the above
Ze Xie (Rhizoma Alismatis Orientalis), stripped of hair

Zhu Ling (Sclerotium Polypori Umbellati), stripped of the black skin
Fu Ling (Sclerotium Poriae Cocos), 2 *fen* [for each of] the above
Huang Lian (Rhizoma Coptidis Chinensis), stripped of hair, 1 *fen*

This formula is an excellent one for modification for wind damp heat impediment condition with concomitant spleen vacuity and liver depression where
dampness is more prominent than heat. As Yan De-xin has correctly noted,
patients with chronic, enduring diseases, such as autoimmune diseases, will have
liver depression whether or not the liver depression was a causative factor in the
development of the chronic disease or not. This is because anyone with a chronic
disease must have many unfulfilled desires.

Slice the above [and take] 3-5 *qian* per dose, boiled in two cups of water down
to one cupful and taken moderately hot after removing the dregs. The dosage
depends on vacuity and repletion. In the presence of signs not mentioned, use
the formula according to the rules of modification.

When the pulse is bowstring, surging, moderate [or relaxed], and occasionally
rough [or choppy] when felt at the deep level, the signs are fullness and oppression of the limbs, vexatious pain in the limbs with difficulty in flexing and stretching, generalized heaviness, heart vexation and restlessness, sometimes gaining
weight and sometimes losing weight, languid, fatigued limbs, the mouth's loss
of taste [for food], difficulty relaxing and stretching the abdomen, and frequent
voiding of clear, uninhibited stools and urine or urinating immediately upon
drinking, possible astringent, stagnant, unmoving stools with no movement for
one or two days, swill diarrhea in summer months with untransformed food in
the stools, or blood and white pus appearing at the end of evacuation, fullness
of the chest, shortness of breath, non-freely flowing diaphragm and throat, or
coughing with sticky phlegm, foaming at the mouth, regurgitation of what is
just taken in, tinnitus, deafness, fire sparks emitting in the eyes, clouded vision,
canthus outcrop with red threads [in the eye], heat congested in the head and
eyes, inability to sleep quietly, somnolence, lack of strength, and no thought of
eating. *Tiao Zhong Yi Qi Tang* (Balance the Center & Boost the Qi Decoction)
governs [all these signs and symptoms].

Tiao Zhong Yi Qi Tang
(Balance the Center & Boost the Qi Decoction)

Huang Qi (Radix Astragali Membranacei), 1 *qian*
Ren Shen (Radix Panacis Ginseng), stemmed, delete in case of coughing

Gan Cao (Radix Glycyrrhizae Uralensis)

Cang Zhu (Rhizoma Atractylodis), 5 *fen* [for each of] the above

Chai Hu (Radix Bupleuri) This ingredient is good for insufficient qi above and pouring downward of the stomach and spleen qi. It is used for the purpose of supplementing the qi in the upper and abducting yin to yang. The lower is yin and the upper is yang. Since the stomach and spleen qi is pouring downward, it is justifiably said that qi should be abducted or conducted from yin to yang.

Chen Pi (Pericarpium Citri Reticulatae), increase by 1 *qian* in case of inability to circulate qi in the abdomen

Sheng Ma (Rhizoma Cimicifugae), 2 *fen* [for each of] the above

Mu Xiang (Radix Auklandia Lappae), 1-2 *fen*

This is an excellent base formula for the treatment of irritable bowel syndrome (IBS) due to a liver-spleen disharmony. If there is concomitant dampness and heat, it may be modified with a variety of added ingredients. Interestingly, patients with fibromyalgia syndrome (FMS) also often suffer from IBS.

Slice the above ingredients to the size of cannabis seeds [and take] as one dose, boiled in two large cups of water down to one cupful and taken while hot after removing the dregs and when food is already dispersed completely [in the stomach. Given] tranquility and repose of mind, this formula will prove miraculously effective. Since this disease lies in the four limbs and the blood vessels, an empty stomach in the dawn is [demanded]. The logic implied is that, since the formula is designed to conduct yin to yang, if taken in the morning, a time when yin is expiring and yang begins to prevail, the formula is believed to be particularly effective.

Frequent appearance of heat and agitation is due to yin fire in the lower origin [*i.e.*, the lower burner, including the kidneys and liver] steaming and effusing. There are only three basic mechanisms for agitation and restlessness of the heart spirit. The first is nonconstruction and malnourishment of the heart spirit. Such construction and nourishment of the spirit are mainly dependent upon th spleen's upbearing of the qi and blood. The second basic mechanism of agitation and restlessness of the spirit is harassment from some kind of heat evils which make the spirit stir frenetically. The third mechanism of agitation and restlessness of the heart spirit is blockage and obstruction by either phlegm turbidity or blood stasis. Because yin fire always involves an element of spleen vacuity as well as heat evils ascending to accumulate in the heart, agitation of the spirit is typically present in patients with yin fire. [For this,] add *Sheng Di* (uncooked Radix

Rehmanniae Glutinosae), two *fen*, and *Huang Bai* (Cortex Phellodendri), three *fen*, and remove these in the absence of such signs. These medicinals enrich yin, nourish the blood, and clear heat. Desire but inability to defecate or a desire to void remaining after evacuation with constant pressure and urgency in the abdomen is due to blood vacuity and blood stasis. [For this,] add *Dang Gui* (Radix Angelicae Sinensis), three *fen*. In case of generalized heaviness, despite frequent urination add *Fu Ling* (Sclerotium Poriae Cocos), two *fen*, *Cang Zhu* (Rhizoma Atractylodis), one *qian*, *Ze Xie* (Rhizoma Alismatis Orientalis), five *fen*, and *Huang Bai* (Cortex Phellodendri), three *fen*. [These are used] to eliminate dampness as a stopgap measure but should not be administered for long. Because the foot tai yin is diseased [with dampness] and its channel links to the heart, dampness and heat combine to give rise to vexation and agitation.

In case of stomach qi disharmony, add boiled water-washed *Ban Xia* (Rhizoma Pinelliae Ternatae), five *fen*, and *Sheng Jiang* (uncooked Rhizoma Zingiberis Officinalis), three slices. In case of coughing, add *Sheng Jiang* (uncooked Rhizoma Zingiberis Officinalis) and *Sheng Di* (uncooked Radix Rehmanniae Glutinosae), two *fen* each, to counteract the toxins of *Ban Xia*. Phlegm reversal with headache can be cured by nothing but *Ban Xia*. Phlegm reversal refers to frigidity of the limbs with asthma and copious phlegm. It is due to the foot tai yin spleen. In case of simultaneous agitation and heat, add *Huang Bai* (Cortex Phellodendri) and *Sheng Di* (uncooked Radix Rehmanniae Glutinosae), two *fen* each. In case of absence of the above signs, administer the preceding formula alone. Slice the above ingredients to the size of cannabis seeds [and take] as one dose, boiled in one large cup of water and taken while hot between meals after removing the dregs.

In summer months, it is necessary to add *Bai Shao* (Radix Albus Paeoniae Lactiflorae), three *fen*. In spring months, especially in case of abdominal pain, it is necessary to add this [also]. In case of aversion to heat with thirst or abdominal pain, increase *Bai Shao* by five *fen* and add *Sheng Di* (uncooked Radix Rehmanniae Glutinosae), two *fen*. In case of aversion to cold and abdominal pain, add debarked *Gui Zhi* (Ramulus Cinnamomi Cassiae), three *fen*, and delete *Huang Qin* (Radix Scutellariae Baicalensis), thereby composing a formula called *Gui Zhi Shao Yao Tang* (Cinnamon & Peony Decoction), [so named because *Gui Zhi*] is decocted together with the *Bai Shao*. In case of abdominal pain in winter months, *Bai Shao* cannot be added for it is a medicinal which is greatly cold. Only add *Gan Jiang* (dry Rhizoma Zingiberis Officinalis), two *fen*, or *Ban Xia* (Rhizoma Pinelliae Ternatae), 5-7 *fen*, processed with a small amount of ginger.

In autumn and winter months, if the four pathways of the stomach channel are caused to counterflow by the penetrating vessel and simultaneously the two pathways of the shao yang below the rib-side contrarily move upward, the disease is called reversal counterflow. Since the stomach channel's transporting point is *Qi Jie* (St 30) which means a thoroughfare leading in four directions in Chinese, the channel is also spoken of as the four pathways of the stomach channel. Since the foot shao yang channel goes bilaterally across the rib-side, it is also spoken of as the two pathways of the shao yang. The *Nei Jing (Inner Classic)* states, "When qi counterflow moves upward, the vessels are filled up and the form is made to depart."[8] [It is] clear [that when] the seven spirits become clouded and expire and the form departs, death arrives. The signs are qi surging up into the throat with inability to obtain breath with panting respiration and inability to lie down. [For this,] add *Wu Zhu Yu* (Fructus Evodiae Rutecarpae), washed with boiled water to rid it of bitterness, five *fen* to 1.5 *qian* depending on [whether there is] a lot or a little reversal qi.

If the pathocondition arises in the summer months, it is [due to] great heat. Following the four seasons, this disease presents itself as cold, hot, warm, or cool. [For it,] it is appropriate to prescribe wine[-processed] *Huang Lian* (Rhizoma Coptidis Chinensis), wine[-processed] *Huang Bai* (Cortex Phellodendri), and wine[- processed] *Zhi Mu* (Rhizoma Anemarrhenae Aspheloidis), in equal amounts, powdered, and made into pills with boiled water the size of Chinese parasol tree seeds, 200 pills a dose, taken with boiled water on an empty stomach. [Then] drink more boiled hot water. A little while later, take delicious food to press [the medicinals] straight down to the lower origin without letting them suspend in the stomach in order to drain the evils in the penetrating vessel. Generally speaking, diseases due to diet and taxation fatigue are all patterns of vacuity taxation and the seven detriments. In fact, there are only five detriments. They are skin and hair detriment causing ruffled skin and falling out hair, blood vessel detriment causing failure to nourish the viscera and bowels, muscle detriment causing inability of food to nourish the flesh and muscles, sinew detriment causing slackening of the sinews, and bone detriment causing bone wilting with inability to get out of bed. However, as a collective term, it is often used to convey a general sense of damage and detriment. [For these,] it is necessary to use warm, moderate, and more sweet than acrid formulas. This is the fundamental method.

If sometimes above there appears cold and heat, this is a seasonal disease. It may be a result of inappropriate methods of nurturing and regulation, dissipation in wine and overeating, a disease started by acrid, hot food or cold food, or living in intensely hot or cold environments. To help this disease, it is necessary to adopt makeshift measures in accordance with the conditions. The treatment method of employing greatly cold and greatly hot [medicinals] for the time being can achieve some effect. This serves, [however,] as just a stop-gap and cannot be used for long in spite of its effectiveness or [the disease] will invariably become recalcitrant.

I take this paragraph to mean that occasional, transient repletions of cold and heat may be treated simply by a single method, such as clearing heat or warming cold. However, these simple, discreet methods should not be used long-term if there are other underlying disease mechanisms, which, in adults, there always are. For instance, while one may use *Long Dan Xie Gan Tang* (Gentiana Drain the Liver Decoction) for damp heat for a couple or a few days to drain these evils, if used much longer than that in a patient with concomitant spleen vacuity, this is likely to give rise to further spleen vacuity without necessarily getting rid of all the damp heat. Now one has a more complicated pattern which is likely to become a chronic, enduring condition. Therefore, it is important to understand that such treatment methods are only stop-gap emergency measures based on the saying, "In acute [diseases] treat the tip (or branch)."

The *Huang Di Zhen Jing (Yellow Emperor's Acupuncture Classic)* states, "That which goes from the lower to the upper can be removed by abducting it [upwards]," and "Insufficient qi in the upper can be raised by pushing."[9] This originally referred to an acupuncture technique. The qi in the upper is the qi of the lungs and heart in the upper burner. For a yang disease in the yin, [the qi] should be abducted from yin to yang, and medicinals able to enter the kidneys and liver in the lower burner are required to abduct more sweet and less acrid medicinals. Thus the spleen and stomach qi can be upraised and emitted [or out-thrust], and thereby the evil qi can be removed from the interstices and the skin and hair. It also says, "The pain seen in the anterior is usually chosen [or treated] first." This implies that the congested channels and network vessels should be drained first with contralateral needling. Since blood is congealed and is not flowing, [the congestion] should be removed first and other diseases [should be] treated afterwards.

Endnotes

1 *Su Wen*, Ch. 9

2 Sun Si-miao (?581-682 CE), one of the most famous Chinese medical scholars, the author of the *Qian Jin Yao Fang (Formulas [Worth] a 1,000 Pieces of Gold)*, *Qian Jin Yi Fang (Subsidiary Formulas [Worth] a 1,000 Pieces of Gold)*, and many other important works.

3 This formula is composed of: *Gan Cao* (Radix Glycyrrhizae Uralensis), *Gan Jiang* (dry Rhizoma Zingiberis Officinalis), *Xing Ren* (Semen Pruni Armeniacae), and *Rou Gui* (Cortex Cinnamomi Cassiae).

[4] This formula is composed of: *Cang Zhu* (Rhizoma Atractylodis), *Shi Gao* (Gypsum Fibrosum), *Zhi Mu* (Rhizoma Anemarrhenae Aspheloidis), *Gan Cao* (Radix Glycyrrhizae Uralensis), and rice.

[5] Zhang Yuan-su, styled Jie-gu, a pre-eminent physician and Li Dong-yuan's teacher

[6] *Huang Qi Ren Shen Tang* (Astragalus & Ginseng Decoction)

[7] *I.e.*, *Bai Zhu* (Rhizoma Atractylodis Macrocephalae) and *Cang Zhu* (Rhizoma Atractylodis)

[8] *Su Wen*, Ch. 5

[9] *Ling Shu*

4

Treatise on the Use of *Qing Shu Yi Qi Tang* (Clear Summerheat & Boost the Qi Decoction) in Case of the Stomach Troubled Particularly Profoundly by Damp Heat in Long Summer

The *Ci Zhi Lun (Treatise on Epigrams [Concerning] Needling)* states, "Qi vacuity with generalized fever results from summerheat damage,"[1] a damage of qi by heat. The *Wei Lun (Treatise on Wilting)* states:

> Long travelling results in taxation fatigue and accidental great hot weather arouses thirst. With thirst, yang qi attacks inward, and inward attacking makes heat lodge in the kidneys, the water viscus. If water is no longer able to conquer fire, the bones become dry, the marrow gets vacuous, and the legs are unable to carry the body. Bone wilting thus arises.[2]

Therefore the *Xia Jing (Lower Classic)* states, "Bone wilting is engendered by great heat."[3] [Thus] it is damp heat that gives rise to wilting, making the bones fatigued and lose their strength. Therefore, to treat wilting, only choose the yang ming alone [to be treated]. The stomach is the sea of water and grain responsible for moistening the gathering sinews and binding the joints. Therefore, wilting due to damage of the qi is concerned mainly with the yang ming and must be treated through it.

Once again, with the word "wilting," the reader is alerted to the relevance of the following information to the treatment of various autoimmune diseases. In my experience, most patients with autoimmune impediment and/or wilting disorders typically do present with some element of internally engendered damp heat and often experience exacerbations when exposed to external heat or damp heat, and summerheat is a species of external damp heat.

Damp heat overwhelmingly prevails in long summer, steaming, steaming, and burning. When people are affected [by damp heat,] they usually have encumbered, fatigued limbs, diminished essence spirit, disinclination to move, fullness in the chest with distressed rapid breathing, heavy, aching joints, or raised qi with

panting, generalized heat with vexation, inflating glomus below the heart, frequent, yellow urination, frequent loose stools or dysentery with chyme-like, yellow or rice water-like stools, the presence or absence of thirst, no thought for
food or drink, spontaneous perspiration, generalized heaviness, or lack of sweating. This is blood that is first diseased, while the qi is not [yet] diseased. The pulse
is felt surging and moderate. Again, the equation of the surging pulse with yin
fire. If blood and qi mutually struggle, [the pulse] must additionally be slow. [If
the pulse is] slow, one should treat with dryness-clearing formulas even though
the disease varies a little [in signs], since summerheat dampness remains [the
pathogenic factor] all the same. The *Nei Jing (Inner Classic)* states, "The yang qi
defends the exterior and makes it secure."[4] And, "Hot weather discharges [or
drains] the qi."[5] Since summerheat evils attack the defensive, generalized fever
and spontaneous perspiration occur. [In that case,] use *Huang Qi* (Radix Astragali
Membranacei), which is sweet and warm, as the sovereign to supplement the
defensive; *Ren Shen* (Radix Panacis Ginseng), *Chen Pi* (Pericarpium Citri
Reticulatae), *Dang Gui* (Radix Angelicae Sinensis), and *Gan Cao* (Radix
Glycyrrhizae Uralensis), which are sweet and slightly warm, as the ministers to
supplement the center and boost the qi; and *Cang Zhu* (Rhizoma Atractylodis),
Bai Zhu (Rhizoma Atractylodis Macrocephalae), and *Ze Xie* (Rhizoma Alismatis
Orientalis), which are percolators and disinhibitors, to eliminate dampness. *Sheng
Ma* (Rhizoma Cimicifugae) and *Ge Gen* (Radix Puerariae), which are sweet, bit-
ter, and balanced, are good not only for resolving muscle heat but for conquer-
ing dampness with their windy [nature]. Prevailing dampness causes inability
to disperse food as well as glomus and fullness. Therefore, stir-fried *Shen Qu*
(Massa Medica Fermentata), which is sweet and acrid, and *Qing Pi* (Pericarpium
Citri Reticulatae Viride), which is acrid and warm, [are used to] disperse food
and expedite the qi. The kidneys are adverse to dryness. [Thus] one should quickly
eat acrid to moisten them. Hence *Huang Bai* (Cortex Phellodendri), which is
bitter, acrid, and cold, [is used to] drain heat and supplement water with the help
of the sweet flavors. [Kidney] vacuity requires enriching the source of transformation. The source of transformation of the kidneys is metal, *i.e.*, the lungs and
large intestine. *Ren Shen*, *Wu Wei Zi* (Fructus Schisandrae Chinensis), and *Mai
Men Dong* (Tuber Ophiopogonis Japonici), which are sour, sweet and slightly
cold, [are, therefore, used] as the assistants to rescue *geng* metal from summerheat damage. The formula is named *Qing Shu Yi Qi Tang* (Clear Summerheat &
Boost the Qi Decoction).

Qing Shu Yi Qi Tang
(Clear Summerheat & Boost the Qi Decoction)

Huang Qi (Radix Astragali Membranacei), reduce by 5 *fen* in case
of scant sweating

Cang Zhu (Rhizoma Atractylodis), soaked with rice water, skinned
Sheng Ma (Rhizoma Cimicifugae), 1 *qian* for each of the above
Ren Shen (Radix Panacis Ginseng), stemmed
Ze Xie (Rhizoma Alismatis Orientalis)
Shen Qu (Massa Medica Fermentata), stir-fried
Chen Pi (Pericarpium Citri Reticulatae)
Bai Zhu (Rhizoma Atractylodis Macrocephalae), 5 *fen* [for each of]
    the above
Mai Men Dong (Tuber Ophiopogonis Japonici), cored
Dang Gui (Radix Angelicae Sinensis)
mix-fried *Gan Cao* (Radix Glycyrrhizae Uralensis), 3 *fen* [for each of]
    the above
Qing Pi (Pericarpium Citri Reticulatae Viride), stripped of the inner
    white skin, 2.5 *fen*
Huang Bai (Cortex Phellodendri), wine-washed, skinned, 2-3 *fen*
Ge Gen (Radix Puerariae), 2 *fen*
Wu Wei Zi (Fructus Schisandrae Chinensis), 9 pieces

Slice the above ingredients [and take] all in one dose, boiled in two large cups of water down to one cupful. Take while quite warm between meals after removing the dregs. The quantities of the formula can be varied according to conditions.

This formula was originally intended for yin summerheat, *i.e.*, summerheat dampness as opposed to summerheat heat. However, it is an excellent formula for the treatment of a liver-spleen disharmony with internally engendered dampness and heat in which dampness is relatively more marked than heat. The *Wu Wei Zi, Mai Men Dong*, and *Ge Gen* artfully keep the acrid, dry and bland, seeping medicinals from damaging yin at the same time as treating any symptoms of thirst due to enduring heat floating upward. *Sheng Ma, Ge Gen, Qing Pi*, and *Chen Pi* work together to rectify the qi and disinhibit the qi mechanism. When combined with *Dang Gui*, they also harmonize the liver. This formula has a wider scope of application than just treating spleen damage due to externally contracted damp heat.

In all cases, this disease is a result of damage of the spleen and stomach by food and drink and taxation fatigue but [its active course is] initiated by summerheat. This formula includes prohibited medicinals like *Ze Xie* (Rhizoma Alismatis Orientalis), *Zhu Ling* (Sclerotium Polypori Umbellati), *Fu Ling* (Sclerotium Poriae Cocos), *Deng Xin Cao* (Medulla Junci Effusi), *Tong Cao* (Medulla Tetrapanacis Papyriferi), and *Mu Tong* (Caulis Akebiae), which are bland, percolating urination-disinhibitors. Since this disease involves loss of fluids by, for example, spontaneous sweating, percolation in this case is tantamount to evacuating vacuity. They are used in accordance with the effulgent qi of the season in order to drain the intruding evils in the spleen and stomach as well as to supplement the insufficiency of metal and water. This is a conventionally prescribed formula, but it should only be used as a makeshift. If it is misused for a pattern devoid of the seasonal signs of effulgent damp heat in the spleen or for a pattern of frequent urination with kidneys and liver unaffected by evils, true yin will for sure be greatly drained, thus exhausting kidney water completely. This will first cause detriment to the two eyes. Variations [of this formula] are given below for transmuted patterns.

If heart fire overwhelms the spleen, this means that blood suffers from fire evils and is unable to upbear and effuse yang qi to send it home into the earth. In humans, earth means the spleen. [Therefore,] it is necessary to use *Dang Gui* (Radix Angelicae Sinensis) to harmonize the blood and a little *Huang Bai* (Cortex Phellodendri) to boost true yin.

The pattern of insufficient spleen and stomach requires a small quantity of *Sheng Ma* (Rhizoma Cimicifugae), a medicinal which conducts to the foot yang ming and tai yin channels. [Yang qi] will thus be made to travel the yang tract and turn right from the spleen and stomach. In ancient times, the right side was regarded more highly than the left. Therefore, turning left was synonymous with taking a wrong turn. In medical works, turning right was often referred to as rising, while turning left as falling. The shao yang governs spring, the root of engenderment and transformation of the tens of thousands of things. To enrich the harmonizing qi of spring, using, in addition, a small quantity of *Chai Hu* (Radix Bupleuri) turns the various channels right to engender and effuse the qi of the yang ming.

Spleen vacuity is the result of hyperactive heart fire which overwhelms earth. Again, it is a seminal concept of yin fire theory that heart fire due to upward counterflow and frenetic stirring of ministerial/life-gate fire can damage and cause detriment to the spleen. Secondly, lung qi is subjected to evils and is damaged by heat. When heat evils ascend from the middle and lower burners, they do not all accumulate in the heart. They also may accumulate in the lungs, the florid canopy. [In that case,] it is necessary to use *Huang Qi* (Radix Astragali Membranacei) most, *Gan Cao* (Radix Glycyrrhizae Uralensis) less, and *Ren Shen* (Radix Panacis Ginseng) the least. These three are all sweet, warm, yang medicinals. When the spleen becomes vacuous, lung qi expires. Therefore, *Huang Qi*, which is sweet and warm, is used to boost the qi of the skin and hair to secure the interstices in order to check spontaneous perspiration from damaging the original qi. [Qi] ascent panting, shortness of breath, and disinclination to speak require *Ren Shen* to supplement [the qi, while] heart fire overwhelming the spleen requires mix-fried *Gan Cao* to drain fire heat and supplement the original qi in the spleen and stomach. This is an interesting point. In contemporary Chinese medicine, we typically use uncooked *Gan Cao* to clear heat and mix-fried *Gan Cao* to supplement the spleen. It would seem that Li is saying that even mix-fried *Gan Cao* retains some ability to clear heart fire. If so, this is an important fine point in formula construction. *Gan Cao* should be used in the smallest amount out of fear it might promote fullness. But, in case of acute pain in the spleen and stomach and extremely severe spleen and stomach vacuity with violent contraction inside the abdomen and of the skin [over] the abdomen, it should be used in large amounts. The classic states, "Tension should be treated by relaxation."[6]As a make-shift measure, it is necessary to add *Sheng Ma* (Rhizoma Cimicifugae) as a conductor for fear that [any] left-turning evils are strong and exuberant enough to refuse to retreat after all. [In this case,] evils may emaciate the flesh in the neck, hips, and sacrococcygeal region and [force yang qi] to embark on the yin tract. Therefore, to harmonize yin and yang qi, *Sheng Ma* is used to conduct the clear qi to the yang tract and turn it right from the earth to ascend. In case of center fullness, delete *Gan Cao*. In case of severe coughing, delete *Ren Shen*. In case of dry mouth and dry throat, add *Ge Gen* (Radix Puerariae).

Since the spleen and stomach are vacuous, unable to upbear and float, their engendering and emission of the qi are damaged by yin fire, the constructive and the blood are greatly depleted, and the constructive qi lies deeply [or is hidden] in the earth. Earth here means the kidneys and liver or the lower burner. If yin fire burns exuberantly, boiling day after day, blood and qi become [more and more] depleted and scanty. In addition, the pericardium and heart rule the blood. [Therefore,] diminished blood leaves no place from which the heart to [receive its] nourishment. This causes the heart to be chaotic and vexed, a disease called disturbance. Disturbance means a confused, vexed, oppressed, and restless heart. This is due to non-upbearing of the clear qi and non-downbearing of the turbid qi. [Instead,] the clear and turbid mutually attack each other, and, being in chaos within the chest, qi and blood move counterflow throughout the body and are in chaos. The *Nei Jing (Inner Classic)* says, "That which goes from the lower to the upper can be removed by abducting it (upwards)."[7] Therefore, one should add acrid, warm and sweet, warm formulas to engender yang. The engenderment of yang leads to the growth of yin. There is a consensus about the three sweet, warm medicinals. This means that *Huang Qi* (Radix Astragali Membranacei), *Ren Shen* (Radix Panacis Ginseng), and mix-fried *Gan Cao* (Radix Glycyrrhizae Uralensis) can all engender yang. It may be questioned why the sweet and warm can engender the blood since they are not blood medicinals. The answer is as follows: Supplementation of blood vacuity with *Ren Shen* (Radix Panacis Ginseng) is [Zhang] Zhong-jing's method. When yang is made effulgent, yin blood is engendered. In addition, one should add *Dang Gui* (Radix Angelicae Sinensis) to harmonize blood and a little *Huang Bai* (Cortex Phellodendri) to rescue kidney water. The sweet, cold is able to drain fire and heat. When fire is decreased, heart qi can obtain calm and is quieted. If vexation and restlessness cannot be stopped, add a small amount of *Huang Lian* (Rhizoma Coptidis Chinensis) to get rid of it. If kidney water is supplemented, thus promoting kidney water effulgence, heart fire will automatically be downborne and the yang qi of earth will be supported.

In case of qi floating and heart chaos, administer *Zhu Sha An Shen Wan* (Cinnabar Quiet the Spirit Pills)[8] to settle and secure [the qi]. Qi floating and heart chaos refers to upward surging of yin fire manifested by restlessness and fidgets with a sensation of something inside disturbed and surging. When vexation is decreased, do not administer [this formula] any more to prevent the draining of yang qi erroneously [resulting in] falling [of the central qi]. In other words, this cold, draining formula should only be used for a short period of time based on the dictum, "In acute [diseases], treat the tip [or branch]." Long-term administration will damage the spleen. In case of glomus below the heart, also add a little *Huang Lian* (Rhizoma Coptidis Chinensis) [to *Qing Shu Yi Qi Tang*]. Qi chaos in the chest is [due to] mutual attack between the clear and turbid. Therefore, it should be rectified by *Chen Pi* (Pericarpium Citri Reticulatae) which is also able to assist the upbearing of yang qi and the dissipation of stagnant qi as well as assist and bring the various sweet, acrid [medicinals] into full play.

When the intruding evils of damp earth are extremely effulgent in long summer, *Cang Zhu* (Rhizoma Atractylodis), *Bai Zhu* (Rhizoma Atractylodis Macrocephalae), and *Ze Xie* (Rhizoma Alismatis Orientalis) can be added as a stratagem to separate and disperse the qi of damp heat above and below. Overwhelming prevalence of damp qi mainly leads to inability to disperse and transform food. Therefore food [intake] is reduced and there is no knowledge of the flavor of grains [*i.e.*, the flavor of food is lost. For this,] stir-fried *Shen Qu* (Massa Medica Fermentata) is added to disperse food. Then *Wu Wei Zi* (Fructus Schisandrae Chinensis), *Mai Men Dong* (Tuber Ophiopogonis Japonici), and *Ren Shen* (Radix Panacis Ginseng) are added to drain fire, boost the lung qi, and help autumn reduction. Excessively effulgent damp heat in long summer damages the lung qi which then becomes insufficient in autumn, the season ruled by the lungs. This kind of insufficiency is called autumn reduction. These are the medicinals in constant use when long summer [qi] is just effulgent in the triple hiding. The triple hiding refers to the three 10 day periods of the hot seasons as described above in Chapter Three.

REPRESENTATIVE CASE HISTORIES

From "Lifting the Borders on the Clinical Use of Dong-yuan's *Qing Shu Yi Qi Tang*" by Guo Jian-sheng *et al.*, *Zhe Jiang Zhong Yi Za Zhi (Zhejiang Journal of Chinese Medicine)*, #6, 2004, p. 237

CASE 1: Hypothyroidism

The patient was a 30 year-old female who was first seen on Dec. 10, 2000 who had been suffering from hypothyroidism for half a year. She had taken Western thyroid medication to raise her hormone level but it had not improved. Therefore, she had sought out Chinese medical treatment. The patient was easily fatigued and had no desire to speak very much. Her appetite was poor, and, after eating, she easily developed duct and abdominal fullness and distention. In addition, the patient was constipated, although her stools were soft. When the patient woke up in the morning, her skin felt swollen and distended. The woman's menstruation tended to be scanty in amount and pale in color and contained a small amount of blood clots. Her tongue was also pale with white, slightly yellowish fur which was slightly slimy at the root. Her pulse was fine and moderate or slightly slow. Therefore she was prescribed *Qing Shu Yi Qi Tang* with additions and subtractions: *Dang Shen* (Radix Codonopsitis Pilosulae), 20g, *Huang Qi* (Radix Astragali Membranacei), 30g, *Bai Zhu* (Rhizoma Atractylodis Macrocephalae), *Dang Gui* (Radix Angelicae Sinensis), *Ze Xie* (Rhizoma Alismatis Orientalis), *Chen Pi* (Pericarpium Citri Reticulatae), *Shen Qu* (Massa Medica Fermentata), *Gu Ya* (Fructus Germinatus Oryzae Sativae), *Mai Ya* (Fructus Germinatus Hordei Vulgaris), and *Hou Po* (Cortex Magnoliae Officinalis), 10g each, *Huang Bai* (Cortex Phellodendri), *Gan Cao* (Radix Glycyrrhizae Uralensis), and *Wu Wei Zi* (Fructus Schisandrae Chinensis), 6g each, *Ge Gen* (Radix Puerariae), 15g, *Mai Men Dong* (Tuber Ophiopogonis Japonici), 8g, and *Xie Bai* (Bulbus Allii), 7g. After taking seven packets of these medicinals, the patient's feeling of fatigue was less and her abdominal distention was greatly reduced. Her stools were now replete and she was no longer constipated. Therefore, the original formula was continued for three whole months, after which time, her T3 and T4 had returned to normal and all her symptoms were eliminated.

CASE 2: Type 2 diabetes mellitus

The patient was a 53 year-old female who was first seen on May 15, 2003. This patient had been diagnosed with type 2 diabetes for 10 years and had already been treated with a number of Chinese and Western medicines, however with poor effects. In recent days, the patient's blood sugar had become elevated. Her fasting blood glucose was 8.9mmol/L. Therefore, she came for a consultation. At that time, she complained of lack of strength, sleepiness which was especially worse after eating, a bland taste in the mouth, torpid intake, abdominal distention, thin, soft stools which occurred three times per day, turbid urination, but no polydipsia, polyphagia, or polyuria. The patient's tongue tended to be fat with white fur, and her pulse was weak. In addition, her cholesterol and blood pressure both tended to be high. Based on these signs and symptoms, the patient was prescribed *Qing Shu Yi Qi Tang* with additions and subtractions: *Dang Shen* (Radix Codonopsitis Pilosulae), 20g, *Huang Qi* (Radix Astragali Membranacei), 30g, *Bai Zhu* (Rhizoma Atractylodis Macrocephalae), *Dang Gui* (Radix Angelicae Sinensis), *Shen Qu* (Massa Medica Fermentata), *Ze Xie* (Rhizoma Alismatis Orientalis), *Hou Po* (Cortex Magnoliae Officinalis), *Chen Pi* (Pericarpium Citri Reticulatae), and *Dan Shen* (Radix Salviae Miltiorrhizae), 10g each, *Wu Wei Zi* (Fructus Schisandrae Chinensis), *Huang Bai* (Cortex Phellodendri), and *Gan Cao* (Radix Glycyrrhizae Uralensis), 6g each, *Ge Gen* (Radix Puerariae), 15g, and *Mai Men Dong* (Tuber Ophiopogonis Japonici), 8g. After taking seven packets of these medicinals, the woman's blood glucose had returned to normal. Therefore, she was continued on the same formula plus 15 grams each of *Shan Yao* (Radix Dioscoreae Oppositae) and *Fu Ling* (Sclerotium Poriae Cocos). The woman then took this formula with additions and subtractions for two more months and her fasting blood glucose remained within normal parameters.

CASE 3: Chronic glomerulonephritis

The patient was a 30 year-old male who was first examined on July 9, 2002. One year previous, due to having caught a cold, the man had developed a fever, facial edema, and scanty urination. At the time, his Western medical diagnosis was acute nephritis. After one month of treatment, his symptoms were eliminated. However, protein in his urine was not able to be eliminated. One month prior to his visit on July 9, the man had been diagnosed with chronic glomerulonephritis. When the patient got up in the morning, his eyelids were slightly swollen and his throat was red and felt blocked or obstructed. He was afraid of wind (or chill), and his low back was sore and distended. The man's stools were soft, and his urination was short, slightly yellow, turbid, and foamy. His tongue was red with thin, yellow fur, and his pulse was floating and slightly bowstring. Proteinuria was triple plus. At first, the man was prescribed *Yin Qiao Ma Bo San* (Lonicera, Forsythia & Lasiosphera Powder) plus *Fang Ji Huang Qi Tang* (Stephania & Atragalus Decoction) with additions and subtractions: *Jin Yin Hua* (Flos Lonicerae Japonicae), *Lian Qiao* (Fructus Forsythiae Suspensae), and *Sang Ji Sheng* (Ramulus Loranthi Seu Visci), 15g each, *Ma Bo* (Fructificatio Lasiospherae Seu Calvatiae), *She Gan* (Rhizoma

Belamcandae), *Fang Ji* (Radix Stephaniae Tetrandae), *Bai Zhu* (Rhizoma Atractylodis Macrocephalae), and *Du Zhong* (Cortex Eucommiae Ulmoidis), 10g each, *Niu Bang Zi* (Fructus Arctii Lappae) and *Gan Cao* (Radix Glycyrrhizae Uralensis), 6g each, *Yi Yi Ren* (Semen Coicis Lachryma-jobi) and *Shan Zhu Yu* (Fructus Corni Officinalis), 12g each, *Yu Mi Xu* (Stylus Zeae Maydis), 1 bunch, and *Huang Qi* (Radix Astragali Membranacei), 25g.

After taking seven packets of these medicinals, the edema, red throat, and feeling of obstruction in the back of the throat were all improved, the tongue was no longer red, and the pulse was no longer bowstring. However, the proteinuria was still triple plus. In addition, the man was easily exhausted, easily caught cold, and his stools were loose and unformed. Therefore, he was prescribed *Qing Shu Yi Qi Tang* with additions and subtractions: *Dang Shen* (Radix Codonopsitis Pilosulae), 20g, *Huang Qi* (Radix Astragali Membranacei), 30g, *Bai Zhu* (Rhizoma Atractylodis Macrocephalae), *Dang Gui* (Radix Angelicae Sinensis), *Ze Xie* (Rhizoma Alismatis Orientalis), *Shen Qu* (Massa Medica Fermentata), *Du Zhong* (Cortex Eucommiae Ulmoidis), and *Chen Pi* (Pericarpium Citri Reticulatae), 10g each, *Sang Ji Sheng* (Ramulus Loranthi Seu Visci), *Yi Yi Ren* (Semen Coicis Lachryma-jobi), and *Ge Gen* (Radix Puerariae), 15g each, *Mai Men Dong* (Tuber Ophiopogonis Japonici), 8g, *Gan Cao* (Radix Glycyrrhizae Uralensis), *Wu Wei Zi* (Fructus Schisandrae Chinensis), *Chan Yi* (Periostracum Cicadae), and *Huang Bai* (Cortex Phellodendri), 6g each, and *Yu Mi Xu* (Stylus Zeae Maydis), 1 bunch. After taking seven packets of this new formula, the proteinuria was only one plus. Thus the man was continued on modifications of this formula for three whole months, after which his urine was normal and all his symptoms had disappeared.

Endnotes

1 *Su Wen*, Ch. 53
2 *Su Wen*, Ch. 44
3 A long lost ancient medical work
4 *Su Wen*, Ch. 3
5 *Su Wen*, Ch. 39
6 *Su Wen*, Ch. 74
7 *Ling Shu*, Vol. 11, Ch. 73
8 This formula is composed of: *Zhu Sha* (Cinnabaris), *Huang Lian* (Rhizoma Coptidis Chinensis), *Dang Gui* (Radix Angelicae Sinensis), *Sheng Di* (uncooked Radix Rehmanniae Glutinosae), and *Gan Cao* (Radix Glycyrrhizae Uralensis).

5

Rules for Adding & Subtracting in the Use of Medicinals Following the Seasons

According to Yang Shou-zhong, unless otherwise indicated, the modifications given in this chapter are all based on *Qing Shu Yi Qi Tang* (Clear Summerheat & Boost the Qi Decoction). I am not convinced of this since summerheat does not strike in the winter. It is a seasonal external contraction. However, if summerheat does not just mean summerheat but also damp heat, whether externally contracted or internally generated, then I can accept this.

Turbid qi [trapped] in the yang and its chaos in the chest causes distention, fullness and obstruction, and constipation. In summer months, it is appropriate to add a little greatly bitter, cold medicinals, such as wine-washed *Huang Bai* (Cortex Phellodendri), while in winter months, it is appropriate to add greatly acrid, bitter, hot medicinals, like *Wu Zhu Yu* (Fructus Evodiae Rutecarpae), as a temporary measure. The use of medicinals should vary in accordance with the seasons to drain and downbear turbid qi. Because greatly cold qi exists within the sweet flavor, sweet, cold [medicinals] are able to drain fire and heat. However, acrid, warm, cold qi-dissipators should be used in larger amounts than *Huang Bai* (Cortex Phellodendri).

Clear qi [trapped] in the yin means decrepit spleen and stomach qi which is unable to upbear and effuse the yang qi. Thus, *Sheng Ma* (Rhizoma Cimicifugae) and *Chai Hu* (Radix Bupleuri) are used to assist the acrid and sweet flavors in abducting [or leading] the original qi upward to check swill diarrhea.

When the throat is obstructed, failure of yang qi to obtain exit is called choking, [and] failure of yin qi to obtain descent and downbearing is called constriction. Choking and constriction bar [qi] counterflow [within the space] between the throat, chest, and diaphragm. Hence there is no movement in the various channels. This leads to an open mouth, fixed gaping, and qi bordering on expiration. [In this case,] one must first administer acrid, sweet, yang medicinals in both qi and flavor to lead the stomach qi to treat the root and to add blockage[-breaking] medicinals to drain the branch. In cold months, when yin qi greatly assists yin evils from the outside, greatly hot, greatly acrid and bitter *Wu Zhu Yu* (Fructus Evodiae Rutecarpae) should be added to the standard formula [*i.e., Qing Shu Yi Qi Tang,* Clear Summerheat & Boost the Qi Decoction] to drain the yin cold qi. In summer months, when yang is exuberant, *Qing Pi* (Pericarpium Citri Reticulatae Viride), *Chen Pi* (Pericarpium Citri Reticulatae), *Yi Zhi Ren* (Fructus Alpiniae Oxyphyllae), and *Huang Bai* (Cortex Phellodendri) should be added to the standard formula to dissipate cold qi and drain the ascending counterflow of yin fire. One can also administer *Xiao Pi Wan* (Disperse Glomus Pills)[1] in combination with *Zi Shen Wan* (Enrich the Kidneys Pills) which is composed of three ingredients, *Huang Bai* (Cortex Phellodendri), *Zhi Mu* (Rhizoma Anemarrhenae Aspheloidis), and a tiny amount of *Rou Gui* (Cortex Cinnamomi Cassiae), or with *Huang Lian* (Rhizoma Coptidis Chinensis) which can be made into pills separately. These two formulas [*i.e., Xiao Pi Wan* and *Zi Shen Wan*] can be taken, 70-80 pills together each time, on an empty stomach at a time when the food from a previous meal is almost completely dispersed. A while later, delicious food should be eaten to press [these medicinals] down and not allow them to stay in the stomach.

In case of low food intake without hunger, add stir-fried *Shen Qu* (Massa Medica Fermentata). In case of glomus appearing after meals, administer *Ju Pi Zhi Zhu Wan* (Citrus, Aurantium, & Atractylodes Pills) separately.[2] In case of a bowstring pulse, fullness and oppression of the four limbs, difficult defecation, and glomus below the heart, add *Gan Cao* (Radix Glycyrrhizae Uralensis), *Huang Lian* (Rhizoma Coptidis Chinensis), and *Chai Hu* (Radix Bupleuri). In case of qi ascending counterflow in the abdomen, which is the counterflow of the penetrating vessel, add *Huang Bai* (Cortex Phellodendri), three *fen,* and *Huang Lian* (Rhizoma Coptidis Chinensis), 1.5 *fen,* to drain. In case of dry, bound stools and glomus below the heart, add *Huang Lian* (Rhizoma Coptidis Chinensis), *Tao Ren* (Semen Pruni Persicae), a small amount of *Da Huang* (Radix Et Rhizoma Rhei), and *Dang Gui* (Radix Angelicae Sinensis). In case of glomus below the heart with heaviness and oppression, add *Bai Shao* (Radix Albus Paeoniae Lactiflorae) and *Huang Lian* (Rhizoma Coptidis Chinensis). In case of glomus below the heart with abdominal distention, add *Wu Wei Zi* (Fructus Schisandrae Chinensis), *Bai Shao* (Radix Albus Paeoniae Lactiflorae), and *Sha Ren* (Fructus Amomi). In cold weather, add a little *Gan Jiang* (dry Rhizoma Zingiberis Officinalis) or barked *Gui Zhi* (Ramulus Cinnamomi Cassiae). In case of glomus below the heart with cold [in the] center, add *Fu Zi* (Radix Lateralis Praeparatus Aconiti Carmichaeli) and *Huang Lian* (Rhizoma Coptidis Chinensis). In case of glomus below the heart with counterflow retching, add *Huang Lian* (Rhizoma Coptidis Chinensis), *Sheng Jiang* (uncooked Rhizoma Zingiberis Officinalis), and *Chen Pi* (Pericarpium

Citri Reticulatae). In winter months, do not add *Huang Lian* (Rhizoma Coptidis Chinensis) but add a little *Ding Xiang* (Flos Caryophylli) and *Huo Xiang* (Herba Agastachis Seu Pogostemi). In case of dry mouth and throat, add *Wu Wei Zi* (Fructus Schisandrae Chinensis) and dry *Ge Gen* (Radix Puerariae). In case of rib-side spasm or severe pain, add *Chai Hu* (Radix Bupleuri) and *Gan Cao* (Radix Glycyrrhizae).

In case of fullness and oppression and depression in the chest, add *Ju Hong* (Pericarpium Citri Erythrocarpae), *Qing Pi* (Pericarpium Citri Reticulatae Viride), and a little *Mu Xiang* (Radix Auklandiae Lappae). In case of headache with phlegm, heaviness, and languor which is a phlegm reversal, tai yin headache, add *Ban Xia* (Rhizoma Pinelliae Ternatae), five *fen*, and *Sheng Jiang* (uncooked Rhizoma Zingiberis Officinalis), 2-3 *fen*. Pricking pain in the abdomen or all over the body is [due to] blood stasis and insufficiency. Add *Dang Gui* Radix Angelicae Sinensis. In case of belching, add a lot of *Wu Wei Zi* (Fructus Schisandrae Chinensis) and a little *Yi Zhi* (Fructus Alpiniae Oxyphyllae). Inability to take in food is (due to) cold existing in the chest and stomach or stagnant qi in them. Add *Qing Pi* (Pericarpium Viridis Citri Reticulatae), *Chen Pi* (Pericarpium Citri Reticulatae), and *Mu Xiang* (Radix Saussureae Seu Vladimiriae). The (combined use of) the three medicinals is an established method. In winter, add *Yi Zhi Ren* (Fructus Alpiniae Oxyphyllae) and *Cao Dou Kou Ren* (Semen Alpiniae Katsumadai). In summer months, do not use much of these but add *Huang Lian* (Rhizoma Coptidis Chinensis). In autumn months, in case of stagnant qi with inability to take in food, add *Bing Lang* (Semen Arecae Catechu), *Cao Dou Kou Ren* (Semen Alpiniae Katsumadai), and/or *Suo Sha Ren* (Fructus Amomi) and a little *Bai Dou Kou Ren* (Fructus Cardamomi).

In the three months of spring, in case of inability to take in food, add, in addition, a little *Qing Pi* (Pericarpium Viridis Citri Reticulatae), and a lot of *Chen Pi* (Pericarpium Citri Reticulatae) besides windy medicinals to clear cold from [the stomach]. In early spring, if it is still cold, add a little acrid, hot medicinals to supplement insufficiency of spring qi as assistants to the windy medicinals. *Yi Zhi Ren* (Fructus Alpiniae Oxyphyllae) or *Cao Dou Kou* (Semen Alpiniae Katsumadai), either will do. In case of a bowstring pulse with signs of stirring wind condition, use windy medicinals to free the flow. This implies that liver wind is stirring with spinning of the brain, visual dizziness, and the like. So-called wind medicinals are those that can calm the liver, for example, *Tian Ma* (Rhizoma Gastrodiae Elatae) and *Ju Hua* (Flos Chrysanthemi Morifolii). In case of a rough [or choppy] pulse with a sensation of qi stagnation, add *Dang Gui* (Radix Angelicae Sinensis), *Tian Men Dong* (Tuber Asparagi Cochinensis), *Mu Xiang* (Radix Auklandiae Lappae), *Qing Pi* (Pericarpium Citri Reticulatae Viride), and *Chen*

Pi (Pericarpium Citri Reticulatae). If there is cold, add *Gui Zhi* (Ramulus Cinnamomi Cassiae) and *Huang Qi* (Radix Astragali Membranacei).

Choking and stuffiness in the chest or blocked qi [in the chest] with oppression and agitation [is due to] obstruction and stagnation of the lung qi. [In that case,] one should break this stagnant qi with *Qing Pi* (Pericarpium Citri Reticulatae Viride) and *Chen Pi* (Pericarpium Citri Reticulatae) with the addition of a little *Mu Xiang* (Radix Auklandiae Lappae) and *Bin Lan* (Semen Arecae Catechu). In winter months, add *Wu Zhu Yu* (Fructus Evodiae Rutecarpae) and *Ren Shen* (Radix Panacis Ginseng). Choking, stuffiness, blockage, oppression, and non-free flow in the chest are [due to] obstruction by external cold which does not allow the qi to exhale smoothly. [In that case,] the inch mouth pulse must be bowstring or a little tight. This shows great cold in the chest. In addition, if the tongue has white, glossy fur, it is evident that heat exists in the cinnabar field [or the lower *dan tian,* the part of the lower abdomen about two *cun* below the navel] while cold [exists] in the chest. [If] there is heat in the cinnabar field, there must be chill in the hips and sacrococcygeal region, chilly genital sweating, and chill in both testicles since evil qi has assailed the root and righteous qi must flee into the channels and vessels. The cinnabar field is regarded as the root of qi. Being caught in the cold leads inevitably to the arising of yin in the yin [or genitals] and pain [in the cinnabar field]. This helps discriminate fire deep-lying [or hidden] in the cinnabar field. [For this,] add *Huang Bai* (Cortex Phellodendri) and *Sheng Di* (uncooked Radix Rehmanniae Glutinosae). Do not treat this by mistake as a cold pattern. In other words, this is a false cold pattern or true heat.

In case of abdominal pain in cool and cold weather in the autumn and winter, add *Ban Xia* (Rhizoma Pinelliae Ternatae), *Yi Zhi Ren* (Fructus Alpiniae Oxyphyllae), *Cao Dou Kou* (Semen Alpiniae Katsumadai), or the like. Fever or heat felt in the exterior flesh is an exterior pattern. [In that case,] merely administer *Bu Zhong Yi Qi Tang* (Supplement the Center & Boost the Qi Decoction). One to two doses suffice to promote a little sweating to cool [the body]. Wilting and limpness of the feet and knees with difficulty or pain in walking is [due to] hidden damp heat in the kidneys and liver. [For this,] add a little *Huang Bai* (Cortex Phellodendri) taken on an empty stomach [together with the standard formula]. If no effect is achieved, increase the *Huang Bai* and add *Han Fang Ji* (Radix Stephaniae Tetrandrae), five *fen,* and the strength of the feet and knees will be restored to normal. Profuse spittle or spitting of white foam is [due to] cold retained in the stomach mouth. [For this,] add *Yi Zhi Ren* (Fructus Alpiniae Oxyphyllae).

Endnotes

1 This formula is composed of: *Gan Jiang* (dry Rhizoma Zingiberis Officinalis), stir-fried *Shen Qu* (Massa Medica Fermentata), mix-fried *Gan Cao* (Radix Glycyrrhizae Uralensis), *Zhu Ling* (Sclerotium Polypori Umbellati), *Ze Xie* (Rhizoma Alismatis Orientalis), *Hou Po* (Cortex Magnoliae Officinalis), *Sha Ren* (Fructus Amomi), *Ban Xia* (Rhizoma Pinelliae Ternatae), *Chen Pi* (Pericarpium Citri Reticulatae), *Ren Shen* (Radix Panacis Ginseng), *Yi Zhi Ren* (Fructus Alpiniae Oxyphyllae), *Huang Lian* (Rhizoma Coptidis Chinensis), *Huang Qin* (Radix Scutellariae Baicalensis), *Jiang Huang* (Rhizoma Curcumae Longae), and *Bai Zhu* (Rhizoma Atractylodis Macrocephalae).

2 This formula is composed of: *Bai Zhu* (Rhizoma Atractylodis Macrocephalae), *Zhi Shi* (Fructus Immaturus Citri Seu Ponciri), *Ju Pi* (Pericarpium Citri Reticulatae), and *He Ye* (Folium Nelumbinis Nuciferae).

6

Treatise on Intestinal Afflux with Blood in the Stools

The *Tai Yin Yang Ming Lun (Treatise on the Tai Yin & Yang Ming)* states:

Yin suffers from dietary irregularity and failure to keep regular hours of life. When yin suffers, [evils] invade the five viscera. Invasion of the viscera results in distention, fullness, and blockage in the chest and swill diarrhea in the lower body which may, over time, develop into intestinal afflux.[1]

What is known as intestinal afflux is the outpouring [*i.e.*, diarrhea] of water and food mixed with blood as from a pump. Today, this is more commonly known as intestinal wind. In long summer, damp heat is immensely exuberant. The guest qi [the external or cosmopathogenic qi, *i.e.*, dampness and heat] is prevailing, while the ruling [or host] qi, [the original qi of the spleen and stomach], is weak. Therefore, the disease of intestinal afflux is severe. [For this,] *Liang Xue Di Huang Tang* (Cool the Blood Rehmannia Decoction) is indicated.

Liang Xue Di Huang Tang (Cool the Blood Rehmanniae Decoction)

Huang Bai (Cortex Phellodendri), debarked, grated, stir-fried
Zhi Mu (Rhizoma Anemarrhenae Aspheloidis), grated, stir-fried, 1 *qian* each
Qing Pi (Pericarpium Citri Reticulatae Viride), with the inner side preserved
Huai Hua Mi (Flos Immaturus Sophorae Japonicae), stir-fried
Shu Di (cooked Radix Rehmanniae Glutinosae)
Dang Gui (Radix Angelicae Sinensis), 5 *fen* [for each of] the above

Slice the above ingredients [and take] all in one dose, boiled in one cup of water down to 7/10 and taken while warm after removing the dregs.

This is a somewhat uncharacteristic formula for Li. As the reader will note, it does not contain any qi-supplements or windy, upbearing medicinals. This is because it is meant as a tip or branch treatment for an acute condition, *i.e.*, bleeding.

Later, in the Qing dynasty, Ye Tian-shi codified that, in all cases of acute bleeding, the first step is to simply stop the bleeding. Although this formula is not commonly used today, it certainly could be. In that case, I would suggest substituting *Sheng Di* (uncooked Radix Rehmanniae Glutinosae) for the *Shu Di* to better cool the blood and stop bleeding.

In case of astringent urination and oppression below the navel or tenesmus after defecation, take while yet a little hot mixed with finely powdered *Mu Xiang* (Radix Auklandiae Lappae) and *Bin Lan* (Semen Arecae Catechu), five *fen* each, on an empty stomach or after a meal. This is still an effective combination for the treatment of tenesmus. In case of interior [*i.e.*, abdominal] cramping and tenesmus which still is not removed, one must precipitate. In case of arising of transmuted [patterns], add and subtract following the symptoms. Stirring and gurgling of water in the abdomen with urinary irregularity [demonstrate] collection of rheum. When the pulse of the involved viscus is identified, [appropriate] water rheum-removing medicinals [can be used] to drain it. For instance, if the pulse is large and surging, use fire-draining and urination-disinhibiting medicinals. [But,] in case of stomach vacuity with inability to eat and great, unstoppable thirst, it is not ok to use bland, percolating medicinals to stop [this], since this is a result of scanty original qi in the stomach. [In that case,] supplement this with *Qi Wei Bai Zhu San* (Seven Flavors Atractylodes Powder).²

Fever, aversion to heat, vexation and agitation, great, unstoppable thirst, flesh so hot there is no desire to dress, a large, surging pulse which becomes forceless when pressed, and possible simultaneous pain in the eyes and dry nose are not a pattern [indicating] *Bai Hu Tang* (White Tiger Decoction). This is blood vacuity emitting [or causing] dryness, [for which] one should [administer] *Huang Qi* (Radix Astragali Membranacei), one *liang*, and *Dang Gui* (Radix Angelicae Sinensis), 2 *qian*, taken after being sliced and boiled in water. [However,] in case of constipation, interior cramping, tenesmus, going to the latrine several times without defecation, or a small amount of white pus or blood in stools, be careful not to use disinhibition. Disinhibition is sure to make the disease more serious, contrarily causing depression, binding, and nonfree flow. [Instead,] use *Sheng Yang Chu Shi Fang Feng Tang* (Upbear Yang & Eliminate Dampness Ledebouriella Decoction). Lifting yang, leads to yin qi automatically being downborne.

Sheng Yang Chu Shi Fang Feng Tang
(Upbear Yang & Eliminate Dampness Ledebouriella Decoction)

Cang Zhu (Rhizoma Atractylodis), soaked with rice water, skinned and cleaned, 4 *liang*

Fang Feng (Radix Ledebouriellae Divaricatae), 2 *qian*
Bai Zhu (Rhizoma Atractylodis Macrocephalae)
Fu Ling (Sclerotium Poriae Cocos)
Bai Shao (Radix Albus Paeoniae Lactiflorae), 1 *qian* [for each of] the above

Slice the above except for *Cang Zhu*. *Cang Zhu* should be sliced separately and boiled in 1 1/2 bowls of water down to two big cupfuls. [Then] put in the rest of the medicinals and continue to boil down to one big cupful. Remove the dregs and take [the decoction] while a little warm on an empty stomach or before a meal.

This formula can be used as a basis for the treatment of liver-spleen disharmony diarrhea complicated with dampness. It contains three of the four ingredients of the more standardly used *Tong Xie Yao Fang* (Painful Diarrhea Essential Formula), *i.e., Bai Zhu, Fang Feng,* and *Bai Shao*. The rationale of its composition is essentially the same.

If there is the pattern of unchecked swill diarrhea, use this formula to abduct [or lead out] the dampness. In case of swill diarrhea or incessant diarrhea, use windy medicinals to upbear yang. *Cang Zhu* (Rhizoma Atractylodis) is able to boost the stomach and eliminate dampness. Abdominal distention, blockage, obstruction, and nonfree flow with a replete pulse [require] more bitter and less sweet medicinals to drain in accordance with particular conditions. If [the bowels] obtain free flow, again use *Sheng Yang [Chu Shi Fang Feng] Tang* to assist yang plus draining and precipitating medicinals.

Endnotes

[1] *Su Wen*, Ch. 29
[2] The ingredients in this formula are: *Ren Shen* (Radix Panacis Ginseng), *Bai Zhu* (Rhizoma Atractylodis Macrocephalae), *Fu Ling* (Sclerotium Poriae Cocos), *Ge Gen* (Radix Puerariae), *Huo Xiang* (Herba Agastachis Seu Pogostemi), *Mu Xiang* (Radix Auklandiae Lappae), and mix-fried *Gan Cao* (Radix Glycyrrhizae Uralensis).

7

Treatise on the Prohibition of Unwarranted Use of Ejecting Medicinals in Spleen & Stomach Vacuity

This chapter deals with the treatment method of ejection. Ejection was one of the three main therapies recommended for the treatment of a variety of conditions by a contemporary of Li Dong-yuan, Zhang Zi-he. To some extent, this chapter is a rebuttal to Zhang Zi-he. However, the bottom line is that, today, professional Chinese medical practitioners rarely use the ejection method. This is another case of the progressive evolution of this medicine. In fact, within only several generations, some Chinese doctors had trouble remembering which Zhang was one of the four great masters of the Jin-Yuan.

The *Liu Yuan Zheng Ji Lun (Treatise on the Orthodox Chronology of the 60 [Year] Cycle)* instructs that depressed wood should [be treated by] out-thrusting.[1] And out-thrusting is accomplished by using acrid, windy, upbearing and effusing medicinals, such as *Chai Hu* (Radix Bupleuri), *Sheng Ma* (Rhizoma Cimicifugae), *Ge Gen* (Radix Puerariae), *Qiang Huo* (Radix Et Rhizoma Notopterygii), etc. The upbearing and out-thrusting of depression, especially liver depression qi stagnation is the basis for using *Chai Hu* as a liver-coursing, qi-rectifying medicinal. This discussion on the out-thrusting of depression is probably the most important part of this entire chapter from today's point of view. Wood ought to be ever-stirring and is disposed to exaltation by nature. This is characteristic of the substance of wood. When it is depressed within earth with nothing to be done, it is the same as saying it is deprived of its nature of wind. This implies that wood is similar to wind in nature. Note also that the liver is at once wood and wind and, therefore, wood and wind are often referred to as the same. [When] the human body exhibits such a pattern of depressed wood, it is necessary to open and free the flow [of wood]. Only then can ejection be used to assist wind wood. This is the meaning [of the statement that] depressed wood should [be treated by] out-thrusting.

[However,] there is another approach to out-thrusting depressed wood. Wood can be said to be depressed in earth at the initial [stage] of losing its nature. Once it is opened and emitted to move within heaven above, it is emitting and not depressed. Wood regains its nature and has a surplus. Having a surplus leads [wood] to prevail over [that which it ordinarily restrains], and thus spleen earth is subjected to evils. [This approach] can be seen in the section on the out-thrusting of depressed wood,[2] and [this substantiation] does not stop there. Another example of this is the jue yin administration in heaven.[3] The heavenly stems and earthly branches can be matched to denote years, and years can also be divided into the three yin and three yang. If a year falls in the jue yin (si [B6] or hai [B12]), jue yin is said to govern heaven. Then, according to a special calculation, one can predict that the weather in such a year will be dominated by wind since jue yin is wood or wind. This is [related to] effulgent wind wood, and [the discussion about] the prevailing jue yin[4] is also related to effulgent wind wood. All the above mentioned sections [of the classic] concern subjection of the spleen and stomach to evils and their arguments are quite consistent with each other. If, due to a lack of awareness of the significance of the four Chinese words, "depressed wood leads to out-thrusting," [emitting or effusing wood] is treated inappropriately as depressed wood, this to doubly replenish repletion. [When] the spleen and stomach are restrained by wood, to reinforce wood is exactly to supplement [that which] has a surplus and to [cause] detriment to [that which is already] insufficient. Since the spleen and stomach qi is already insufficient, how can they escape from double expiration due to [such wrong treatment]?

Proceeding on to the necessity of ejection in case of choking and constriction in the chest, a qi mouth [pulse, *i.e.*, the radial pulse at the styloid process of the wrist] four times as large as the *Ren Ying* (St 7) pulse indicates food damage of the tai yin. If the pulse is present in the upper section but absent from the lower section, the patient requires ejection. The qi mouth, a.k.a. inch mouth, pulse is divided into three sections: As mentioned above, the section immediately proximal to the wrist is called the upper section or inch. The section proximal to the styloid process is called the lower section or cubit. Between these two is the barrier section. However, some scholars interpret the lower and upper sections spoken of here as the inch mouth and the *Ren Ying* pulses. Without ejection, death [is certain]. Absence of a pulse in the lower section indicates that wood is depressed below. Since its pathway is blocked, liver qi is expiring in the lower. In addition, lung metal governs blockage and non-descent. Something bars the pathway there. Because metal restrains wood, liver wood is subjected to evils, and wood congests the throat and chest. It is [thus] reasonably said that that which is above should be surmounted. [Zhang] Zhong-jing instructs, "Repletion vexation should be treated by ejection with *Gua Di San* (Melon Pedicle Powder)."[5] Vexation arising after diaphoresis and precipitation is known as vacuity vexation or annoying oppression. Vexation, agitation, and sleeplessness show that wood is depressed. It is necessary to use ejection with *Zhi Zi Chi Tang* (Gardenia & Soybean Decoction).⁶ Unintelligent physicians use ejection to [treat] distention in the chest due to turbid qi [lodging] in the upper [with] constricted diaphragm and throat, propping up against the rib-sides, abdominal distention, and stomach vacuity and insufficiency. Moreover, [if] there is stomach vacuity, there must be anger [or irritability]. Since anger is the affect associated with the liver, this sentence implies that overwhelming liver qi restrains the stomach. For wind wood that already overwhelms and oppresses the stomach, the *Nei Jing (Inner Classic)* prescribes *Tie Luo* (Frusta Ferri) to settle and downbear it. Then how can it be treated with ejection to assist evil wind wood? [Using] ejection for a pattern indicating other than ejection is as monstrous a blunder as the gap between heaven and earth. Roughly speaking, choking and constriction in the chest with incessant vexation and oppression calls for ejection.

Endnotes

¹ *Su Wen*, Ch. 71
² *Ibid.*
³ *Su Wen*, Ch. 74
⁴ *Ibid.*
⁵ This is composed of: *Gua Di* (Pediculus Cucumis Melonis) and *Chi Xiao Dou* (Semen Phaseoli Calcarati) in equal amounts taken after being ground and boiled with *Dan Dou Chi* (Semen Praeparatus Sojae).
⁶ This is composed of: *Zhi Zi* (Fructus Gardeniae Jasminoidis) and *Dan Dou Chi* (Semen Praeparatus Sojae).

8

Treatise on Quieting & Nourishing the Heart Spirit [by] Regulating & Treating the Spleen & Stomach

Although Li does not include any specific protocols in this chapter, it is an extremely important one for anyone interested in the heart spirit. Readers should note that, because of the connection or "ligation" between ministerial/life-gate fire and the heart/pericardium, yin fire virtually always involves some element of spirit disquietude from a combination of 1) nonconstruction and malnourishment and 2) harassment by heat evils.

The *Ling Lan Mi Dian Lun (Treatise on the Secret Classics in the Exquisite Orchid Library)* states, "The heart is the ruler from whence the spiritual brilliance emanates."[1] Spirit brilliance refers to the functions of consciousness, thinking, and feeling. Anger, indignation, sorrow, worry, fear, and fright can all cause detriment to the original qi. In other words, Li is saying that any of the affects can cause detriment and damage to the spleen qi. Raging, exuberant yin fire is the result of congelation and stagnation arising in the heart and disturbances of the seven affects, [*i.e.,* joy, anger, worry, thought, sorrow, fear, and fright]. It is a statement of fact in Chinese medicine that any of the seven affects may transform into fire if extreme. The heart and vessels are the abode of the spirit. When the sovereign heart is not calm, fire is transformed. Fire is the foe of the seven spirits.[2] Fire and heat evils harass the spirit and make it stir frenetically. In addition, fire eats the qi, and the spirit is nothing other than the accumulation of qi in the heart nourished by blood and yin essence. Therefore, it is said that when yin fire is too effulgent, channel qi is unable to keep fit and nourish the spirit. The channels qi is the constructive qi. This is a disease of the vessels. The spirit has nothing more to nourish it, and fluids and humors stop circulating. Hence the blood vessels are no longer engendered. The spirit of the heart is [nothing other than] the true qi by another name. This is an unequivocal statement equating the heart spirit with qi. This has huge implications in clinical practice. If one understands the functions, characteristics, and behavior of qi, then one can easily understand the spirit both physiologically and pathologically. [The spirit] is engendered as long as it is supplied with blood, and, when blood is engendered, the vessels are effulgent. The vessels are the abode of the spirit. If congelation and stagnation arise in the heart, the seven spirits will leave the form and, in consequence, there is nothing but fire left in the vessels.

Those who are proficient in treating this kind of disease simply regulate and harmonize the spleen and stomach. When the heart is rid of congelation and stagnation, owing to delight, gratification, favorable weather, a balmy living environment, delicious food, or a treat to the eye, [the patient] will cheer and recover from this disease. This is because the original qi in the stomach is soothed and eased. I likewise believe that the key to keeping the spirit healthy and quiet is making sure the spleen is well fortified and that heat evils are not transformed from depression.

Endnotes

[1] *Su Wen*, Ch. 8

[2] *I.e.*, the ethereal soul, corporeal soul, essence, spirit, reflection, wisdom, and will

9

The Necessity of Inquiring About Inclinations Before Treating Any Disease

The *Huang Di Zhen Jing (Yellow Emperor's Acupuncture Classic)* states:

Center pure heat wasting thirst justifies cold [therapy], while cold center type justifies heat. Heat existing in the stomach means swift digestion. It causes the heart to be suspended with constant hunger and heat in the skin above the umbilicus. Heat existing in the intestines results in chyme-like yellow stools and cold in the skin below the umbilicus. Cold existing in the stomach results in abdominal distention, while cold existing in the intestines results in borborygmus with swill diarrhea.[1]

Another theory [says that]:

With cold in the intestines, there arises cramping and pressure [*i.e.*, an urgent desire to defecate] after meals, rumbling of the intestines, lancinating [intestinal] pain, and white stools. While with cold in the intestines and heat in the stomach, there is rapid hungering [after eating] and lower abdominal pain and distention. But with heat in the intestines and cold in the stomach, there is distention with diarrhea.

It is true that with heat in the intestines there arises diarrhea, but cold existing in the stomach can also transmute into diarrhea.

The stomach desires hot drinks, while the intestines desire cold drinks. [Despite] this difference in liking and aversion, the tip [or branch] is treated first in the spring and summer, whereas the root is treated first in autumn and winter. Clothing should never be [so thin] as to be chilly in cold weather or [so thick] in summer to cause perspiration. [Food] should never be burning hot or chilly cold but of a moderate temperature. [Then] qi will be well sustained so as to prevent evils from assailing.

These [principles] are [like] a square, a compass, or laws. A square and a compass are necessary instruments for drawing a design according to established proportions and thus the simile employed here. They are a standard pathway [or established knowledge], a rational approach, and a compulsory requirement. [However,] one should act in accordance with the particular situation in using [these laws] of interchange between normality and abnormality.

Endnote

¹ *Ling Shu,* Vol. 6, Ch. 29

10

Treatise on Downward Pouring of Stomach Qi, Chaos of All the Five Viscera Qi & the Consequent Simultaneous Manifestation of Various Diseases

Li Dong-yuan was one of the few great practitioners of herbal medicine who was also an accomplished acupuncturist. The following chapter describes what has come to be known as "Dong-yuan acupuncture." Basically, Li has applied five phase and 10 stem theory to choosing points consistent with the Jin-Yuan doctors' interest in and emphasis on these theories. For me personally, this is all building castles in the sky.

The Yellow Emperor asked: What is meant by stomach counterflow and chaos?

Qi Bo answered: The clear qi is in the yin, [while] the turbid qi is in the yang. The constructive qi flows in the same direction as the vessels, [while] the defensive qi moves counterflow [*i.e.*, in the opposite direction]. When the clear and turbid interfere with each other and are in chaos in the chest, this is [called] major disturbance. Therefore, chaotic qi in the heart leads to heart vexation, taciturnity, bowing one's head [in submission], stillness, and hiding. Chaotic qi in the lungs leads to panting with inability to catch the breath in lying either supine or prone and the hands pressing against the chest [to facilitate breathing]. Chaotic qi in the stomach and intestines results in sudden turmoil disease [*i.e.*, acute gastroenteritis]. Chaotic qi in the forearms and lower legs results in reversal of the four [limbs]. Chaotic qi in the head leads counterflow reversal [with] heavy-headedness, dizziness, and collapse.[1]

The great [or basic] method [or principle] is, "That which goes from the lower to the upper should be removed by abducting it," and, "That which is in the channels requires emission."[2]

The Yellow Emperor asked: [In relation to] the five chaoses, is there a way of needling?

Qi Bo answered: [Evils] take a [certain] path to come and take a [certain] path to leave. Deliberate study of these pathways is a treasure to the body.

The Yellow Emperor asked: I would like to know these pathways.

Qi Bo answered: When qi is in the heart, select the stream points of the hand shao yin and heart governor (*Shen Men*, Ht 7, and *Da Ling*, Per 7 [later editor]).[3]

To enrich the source of transformation, the sweet and warm is used to supplement, the sweet and cold to drain, the sour to astringe, and the moderately bitter to free the flow. A light formula composed of slightly bitter, acrid, and sweet (ingredients) should be used to communicate the essence and abduct the qi, thus restoring [chaotic qi] to normal. Abducting the qi is an acupuncture term. It refers to slow insertion and slow extraction of the needle. Needling in such a way as to neither tangibly supplement nor drain is called communicating the essence or essence communication. This is a method applicable to disharmony between the constructive and defensive or the qi and blood. Therefore, these terms can be interpreted as harmonizing the constructive and defensive. Li gives further explanation in the following passage.

When [chaotic] qi is in the lungs, select the spring point of the hand tai yin [*Yu Ji*, Lu 10] and the stream point *Tai Yuan* (Lu 9) and the stream point of the foot shao yin (*Tai Xi*, Ki 3 [Later editor]).[4]

[Concerning] the tai yin, bitter, sweet, and cold, which are separating and transforming flavors, are used to remove chaotic qi from the chest. If wilting has developed, damp heat should be abducted. Again there is the mention of damp heat as a causative factor of wilting. In case of profuse nasal mucus, acrid, hot [medicinals] should be used as a stop-gap treatment. Such as *Xi Xin* (Herba Asari Cum Radice). Nevertheless, [one should try to] conduct the stomach qi out onto the yang tract in order not to let damp earth restrain the kidneys. The yang tract means the upper burner or the heart and lungs. The acupoint [for this] is *Tai Xi* (Ki 3).

When [chaotic] qi is in the stomach and intestines, select the foot tai yin and yang ming. [If there is] no effect, [then] select [*Zu*] *San Li* (St 36) (*Zhang Men*, Liv 13, *Zhong Wan*, CV 12, and [*Zu*] *San Li*, St 36 [later editor]).[5]

In case of foot tai yin vacuity, the alarm point is needled to abduct [or lead the qi] into the blood. *Zhang Men* (Liv 13) is the alarm point of the spleen. There is a theory that the transporting points of the bowels eliminate diseases of the bowels. If stomach vacuity is why the tai yin is provided with no supplies, abduction can be performed at the alarm point of the foot yang ming [*i.e.*, *Zhong Wan* (CV 12)]. If qi counterflows upward, giving rise to sudden turmoil, select [*Zu*] *San Li* (St 36) and needle it till the qi descends. If qi refuses to descend, continue needling.

When [chaotic] qi is in the head, select *Tian Zhu* (Bl 10) and *Da Zhu* (Bl 11). [If there is still] disharmony, select the spring and stream points of the foot tai yang. (*Tong Gu*, Bl 66, with deep insertion; *Shu Gu*, Bl 65, with deep insertion [later editor].)[6]

Tian Zhu and *Da Zhu* are needled first, neither supplementing nor draining but merely abducting [or guiding] the qi. Next needle the foot tai yang urinary bladder channel, neither supplementing nor draining, inserting deep at *Tong Gu* and *Shu Gu*. [Needle the points] *ding* (S4), heart fire, and *ji* (S6), spleen earth, to abduct and remove [the chaotic qi]. In terms of using medicinals to abduct and remove [the chaotic qi], select and add some tai yang channel-guiding medicinals as well as small [quantities] of bitter, cold and sweet, cold [medicinals]. Cool, clearing medicinals can serve as assistants and envoys.

When [chaotic] qi is in the forearms and feet, first remove blood from the vessels and then needle the spring and stream points of the yang ming and shao yang. (*Er Jian*, LI 2, and *San Jian*, LI 3, with deep insertion; *Nei Ting*, St 44, and *Xian Gu*, St 43, with deep insertion [later editor].)"[7]

The shao yang includes the foot and hand shao yang, and the points suggested are the spring point *Ye Men* (TB 2) and the stream point *Zhong Zhu* (TB 3) of the hand *shao yang* and the spring point *Xia Xi* (GB 43) and the stream point *Lin Qi* (GB 41) of the foot shao yang.

Let blood from the network vessels found on the lower legs and forearms and then treat wilting and reversal by neither supplementing nor draining but needling deep to abduct [the qi] up from the yin. [Conducting] upward means leading out and eliminating. [It is appropriate if] yin fire has a surplus [but] yang qi is insufficient. [As for what] lies deeply [or hidden] in the earth, [that is] blood or the constructive. To abduct it from yin to yang, it is necessary first to upbear and lift the yang qi from the earth and [then] to drain yin fire. This is the method of qi abduction and essence communication.

The Yellow Emperor asked: How to apply supplementation and drainage?

Qi Bo answered: Slow insertion and slow withdrawal [of the needle] are called qi abduction, while intangible supplementation and drainage are called essence communication. [These are appropriate] for the abnormal [condition] of chaotic qi rather than for surplus and insufficiency.

The Emperor said: What a logical way! What an enlightening instruction! Pray inscribe it on the jade plate and entitle it *The Treatment of Chaos.*[8]

Endnotes

[1] *Ling Shu,* Vol. 6, Ch. 34
[2] *Ling Shu,* Vol. 11, Ch. 73
[3] *Ibid.*
[4] *Ling Shu,* Vol. 1, Ch. 1
[5] *Ibid.*
[6] *Ibid.*
[7] *Ibid.*
[8] *Ibid.*

11

Yin Disease Treated [Through] Yang, Yang Disease Treated [Through] Yin

This chapter also discusses Li's methods of acupuncture. In particular, he discusses the role of network vessel pricking or bleeding in the treatment of yin fire as well as the fine needle treatment of *Zu San Li* (St 36) and the front alarm points of the bowels. These materials I find quite useful in clinical practice.

The *Yin Yang Ying Xiang Lun (Treatise on the Mutual Correspondences of Yin & Yang)* states:

> Examine yin and yang to identify the pliant from the rigid. Treat yang disease through yin and yin disease through yang so as to settle the blood and qi and keep them in their own homes. Blood repletion requires breaking, while qi vacuity requires drawing and abducting.[1]

Yin disease in the yang is caused by wind cold evils of external heaven. These take advantage of center [vacuity] to invade from the outside through the bowels and visceral points on the back. This refers to the back transport points of the foot tai yang channel, such as *Fei Shu* (Bl 13), *Xin Shu* (Bl 15), *Gan Shu* (Bl 18), and *Wei Shu* (Bl 21). Again Li says that if external evils are able to invade the body and cause disease, this is because there is a prior central or spleen qi vacuity. This is a human suffering from the guest evils of external heaven. There are two theories concerning this.

[Evils may] strike yang and then flow to the channels. This kind of disease begins with external cold and ends in external heat. Therefore, to treat wind cold evils, treat the [associated] points of the various viscera. [This method] should not be limited to [treating] only wind and cold. All six environmental excesses, including dampness, summerheat, dryness, and fire, can each affect the five viscera. [In that case,] the sinews, bones, blood, and vessels suffer from these evils. [These various affections] can be eliminated through the [associated] points of the five viscera. This is the theory of cold damage advocated by [Zhang] Zhong-jing.

There is [also] a [special] wind theory concerning the strike of the eight winds. The eight winds are the winds from the north, south, west, east, northwest, north-east, southwest, and southeast. The wind theory referred to here is found in *Ling Shu*, Vol. 11, Ch. 77. According to this theory, winds can never hurt people unless they come from a vacuity home, *i.e.,* unless they blow untimely *vis à vis* the pro-gression of the seasons based on five transport and six qi theory. Summerheat stroke can be treated through *Xiao Chang Shu* (Bl 27) on the back. Damp stroke can be treated through *Wei Shu* (Bl 21). Dry stroke can be treated through *Da Chang Shu* (Bl 25). All these are diseases of intruding surplus evils of the six envi-ronmental excesses and should be treated by drainage at the bowel [associated] points on the back. If the disease has persisted for a long [time] and shifted, there may be vacuity or repletion. Supplementation and drainage should be practiced in accordance with shifts in the disease. [However,] the treatment should be per-formed at the bowel [associated] points on the back nonetheless.

There is another [pattern of] heat above and cold below. Usually this implies vacuity heat floating upward and vacuity cold below due to kidney yang vacuity. The classic states that yin disease in yang requires abducting [or leading] it from yang to yin by first bleeding the network vessels and the channel tunnels.[2] If fire is effulgent in yin, soaring to heaven above, the six yang will be replenished above instead of diminishing. The six yang are the six yang channels, *i.e.,* the channels of the hand and foot yang ming, tai yang, and shao yang. First, let blood from the network vessels of the five viscera to abduct [yin fire] downward. Once qi is downborne from heaven, the disease of cold below will naturally disappear. This is because the lower source is only cold due to ministerial/life-gate fire's upward counterflow. Once ministerial/life-gate fire is led back down to its lower source, there is no further vacuity cold. Be careful not to merely drain the six yang. This disease of yang hyperactivity is due to the enriching of yin fire evils. [Thus,] remove yin fire alone. Merely remove these evils from the blood network vessels and the channel tunnels. Make no mistake [about this]. Yin fire means that there are heat evils in the heart, and the heart governs the blood. Network vessel prick-ing or bleeding is a method of clearing heat evils from the blood aspect. Therefore, it is also a method of treating yin fire.

Yang disease in the yin requires abduction from yin to yang. "The cold and heat of water and grains harm the six bowels once they strike people."[3] It is added that, because of dietary irregularity and overtaxation of the formal body, yin fire may overwhelm *kun* earth, impeding the grain qi, constructive qi, clear qi, stom-ach qi, and original qi from ascending to enrich the yang qi of the six bowels. *Kun* is one of the eight trigrams of the *Yi Jing (Classic of Change)*. It is symbolic of earth and, therefore, *kun* used either alone or in combination with earth refers medically to the spleen and stomach, the organs corresponding with earth. **Thus the five yang qi expire first in the external.** The five yang qi are the qi of the five viscera. What is known as the external is heaven. Here, heaven refers to the upper part of the body or the heart and lungs. The sentence implies that it is the qi of the heart and lungs which is the first affected by lack of nourishment from the grain qi. Because of this, then the other viscera are affected. **The downward flowing [of the five yang qi] into and their confinement with yin fire in** *kun* **earth is always due first to damage done by the five thieves—joy, anger, sorrow, worry, and fright—followed by stagnation of stomach qi. Finally, overtaxation and dietary irregularity succeed in damaging the original qi. [In this case,] it is necessary to use the method of pushing to upraise at the sea point of the stomach, [***Zu***] *San Li* (St 36), to release the original qi. Thus this is called abducting from yin to yang.**

Should the healing of the original qi be insufficient [after such treatment], the remedy lies in the alarm points of the bowels on the abdomen. The alarm points of the stomach, large intestine, small intestine, gallbladder, urinary bladder, and triple burner are *Zhong Wan* (CV 12), *Tian Shu* (St 25), *Guan Yuan* (CV 4), *Ri Yue* (GB 24), *Zhong Ji* (CV 3), and *Shi Men* (CV 5) in that order. If [the disease] is transmitted to the five viscera, the nine orifices will be blocked and the treatment lies in the abdominal alarm points of the viscera pertinent to the diseased orifices. The alarm points of the heart, lungs, kidneys, spleen, liver, and pericardium are *Ju Que* (CV 14), *Zhong Fu* (Lu 1), *Jing Men* (GB 25), *Zhang Men* (Liv 13), *Qi Men* (Liv 14), and *Tan Zhong* (CV 17) in that order. The interrelationships between the nine orifices and the five viscera are eyes/liver, nose/lungs, tongue/heart, ears, anus, & genitals/kidneys, mouth/spleen. It is reasonably said that disquietude of the five viscera is engendered by blockage of the original qi of the six bowels. It is further said that disharmony of the five viscera with blockage of the nine orifices is always attributed to insufficient yang qi and surplus yin qi. Hence it is concluded that yang fails to restrain yin. In all [such] cases, insufficiency of the original qi should be treated by needling at the abdominal alarm points through abduction from yang to yin. Make no mistake [about this].

The famous 20th century northern Chinese acupuncturist, Wang Le-ting, based his Old 10 Needles formula on these paragraphs. For more information on Wang's use of Li's theories in the contemporary practice of Chinese acupuncture, see *Golden Needle Wang Le-ting* also available from Blue Poppy Press.

Inappropriate supplementation and drainage and particularly inappropriate drainage at the points on the four extremities is, as warned by Qi Bo, a gross mistake, to say nothing of selecting points in the heaven, meaning the back. The points on the four extremities are the points found below the knees and elbows referred to as the five transport points. If the [associated] points of the five viscera and six bowels on the back are [mistakenly] needled, survival is the last thing that can be expected. When speaking of this, one cannot help deploring and shuddering apprehensively. In case of intruding evils of the six environmental excesses, upper heat and lower cold, or a disease of the sinews, bones, skin, flesh, and blood vessels, inappropriate selection of the sea point of the stomach and the abdominal alarm points will never fail to cause dangerous situations as is also warned by Qi Bo. Inferior physicians must be, by all means, very careful about this.

Perhaps such dire warnings were necessary in Li's time due to inferior needle technology. However, given the state of fine needles today, they seem excessive and unnecessary.

Endnotes

[1] *Su Wen*, Ch. 5
[2] *Ibid.*
[3] *Ibid.*

12

Debility & Effulgence of the
Original Qi of the Triple Heater

The *Huang Di Zhen Jing (Yellow Emperor's Acupuncture Classic)* states:

> [When] the upper [burner] qi is insufficient, the brain is not full, the ears
> are bitter [or tormented due to] ringing, the head is drooped (tormented
> by drooping [later editor]), and the eyes are heavy (dizzy [later editor]).
> [When] the middle [burner] qi is insufficient, defecation and urination
> become abnormal and the intestines are tormented by borborygmus.
> [When] the lower [burner] qi is insufficient, this leads to wilting, rever-
> sal, and heart oppression. [In this case,] supplement [the point] under the
> lateral malleolus [*i.e., Kun Lun*, Bl 60] without retention [of the needle].[1]

Debility of the true qi of the three origins [*i.e.*, the three burners] is always due to
prior vacuity of the spleen and stomach and failure of the qi to move upward. [If,]
in addition, there is joy, anger, sorrow, worry, or fright, danger or death is hastened.

Here Li is saying that any source qi vacuity of any of the three burners is typically preceded by spleen qi vacuity since the spleen-stomach are the latter heaven
source of the qi of all three burners. Because spleen qi vacuity results in non-
upbearing of the clear, there are vacuity signs and symptoms in the upper burner,
including the uppermost extremity. Because non-upbearing of the clear results
in simultaneous non-downbearing of the turbid, there are problems with urination and defecation.

Endnote

[1] *Ling Shu*, Vol. 5, Ch. 28

脾胃论

Book Three

1

Treatise on the Ascription of the Large Intestine, Small Intestine & All Five Viscera to the Stomach And Stomach Vacuity Leading to Disease of Them All

The *Huang Di Zhen Jing (Yellow Emperor's Acupuncture Classic)* states, "The hand yang ming large intestine and hand tai yang small intestine are both ascribed to the foot yang ming stomach."[1] The point of the small intestine is located at the lower ridge of the great hollow [*Xia Ju Xu*, St 37] and the point of the large intestine is located at the upper ridge of the great hollow [*Shang Ju Xu*, St 39]. Both these two points are below the point [*Zu*] *San Li* (St 36) of the foot yang ming stomach [channel]. The large intestine governs fluids, while the small intestine governs humors. [However,] the large intestine and small intestine must receive the constructive qi from the stomach before they can move fluids and humors to the upper burner to irrigate the skin and hair and fill and replete the interstices. If stomach qi becomes inadequate due to dietary irregularity, the large intestine and the small intestine will have nowhere from which to be endowed [with supplies], and, as a result, fluids and humors will become exhausted. The *Nei Jing (Inner Classic)* says, "Tinnitus, deafness, and inhibition of the nine orifices are engendered by the intestines and stomach."[2] Stomach weakness unable to enrich and nourish the hand tai yang small intestine and hand yang ming large intestine [channels] is the cause of these conditions. However, in the final analysis, stomach weakness is the cause. Thus the sage's confusing statement about the engenderment of [conditions] by the intestines and stomach.

This passage is an attempt to explain the above quote from the *Huang Di Zhen Jing* about the relationship of the intestines to the stomach at the same time as underlining the stomach's primacy over these other two bowels. While it was Li's arguments such as the above which elevated the stomach to its current pre-eminent position above the large and small intestines in standard professional Chinese medicine, I do not find the above passage otherwise particularly important in terms of clinical practice. In fact, its argument seems a bit casuistical.

Some people may ask, "Can you produce evidence to prove your conclusion that these [conditions] are, on the whole, generated by the stomach and intestines?" My answer is as follows. The *Yu Ji Zhen Zang Lun (Treatise on the True Visceral [Pulse Observed through the] Jade Mechanism)* states, "Inadequacy of the spleen causes the nine orifices to not flow freely."[3] It is said that the spleen is dead yin. [Only] after receiving yang qi from the stomach is it able to ascend and upbear the qi of water and grains to the lungs to fill the skin and hair above and dissipate [or spread] it to the other four viscera. If the spleen is not endowed with [such] supplies [by the stomach], it is not able to move the qi to the viscera and bowels. Thus this condition arises [*i.e.*, non-free flow of the nine orifices]. This is what is meant by spleen vacuity resulting in non-free flow of the nine orifices. Although spleen vacuity is spoken of, it is the result of stomach insufficiency. Then what about the ascription of the five viscera to the stomach instead of the spleen? I would say that this also is no different from the above. This theory is based on [the fact] that, if the spleen is not endowed with life by the stomach, the nine orifices governed by the five viscera are unable to communicate above with the heavenly qi. Thus they become blocked, obstructed, and inhibited. Hence the five viscera are [by extension also] ascribed to [the stomach]. These three [*i.e.* blockage, obstruction, and inhibition] are caused by nothing but stomach vacuity. However, [stomach vacuity is capable of] far more. [For, if] the stomach is vacuous, the five viscera, six bowels, 12 channels, 15 network vessels, and the four limbs all will fail to obtain [their supply of] constructing and moving [as in transporting] qi. As a result, hundreds of diseases arise. This is how the few can cover the many. Each of the 12 regular channels plus the governing and conception vessels have a great network vessel. There is also the so-called great network vessel of the spleen. Thus there are 15 great network vessels in all. To paraphrase this last line, one might say: How can a simple study cover them all? They need a thorough study. There is disease upon disease caused by stomach vacuity.

Endnotes

[1] *Ling Shu,* Vol. 1, Ch. 2
[2] *Su Wen,* Ch. 28
[3] *Su Wen,* Ch. 19

2

Treatise on Stomach Vacuity's Leading to Non-free Flow of the Nine Orifices

The true qi is also called the original qi. It is the essence qi prior to the birth of the body. Nothing except the stomach qi can enrich it. The stomach qi is the grain qi, the constructive qi, the moving qi, the engendering qi, the clear qi, the defensive qi, and the yang qi. Besides, the qi of heaven, the qi of humanity, and the qi of earth are the qi of the three heaters. Treated separately, they are different, [but,] as a matter of fact, they are one [and the same thing] and should not be looked upon as different things with different names.

While Li says that the original qi is the former heaven essence qi, he also says that nothing but the latter heaven qi can enrich it. He then goes on to equate this latter heaven qi exiting from the middle burner spleen and stomach with the constructive and defensive qi as well as the yang qi. In fact, yang is nothing other than a lot of qi in one place, enough qi to produce warmth as well as movement, transformation, defense, and containment. Thus the above paragraph helps to clarify Li's use and conception of the term "original qi."

Damage done by food and drink, taxation, and overwork [may lead to] spontaneous perspiration, frequent urination, yin fire overwhelming the earth phase, non-engenderment of the clear qi, and nonmovement of the yang tract. [In that case,] fire is deeply-lying [or hidden] in yin blood. This is a clear statement that yin fire may enter and lie deeply in the yin and blood aspects. This is because yin fire travels upward through the chong mai, the sea of blood, and accumulates in the heart and vessels, the governor and abode of blood. In addition, yang ming stomach earth is dry on the right and hot on the left. Here, right means the large intestine which governs fluids. Left means the small intestine which governs humors. Since the large intestine is associated with the lungs which is dry metal, while the small intestine is associated with the heart which is fire heat, the stomach is said to be dry and hot at its sides. [Therefore,] it transforms dryness and fire, not allowing fluids and humors to collect. Furthermore, urination and sweating can both lead to collapse of fluids and humors. Fluids and humors should transform into blood when they arrive in the central palace [*i.e.*, the spleen and stomach]. The vessels are the mansion of the blood. [If] blood collapses, upon what can the seven spirits rely? The hundreds of vessels are all derived from [blood]. This passage helps explain the tendency for the stomach to become hot and dry even though the spleen is vacuous and damp. If a hot, dry stomach and intestines cause polyuria and constipation at the same time there is spleen vacuity, this is called a straitened spleen. This passage also explains at least one disease mechanism for yin, blood, and humors becoming simultaneously vacuous and insufficient if there is yin fire. The worst of the hundreds of diseases humans are subject to is wind stroke. When one sweats, wind evils may invade. When one does not sweat, yang qi is solid and tight and the interstices are blocked and resistant. Thus the various evils are not able to [do] damage.

Some people quote the classic, saying, "[When] yang is unable to prevail over [or restrain] yin, the qi of the five viscera will be in conflict, causing the nine orifices to be non-freely flowing,"[1] "Inadequacy of the spleen leads to non-free flow of the nine orifices, [a condition] called superimposition disagreement,"[2] "Disharmony of the five viscera leads to non-free flow of the nine orifices,"[3] and, "Headache, tinnitus, non-free flow, and inhibition of the nine orifices are generated by the intestines and stomach."[4] They [then] ask for an analysis and explanation. The answer is as follows: The spleen is yin earth, the qi of ultimate yin. [It] governs stillness and not stirring. The stomach is yang earth. [It] governs stirring and is never at rest. [However,] only when yang qi resides under earth is it able to engender and transform the tens of thousands of things. This line means that only when yang qi or stomach qi is received by spleen-earth can it engender things. This is why the five movements are above and the six qi are below. The five movements or transports are the five phases of wood, fire, earth, metal, and water. They represent the movement of heaven. The six qi are wind, fire, heat, dryness, dampness, and cold. They represent the influences of earth. The spleen is one cubit long, screening the great granary which is the upper mouth of the stomach. The spleen receives its endowment from the stomach and then, and only then, can it fume and steam, ferment and mash [or rotten and ripen] the five grains. The stomach is the source of the 12 channels, the sea of water and grains. [When it is] normal, the transformation of the tens of thousands of things is guaranteed. [When it is] diseased, the transformation of the tens of thousands of things is in danger. The qi of the five viscera ascend to flow freely to [or communicate with] the nine orifices above. Above here means the exterior. The five viscera receive their endowment of qi from the six bowels, while the six bowels receive their qi from the stomach. The six bowels [resonate or correspond with] wind, cold, summerheat, dampness, dryness, and fire in heaven which are [species of] formless qi. [When] stomach qi is harmonious and level [or calm], the constructive qi ascends and is upborne, initiating the engenderment of warmth and heat. Warmth and heat are spring and summer. [The constructive qi] travels 25 circuits in the yang. Yang here means both day as opposed to night and the route the constructive qi travels during the day. When the six yang are at the summit of upbearing and dissipating, they descend to engender yin. The six yang are the six yang channels, *i.e.,* the hand and feet units of yang ming, tai yang, and shao yang. This downbearing of yin leads to the downbearing and descension that is autumn and winter, and, when the yin tract moves, this is cool and cold. If the stomach is diseased and is unable to enrich and nourish, the qi of the six bowels expires. As a result, the intestinal tract does not move and yin fire moves upward. The qi of the five viscera are unable to enrich and nourish the skin, blood vessels, sinews, or bones unless they each benefit from the transformation of one bowel [*i.e.,* the stomach]. On that account, the statement that the qi of the five viscera expire in the exterior means that the vital qi of the six bowels have first expired. The five viscera have no place from which to receive endowment, and their qi consequently expire.

This paragraph explains that the upbearing of the clear and the downbearing of the turbid are interdependent and that nondescension of the stomach may be a cause for the engenderment and upward movement of yin fire. In addition, it states that disease commonly first begins in the yang bowels and especially the stomach before it goes on to cause damage and detriment to the five viscera. This may or may not be true, but does underscore the necessity of treating the spleen and stomach at the same time, even when their diseases are of an opposite nature. By this I mean a vacuous, cold, damp spleen at the same time as a replete, disharmonious, hot, and dry stomach (and intestines).

By nature the lungs are gathering and downbearing. [They] also govern the five qi, [*i.e.,* urine-like, acrid, aromatic, fishy, and decaying smells. If their] qi expires, it flows downward to superimpose on spleen earth in the lower burner. Thus it is called superimposition disagreement. If the stomach qi becomes diseased, it [also] pours downward. The classic states that the lower is the first to suffer from dampness.[5] The spleen is ultimate yin. Its root is the earth. [In this case,] formal [or tangible] earth, [*i.e.,* damp stomach qi] descends to fill the sources of the nine orifices and is not able to ascend and flow freely to [or communicate with] heaven. Therefore, it is said that disharmony of the five viscera leads to non-free flow of the nine orifices. The stomach moves the clear qi upward, namely, the yang qi of earth. [When this] has accumulated [sufficiently,] yang [qi] produces heaven. This is called the clear yang emerging in the upper orifices. This is called clear yang repleting [or replenishing] the four limbs. This is called the clear yang effusing through the interstices. [If] the spleen and stomach are overwhelmed by yin fire and the grain qi is blocked, obstructed, and flows downward, clear qi stops being upborne and the nine orifices are inhibited. [When] the single bowel of the stomach is diseased, the original qi of all 12 channels becomes insufficient. Scant qi [then], leads to fluids and humors not moving. Fluids and humors not moving leads to blood depletion. Therefore, the sinews, bones, skin, flesh, blood, and vessels all become weak. This is [due to] impoverishment and weakness of the qi and blood. How can [one] not be cautious about taxation, labor, and activity as well as hunger and surfeit? Even though this kind of disease does not give rise to transmuted disorders, it [causes] detriment to one's heaven[-decreed span of] years. If, in addition, acupuncture-moxibustion or medication are used in an inappropriate way, how is it possible to avert the expected premature death?

This passage shows how a spleen-stomach disharmony associated with yin fire can damage and cause disease in any or all of the body's tissues. As Li points out, the yang qi which flows to the clear orifices and the four limbs and effuses from and defends the exterior are all derived from the integrated function of the spleen and stomach.

Endnotes

[1] *Su Wen*, Ch. 3
[2] *Su Wen*, Ch. 19.
[3] *Nan Jing*, 37th Difficulty
[4] *Su Wen*, Ch. 28
[5] *Su Wen*, Ch. 29

Treatise on the Viscera & Bowels, Channels & Network Vessels Having Nowhere from Which to Receive Qi and [thus] Contracting Disease When the Stomach Is Vacuous

Spleen-stomach vacuity leads to the qi of damp earth pouring downward below the umbilicus, and the kidneys and urinary bladder suffering from evils. This sentence says two things. First, that when the spleen and stomach are vacuous and weak, dampness is engendered. This dampness, being a turbid, yin evil, tends to pour downward from the middle to the lower burner. Secondly, this dampness may damage the kidneys and bladder. The urinary bladder governs cold, whereas the kidneys are yin fire. According to the five phase theory, the urinary bladder is cold water. If both of them are weak, the qi of moistening fluids will stop moving. The large intestine is *geng*, the dry qi which governs fluids, while the small intestine is *bing*, the hot qi which governs humors. Both of these pertain to the stomach. As described in a previous chapter. Stomach vacuity leads to [these two] having nowhere from which to receive qi and [thus, they also] become vacuous. In contemporary Chinese medicine, a spleen qi vacuity and a small intestine vacuity are essentially identical. As this line states, once the stomach becomes vacuous, the small intestine and large intestine commonly do too. [Because, in this case,] fluids or humors do not moisten, during sleep one sees dryness of the mouth and parching of the throat and the skin and hair lack luster. *Jia*, the gallbladder which is wind and warmth, governs the engenderment and transformation of blood and qi in the whole body. *Bing*, the small intestine which is hot, governs the growth and nourishment of yang qi in the whole body. Both of them also are endowed with qi from the stomach before they can float and dissipate, upbear and effuse. Stomach vacuity leads to the warm and hot engendering, and growing qi of the gallbladder and small intestine become insufficient. [Instead, these] lie deeply and lodge within the blood vessels which have form, causing hot diseases, wind stroke, and countless other diseases. The five viscera, the cyan [or blue-green], red, yellow, white, and black, may all become stagnant. The five colors correspond to the five viscera by way of the five phases. The triple burner is the root of engendering and effusing of the original qi of the lower burner. [Therefore, if it] is overwhelmed by fire, all the qi of the six bowels become debilitated.

While I no longer take the 10 stem and 12 branch correspondences seriously, this paragraph again reaffirms the ability of yin fire to lie deeply within the blood. Li also sates yin fire can result in stagnation of any of the five viscera.

The bowels are dwelling houses and places of storage. They embrace the five viscera and store substances and materials. In addition, in the exterior, the qi of the six bowels have nothing to govern. This implies that the exterior parts, the skin and hair, the blood vessels, and the orifices for example, are governed by the viscera instead of the bowels. In the interior, they have to have their supplies. *Jia*, the gallbladder, is engendered in response to the windy qi of heaven. This means that the gallbladder corresponds to *jia* and resonates with wind. The following sentences can each be interpreted in the same way. *Bing*, the small intestine, is engendered in response to summerheat qi. *Wu*, the stomach, is engendered in response to the transformation of dampness. *Geng*, the large intestine, is engendered in response to dry qi. *Ren*, the urinary bladder, is engendered in response to cold qi. The triple burner, which, being without form, is the paternal qi, is engendered in response to the qi of heaven unique [*i.e.*, water qi, including dew, mist, etc.].Wind, cold, summerheat, dampness, dryness, and fire are the same as warm, hot, cold, and cool but by other names. [The constructive and defensive qi] travel 25 circuits [around the body] in yang. They turn right and then they are upborne, float, are downborne, and sink. Here, the four movements do not merely mean the change in direction of the flow but also changes such as warmth and coolness, hot and cold. Their vacuity always is due to weakness of the spleen and stomach.

In terms of the five viscera, extremely hyperactive heart fire overwhelming spleen earth is called center heat [as manifest by] a surging, large pulse and vexation and oppression. According to the *Nan Jing (Classic of Difficulties)*, when the spleen is diseased, there is "a stirring qi around the umbilicus which feels firm and painful upon pressure." This stirring qi is solid and fixed, as hard as if an accumulation, with vague pain or, in the extreme, even great pain. Presence [of this stirring qi] leads to the disease of spleen vacuity. Absence [of it] leads to no [such condition. However,] there is another differentiation. While the presence of a hard lump around the umbilicus may be a sign of spleen disease, its absence does not mean there is no spleen disease. Encumbrance and fatigue arising upon eating with clouded essence spirit and a desire to sleep indicate a depleted, weak spleen. These are much more dependable symptoms of spleen qi vacuity. Moreover, when heart fire is extremely effulgent, [the qi of the stomach] goes down to enter the aspect [or precinct] of liver wood. In other words, internally engendered damp evils pour downward into the lower burner. Thus wind and dampness mutually struggle and [hence there is] pain all over the body along with a surging, large, bowstring, occasionally moderate pulse or dizziness, trembling and shaking, and insensitivity. All these [are due to] wind. Wind in this case refers to the wind of wind dampness or rheumatic disorders. Spleen disease with generalized heaviness and pain in the joints may develop into painful impediment, cold impediment, various types of damp impediment, wilting, limpness, and lack of strength, or great welling and flat abscesses. In clinical fact, most patients with chronic rheumatic disorders manifest a liver-spleen disharmony with either wind damp cold or wind damp heat. If the evils are assisted by acrid, hot [medicinals], it may develop into a hot disease or wind stroke. There are countless transmuted patterns.

Effulgent wood moves and travels toward the north and turns left into the earth to assist kidney water. The kidneys are north according to five phase correspondence theory. Therefore, turning towards the north means going to the kidneys. With the help of its child, [the liver] water turns into phlegm and drool if it enters the spleen, into spittle if it enters its own [viscus], into tears if it enters the liver, and into snivel if it enters the lungs. "Own [viscus]" here means the kidneys. Although the kidneys govern all five fluids, only spittle is ascribed to them specifically in terms of five phase correspondences. [In that case,] it is evident that [kidney water] is counter-restraining spleen earth by the strength of liver wood. Earth is expected to restrain water, but, in this case on the contrary, the restrained water restrains earth instead. This is but a convoluted five phase explanation for a liver-spleen disharmony. [To treat this,] it is first necessary to supplement yang qi at the yin aspect and make it upbear and soar. This is still a most important principle for the treatment of such a liver-spleen disharmony. [Thus yang qi will] move in the yang tract and penetrate to the cavities and orifices. [In this case,] drink medicinals of cold and watery [nature] to downbear yin fire, such as *Huang Bai* (Cortex Phellodendri) and *Huang Lian* (Rhizoma Coptidis Chinensis). In other words, if there is a liver-spleen disharmony with damp or depressive heat, one must also clear heat with bitter, cold medicinals. Supplement yang first and drain yin later, and the spleen and stomach will both become effulgent and be restored to their position in the middle burner. Thus yin qi and yang qi are leveled [or balanced].

Fire [is that which is] called flaming upward. Water [is that which is] called moistening and descending. [Therefore,] why, in discussing the kidneys' governing the five fluids, are [those fluids] said to go up to the head and emerge from the cavities and orifices as tears, snivel, sweat, drool, and spittle? The answer is as follows: [Imagine] the epileptic foaming at the mouth, chilly sweat exiting from their body, and clear snivel exiting from their nose. All this is due to the evils of the four vessels, the yang motility, yin motility, governing, and penetrating [vessels. When these evils] move upward, kidney water is unable to bear their cooking and burning. [Instead, its fluids] start to boil and move upward to cause [these problems]. This kind of disease caused by peculiar evils does not keep to [the laws] concerning the five phases, yin and yang, and the 12 channels. It requires treatment of the four points that cure the peculiar evils of the governing, penetrating, and two motility vessels, [*i.e., Ren Zhong* (GV 26), *Yin Jiao* (CV 7), *Shen Mai* (Bl 62), and *Zhao Hai* (Ki 6)].

Because of the Jin-Yuan preoccupation with yin-yang and five phase theory, Li is forced or, perhaps, seduced into making some convoluted arguments that are no longer of any particular use today.

The five viscera [each] govern something in the exterior, but, in the interior, they have nothing to receive. This implies that the six bowels receive qi from the stomach, whereas the five viscera receive their supplies from the bowels. This means that what they govern in the exterior are the skin and hair, blood vessels, muscles and flesh, sinews and bones, and the various cavities and orifices. If stomach qi alone becomes vacuous, the four viscera and their channels and network vessels will have no place from which to receive their endowment [and, consequently, may] all [become] diseased. More importantly, it is by dint of level and harmonious stomach earth that the spleen is supplied in order to engender the constructive. Thus the other four viscera in the body are effulgent, the 12 spirits [*i.e.,* the spirits in the 12 viscera and bowels,] fulfill their responsibilities, the skin and hair are solid and strong, the sinews and bones are flexible, and the nine orifices are freely flowing and uninhibited. The word "level" within Chinese medicine in general and in Li-Zhu medicine in particular always has a spatial meaning as well as a more abstract meaning of balance and calmness. Level means that the qi is not counterflowing, usually upward, and especially upward in the case of the stomach. In addition, Li says that the spleen qi cannot be healthy and correctly functioning if the stomach qi is not level and harmonious. [Thus,] external evils are incapable of inflicting harm. If the spleen-stomach are healthy and well, then the production of constructive and defensive qi should be normal and sufficient. If the defensive qi is sufficient and does its job of securing and defending the exterior, then evil qi cannot enter and cause disease.

4

Treatise on the Engenderment of Various Diseases Due to Stomach Vacuity [&] Insufficient Original Qi

Whenever eating, drinking, taxation, and labor, result in spontaneous perspiration, this is due to the yang ming transforming dryness and fire. [Thus,] fluids and humors are unable to collect, resulting in perspiration and frequent urination. No other evil is worse than wind stroke. Wind is the chief of the hundreds of diseases. [Its] predilection [or nature] is to move and frequently change. However, without vacuity evils, wind, rain, or cold alone cannot damage [or harm] people. Vacuity evils do not imply some kind of internally engendered evils. Vacuity evils simply mean pathological vacuity or the evil of vacuity. Thieving evils have no way to enter [the body] unless vacuity evils have [already] struck. Wilting and counterflow reversal both result from exiting of sweat. In winter, yang qi lies deeply [or is hidden] and stored beneath water and earth. If there is extraordinary drainage of essence, yang qi [may become] exhausted. Extraordinary drainage of essence refers to abnormally warm weather in winter manifested by warm springs surging up and rivers breaking up prematurely. Then how can spring exercise its government [in due time]? Spring here means the engendering qi in the body as well as seasonal warmth and engendering qi in outside nature. Then the transformation of the tens of thousands of things cannot occur. [Therefore,] in humans, various diseases may arise from frequent exuding of perspiration [in turn due to damage by] eating, drinking, taxation, and labor. I am repeatedly reminding [the reader] of this because I wish people to learn to be careful.

Basically, this chapter is another refutation that externally contracted wind evils are the main cause of disease. Up till Li's time, this had been the cornerstone of pathogenesis in Chinese medicine. Li clearly and unambiguously argues that external evils cannot enter the human body until or unless the body's righteous qi is vacuous and insufficient. The righteous qi is derived primarily from the finest essence transformed and transported by the spleen and stomach, thus Li's insistence on keeping a strong and healthy middle burner. As I have said above, I find this particular teaching of Li (founded in the *Nei Jing*) to be extremely important in clinical practice.

5

Treatise on Suddenly [Becoming] Fat
& Suddenly [Becoming] Thin

The *Huang Di Zhen Jing (Yellow Emperor's Acupuncture Classic)* states, "With cold and heat and diminished qi, blood moves up and down."[1] Qi vacuity [leads to] inability [to bear] cold, blood vacuity to inability [to bear] heat, and vacuity of both qi and blood to inability [to bear] either cold or heat. The stomach, when vacuous, is unable to move upward. In consequence, the lungs lose their nourishment. Thus qi is diminished. If the defensive qi is vacuous, [one is] unable [to bear] cold. Because [the stomach qi or dampness] moves downward to assail the kidneys and liver, assisting [the transformation of] fire into toxins, qi becomes debilitated and blood depleted in the yin aspect. Hence, cold and heat [arise] with diminished qi. The cause of blood moving upward [at one time] and downward [at another] is that the foot yang ming stomach vessel is debilitated. Consequently, the penetrating vessel joins the yang ming channel to travel up to the yang aspect. It counterflows 72 circuits [around the body]. The fire in it is immensely effulgent, flowing counter to the yang ming channel. While moving upward, blood surges into and fills the upper. When this fire retreats and lies deeply in the lower [body], the blood moves downward. This is what is called blood traveling [sometimes] upward and [sometimes] downward. This is popularly known as suddenly [becoming] fat [at one time] and suddenly [becoming] thin [at another].

The practical implication of the above paragraph, at least to my mind, is that spleen vacuity may allow the penetrating vessel to counterflow upward and become filled with heat evils. It also seems to me that this theory may help explain polycystic ovarian syndrome (PCOS). Polycystic ovarian syndrome is characterized by obesity, acne, hirsutism, amenorrhea, and infertility and it typically does present the elements of a yin fire scenario: liver-spleen disharmony with depressive heat in the liver and stomach with underlying kidney vacuity, either yin, yang, or both. In Chinese medicine, acne is heat in the blood aspect in the upper part of the body. Amenorrhea may be either due to insufficient blood and yin or blockage and obstruction of the flow of blood to and out from the uterus.

While hirsutism is an excess of blood since the hair is the surplus of the blood. The kidneys govern reproduction and fertility, and dampness pouring downward damages the liver and kidneys. Thus it appears to me that the above explanation may cover all of the main clinical symptoms of PCOS, including obesity, remembering that Li has also said that yin fire also causes or aggravates stasis and stagnation within the body.

The classic states, "Heat damages qi."[2] It also says, "Vigorous fire eats the qi."[3] These two sayings may be enough to explain why upwardly stirring ministerial/life-gate fire damages the spleen qi, causing or aggravating its vacuity. When the spleen and stomach are vacuous and evil fire is overwhelming, qi must become lessened and [therefore] unable to defend and protect the skin and hair. This means that the qi that flows freely to and through the upper burner becomes short and scanty. This reiterates that a yin fire scenario typically involves vacuity of the heart, lung, and defensive qi. This helps explain why yin fire scenarios are so complicated by psychiatric and immunological complaints. [Since] blood is depleted in the yin aspect and qi is frittered away in the yang aspect, blood and qi both become scanty in either the yin or yang aspects throughout the entire body. [Since the body] cannot stand either cold or heat, [the disease is] called cold and heat. The Ling Shu Jing (Spiritual Axis Classic) says, "The upper burner opens and effuses, diffusing the flavors from the five grains to fume the skin, fill the body, and moisten the hair as the mist and dew irrigate."[4] This is the result of stomach qi [being] level and moving upward.

Personally, I would say it is the result of the stomach qi being level and the spleen qi upbearing.

Endnotes

[1] *Su Wen,* Ch. 6
[2] *Su Wen,* Ch. 5
[3] *Ibid.*
[4] *Ling Shu,* Vol. 6, Ch. 30

6

Treatise on the Laws of Engendering & Killing of Yin & Yang in Heaven & Earth Consisting of Upbearing & Downbearing, Floating & Sinking

The *Yin Yang Ying Xiang Lun (Treatise on the Mutual Correspondences of Yin & Yang)* states:

> Heaven sees yin grow when yang engenders. Earth sees yin store when yang kills.[1]

Heaven here is synonymous with spring and summer. Earth here is synonymous with autumn and winter.

The first season of the year is spring. *Zheng*, the correct, means the beginning, and *yin* (B3) means drawing out. Usually the correct refers to the first month of the Chinese lunar calendar, but here to the beginning of a new year in terms of spring being the beginning of a new cycle of four seasons. According to the Chinese calendar, spring, the first season of the year, does not necessarily begin with the first day of the first month or the spring festival but rather on the day called the beginning of spring which may fall even in the last month of the previous year. Hence the term "correct" becomes understandable. In other words, there are two kinds of Chinese calendar. According to one, the year begins on the first day of the first month. According to the other, it does not. The qi of the shao yang starts from the under[ground] spring. It draws yin, upbearing [till it rises] above heaven, humanity, and earth. During this aspect of heaven, the hundreds of grains, grasses, and trees sprout and send up shoots. When the beginning of summer comes, the fire of shao yin is raging in the great vacuity [*i.e.,* heaven or the sky] and plants thrive with their twigs waving and leaves spreading. This is yang acting [on] the substance of yin and is what is meant by [the statement that] heaven sees yin grow when yang engenders. "The heavenly qi governing the first half of the year"[2] mentioned in the classic is embodied by upbearing and floating. When autumn comes, the movement of tai yin hurls down from the heaven and yin descends into the earth. Here, tai yin refers to autumn. Now metal vigorously exercises its dry government. In terms of the five phases, autumn is metal and, in terms of the six qi, it is dryness. Dryness originates in the west and gives birth to metal. Wind is relentless, frost is seen everywhere, various [living] things are all dying, and, [on the trees,] nothing but branches stand out like fine hair. When winter comes, the qi of shao yin is hidden in the under[ground] spring again, water becomes ice, and the ground is frozen. The tens of thousands of things are sealed close and tight. This is yin acting [on] the substance of yang and is what is meant by [the statement that] the earth sees yin store when yang kills. "The earthly qi governing the second half of the year" mentioned in the classic is embodied by downbearing and sinking.

Here Li is stating the various correspondences of the four seasons with the four movements of the qi: upbearing, downbearing, floating, and sinking.

The orderly [progression of] the righteous qi is such that spring qi is warm, summer qi is intensely hot, autumn qi is clear and cool, and winter qi is bitterly cold. Therefore, it is said that if the beginning [of the year] is set right, the order will never go wrong. According to the explanation given by the author in a later place in this passage, it is understood that one should act prudently, trying to follow and adapt to the changes in weather in the four seasons if one wants to keep fit. But some scholars interpret it in another way. According to them, if the beginning of the year is correctly calculated, then one will not lose record of the month, the season, etc. Downbearing follows upbearing, and upbearing follows downbearing in an endless cycle. To move and transform the tens of thousands of things is the very identity of qi. Qi is the movement of yin and yang. Yin and yang [however,] may become involved in complicated relations and out of this arise the various [conditions of] victory and retaliation. In summer, for instance, if intense heat prevails, this is called victory of heat, the heart, or fire. In this case, according to five movements and six qi theory, we may experience an abnormally cool autumn. This is called retaliation.

Humans are one of the tens of thousands of things. Inhaling and exhaling, [our qi] upbearing and downbearing, we are similar to heaven and earth and [behave in compliance with] the norms of yin and yang. This is a basic statement of the microcosmic/macrocosmic holism upon which Chinese medicine is founded. The stomach is the sea of water and grains. [After] food and drink enter the stomach, essence qi is first transported to the spleen and sent home to the lungs, moving upward to exercise spring and autumn government to enrich and nourish the whole body. This is the clear qi forming heaven. [Following] this upbearing, it is transported downward to the urinary bladder to exercise autumn and winter government. It conveys and transforms the wastes, conducts their flavors [to the viscera], and [then] discharges [the wastes]. This is turbid yin becoming earth.

[Humans enjoy] quiet [if we] follow the qi in the four seasons normaly and keep [definite] times for sleeping and arising so as to guard against cold and summerheat, [if our] eating and drinking are regulated, [if we] refrain from sudden joy and anger to nurture our spirit mind, and [if we] try to maintain moderation in all the four seasons with no one [phase] prevailing over another. If not, [there will be] detriment and damage to the spleen (and stomach [later editor]), the true qi will pour downward possibly giving rise to diarrhea, and [the clear qi] will be unable to be upborne for a long time. This is [similar to] the presence of autumn and winter and the absence of spring and summer. Thus do the actions of engendering and growing sink into the qi of reducing and killing. Out of this, hundreds of diseases arise. Vice versa, [if the true qi] continues to be upborne for a long time without downbearing, this also leads to disease. Examining things from this point of view, [one] will come to know the significance of setting the beginning right.

In this chapter, Li is using the four seasons and the four movements of qi in order to teach his readers how to lead a regular, well-ordered lifestyle. Although such admonishments were already present in the *Nei Jing*, Li was responsible for raising them to the prominence they hold today.

Endnotes

1 *Su Wen*, Ch. 5
2 *Su Wen*, Ch. 71

7
Treatise on Yin & Yang, Longevity & Premature Death

The *Wu Chang Zheng Da Lun (Great Treatise on the Government of the Five Constants)* states:

> When yin essence mounts, people [enjoy] long life. When yang essence is downborne, people die prematurely.[1]

Yin essence refers to earthly qi. Yang essence refers to heavenly qi.

Yin essence mounting means yin essence mounting to yang [or heaven]. This refers to the engendering and growing qi of spring and summer. Yang essence being downborne means [yang essence] descending and being downborne to yin [or earth]. This refers to the gathering and storing qi of autumn and winter. Take the deep-lying [or hidden] yin of the earth for an example. With the arrival of spring, its essence undergoes change and stirring and begins to soar and be upborne above. This is none other than the engendering and effusing qi. Upbearing to the extreme, it floats. This is nothing other than flourishing qi. The six qi thus turn right to heaven to form the clear yang of heaven. Yang governs life and, therefore, long life. [In terms of] the original yang of heaven, its essence retreats with the arrival of autumn. It is downborne and falls downward to form the gathering, constraining, reducing, and killing qi. Being downborne to the extreme, it becomes the sealing and storing qi. The five movements [or five phases] thus turn left into the earth to form the turbid yin of earth. Yin governs killing and, therefore, administers premature death.

That which takes root in the external [*i.e.*, the outside world and particularly the atmosphere] is called the qi institution. The qi institution refers to the function of respiration and other such metabolic processes. When qi stops, transformation is at an end. That which takes root in the internal [*i.e.*, the spleen and stomach or rather their functions] is called the spiritual mechanism. Spiritual mechanism means the mental-emotional activities. When spirit is gone, this mechanism is at a standstill. Both [of these] are [problems of] downbearing without upbearing. What is known as the earthly qi in humans is the spleen and stomach. The spleen governs the qi of the five viscera, whereas the kidneys govern the essence of the five viscera. Both mount upward to heaven and govern engenderment and transformation to support raising, upbearing, and floating. Heaven here means the upper burner or rather the heart and lungs. It is known that what makes spring engender and summer grow is the product of the stomach. Because of this, one's stirring and stopping [*i.e.*, activity and rest] as well as eating and drinking should be managed in an appropriate way. There must be clearness [or tranquility] and there must be stillness [or quiet]. Thus the original qi of the stomach does not [suffer] detriment nor does it descend to overwhelm the kidneys and liver. [If] the reducing and killing government of autumn and winter is not imposed, one's heaven[-decreed] number will accord with [their actual lifespan].

In this chapter, Li makes a case for promoting the upbearing of the clear and disinhibition of the qi mechanism as the keys to achieving longevity.

Endnote

[1] *Su Wen*, Ch. 70

8

Treatise on the Intricate Changes
of the Qi of the Five Viscera

The *Wu Zang Bie Lun (Divergent Treatise on the Five Viscera)* states, "[After] the five qi enter the nose, [they] are stored in the heart and lungs."[1] The five qi are the five smells: urine-like, acrid, aromatic, fishy, and putrid. The *Nan Jing (Classic of Difficulties)* says, "The lungs govern the nose, and, when harmonious, the nose knows [or distinguishes] fragrance from fetor."[2] Jie-gu says, "Acute vision and hearing show clearness and coolness, [while ability to] differentiate fragrance from fetor shows warmth." This implies that the ears and eyes are free from hot evils and that the nose is free from cold evils respectively. This is [the normal condition when] the interior receives qi from heaven and the exterior's nine orifices are uninhibited. The triple burner orifice opens into the throat and emerges at the nose. As the orifice of the lungs, the nose is a bodily [substance], and the smelling of fragrance and fetor is its function. The heart governs the five smells which are housed in the nose. This means that the heart governs the sensation or consciousness of the five odors or smells. Each of the nine orifices function in the service of that which is in longevity in relation to it. Longevity here does not mean long life in the ordinary sense. It is a technical term describing the complicated relationship between various pairs of the twelve earthly branches. These pairs are numerous, but they are classified into eleven categories figuratively named after the eleven stages of the life process from birth to death. Longevity is one of these eleven symbolizing fresh birth. These categories can be used to represent various things and their relations. Regarding the five viscera, the lungs, for example, are *you* (B10). In that case, *zi* (B1) is its longevity since, according to this scheme, the pair *you/zi* corresponds to the stage called longevity. Since *zi* is the kidneys with their orifices the ears, based on this pairing, one can say that the ears work at the service of the lungs. [Therefore,] the heart has its longevity in *you* (B10) which is the lungs. The associations between the viscera and the earthly branches are as follows:

Earth	Water	Wood	Fire	Metal
Spleen	Kidneys	Liver	Heart	Lungs
B2 12th	B1 11th	B4 2nd	B7 5th	B10 8th
B5 3rd	B12 10th	B3 1st	B6 4th	B9 7th
B8 6th				

From this it is known that the nose functions in the service of the heart in smelling fragrance and fetor. The ears ascend and flow freely to the heaven qi. They are the orifices of the kidneys. [The ears] are the bodily [substance] of the kidneys but function in the service of the lungs. The lungs have their longevity in zi (B1). Zi is the abode of the kidneys but, in it, dwell the lungs. Therefore [the ears] are able to hear.

There is yet another approach. Tone is heavenly yang, while volume is heavenly yin. These have the five standard pitches on earth. This refers to the fact that in ancient China the standard pitches were produced and measured by bamboo pipes which are the produce of the earth. In humans, their orifice is the throat. They function in the mouth at the service of the triple burner. The lungs and heart combine to produce speech which issues from the mouth. The mouth is the orifice of the heart and the tongue is its bodily [substance] into which it opens. [However,] the triple burner [in turn] functions in the service of the lungs. It is not ok not to also know this.

The orifice of the liver flows freely to the eyes. Here orifice means the qi of the liver. Without being fire, they are able to shed light and see things. According to some scholars, this section should be rendered as follows: Bright is heaven which sheds light and make things visible. Therefore, they are able to distinguish the five colors. The liver is the abode [of the blood]. The Chinese implies that the liver governs the blood and the eyes can see only when they are provided with a supply of blood. The kidneys govern the five essences [i.e., the essences of the five viscera]. The nose stores qi in the heart and lungs. Therefore, it is said that [the heart and lungs] govern the hundreds of vessels and move the yang tract. The classic states, "Those with qi desertion are blind, and those with essence desertion are deaf."[3] When the heart and lungs are diseased, the nose becomes inhibited. All this suggests explicitly that the ears, eyes, mouth, and nose are heaven [within the human body] supported by yang qi and that taxation of the heart and detriment to the stomach subjects them to evils.

It is interesting to me that Li is so concerned with explaining the function of the sensory orifices in terms of the stomach (and spleen). While using the yin-yang and five phase systems of the 10 heavenly stems and 12 earthly branches, he is nevertheless arguing against the equality of the viscera and bowels otherwise implied by these systems. Therefore, although the doctors of the Jin-Yuan dynasties have been criticized for overemphasizing these extremely abstract and theoretical aspects of Chinese medicine and applying them to internal medicine, Li actually sets the stage for seeing the functioning of the viscera and bowels independent of five phase theory.

One other thing I would point out is Li's juxtaposition of bodily substance and function or use throughout the above passage. This remains an extremely important dichotomy in Chinese medicine to this day. As soon as we see the word function, we know we are talking about the function of yang qi.

Endnotes

[1] *Su Wen*, Ch. 11
[2] *Nan Jing*, 37th Difficulty
[3] *Ling Shu*, Vol. 6, Ch. 30

9

Treatise on the Upbearing & Downbearing of Yin & Yang

The *Yi (Jing, Classic of Change)* states that the two antipodes [or yin and yang] engender [or ramify into] the four manifestations. The four manifestations or signs are tai yin, tai yang, shao yin, and shao yang. It describes the intercourse of qi between heaven and earth in terms of the eight trigrams. The *ba gua* or eight trigrams consist of three broken or unbroken lines in varied combinations. These eight three-lined patterns represent eight phases of variation in yin and yang and correspond or resonate with innumerable phenomena, processes, and objects analogous to five phase correspondence theory. By the Jin-Yuan dynasties, these eight trigrams and five phase theory had been integrated. Li opens with these lines because he is going to use a four-part yin-yang division in the following passage where he talks about the clear of the clear and the turbid within the clear, the clear within the turbid and the turbid within the turbid. In humans, both the clear and turbid qi exit from the spleen and stomach. The constructive qi, which is transformed from the qi and flavor of water and grains, constructs and nourishes the whole body. Construction and nourishment are important technical terms in Chinese medicine. When used as a compound term, they imply the construction of the physical body (including the qi which is seen as a fine or the finest essence) and the nourishment of the tissue of that body. Only if the bodily tissue or substance obtains sufficient nourishment, can the qi associated with that tissue or organ do its function. The clear yang forms heaven. (The clear yang develops to heaven, [*i.e.,*] the earthly qi ascends, turning into clouds; the heavenly qi descends, turning into rain. These are the essence qi of water and grains, the sea of qi, the seven spirits, and the original qi. They are the paternal [qi]. [Author]) The parenthetic inclusions in this section say they are by the author, but it is suspected that they are the work of some later editor(s). The clear of the clear clears the lungs to assist the heavenly true. This refers to the combination of prenatal essence qi and postnatal grain qi. This clear yang issues from the upper orifices (the seven orifices, [*i.e.,*] the ears, eyes, nostrils, and mouth. [Author]) The turbid within the clear constructs and [makes] lustrous the interstices. This clear yang issues from the interstices ([*i.e.,*] the hair pores [Author]) and repletes [or replenishes] the four limbs. (The true qi fills and repletes the four limbs. [Author]) Turbid yin forms the earth. (Yin accumulates to form the earth. Clouds produce the heavenly qi, while rain produces the earthly qi. The essence of the five flavors of the five grains, which is transformed from the five flavors, it is the blood and constructive [which] sustains the spirit brilliance and nourishes blood. It is the maternal [qi]. [Author]) The clear within the turbid constructs and nourishes the spirit. (It becomes blood when it is downborne to the middle duct. Therefore, it is said that the heart governs the blood and stores the spirit. [Author]) Today, we say that the turbid, meaning the clear part of the turbid, returns to or gathers in the heart where it is transformed into blood by the fire of the heart. The blood then constructs and nourishes the spirit. This turbid yin exits through the lower orifices. (The front yin is the orifice of the urinary bladder. [Author]) The front yin means the urethra in males and urethra cum vagina in females. the rear yin is the anus in both sexes. The turbid of the turbid hardens and strengthens the bones and marrow. This turbid yin penetrates the five viscera. (It is the blood that dissipates in the five viscera. It nourishes the blood vessels, moistens the skin, and fattens the muscles, flesh, and sinews. There appears to be a misprint in the Chinese version used in the preparation of this translation. Literally the Chinese reads, ". . . moistens the skin and muscles are fat with flesh and sinews." Since that makes no sense nor is this grammatically acceptable in English in terms of the parallel structure of this sentence, we have preferred to give what we presume the author intended. This is what is meant by [the statement] that blood engenders flesh. [Author]) [Then, this] turbid yin returns to the six bowels. (This implies that the hair[-like] vessels, after taking in essence, send essence qi home to the bowels. [Author]) The meaning of this line is ambiguous and has led some people to another interpretation. According to this alternative reading, the sentence should be translated as follows: "When the hair and vessels combine the essence, they send..." Because the hair is governed by the lungs and the vessels by the heart, this sentence is further interpreted by these readers as, "When the heart and the lungs combine..."

If qi of heaven is clear, still, luminous, and bright. [Its] virtue is stored and not stopped [or exposed]. Thus it does not descend [or does not stop working]. If heaven is bright, the sun and the moon will not be bright. [As a result,] evils will harm the cavities and orifices. Yang qi will be blocked and obstructed, and the qi of earth qi will be obscured. Clouds and fogs will not disperse. The responses from above are the white dew's non-precipitation and unclear intercourse and communication [or free flow between heaven and earth. As a result,] the life of the tens of thousands of things will not be operated, and this failure to operate sends many famous trees [or plants] to death. Malign qi will not be vented and wind and rain will be unregulated. Because the white dew is not precipitated, [everywhere there is] depression and withering without flourishing. Numerous thieving winds occur. Torrents of rain pour frequently. Heaven and the earth in the four seasons are in disorder. The (natural) laws will be out of practice. In consequence, (everywhere there are) premature deaths and extinction. The sages alone can adapt themselves (to such a situation) and, therefore, be free from serious disease. They never go counter to (the natural laws governing) the ten thousand things and enjoy inexhaustible vital qi.[1]

Virtue in the above passage means the natural power to engender and transform the tens of thousands of things. It is the virtue of the *dao* as in the *Dao De Jing*. This power is expected to be exercised in a peaceful, unnoticeable way. Storms, for example, are an expression of this power. However, they expose it or, we can say, they turn virtue into evil. The phrase, "If heaven is bright...," has also been interpreted as, "If heaven is laid bare..." Or, "If heaven is ostentatious..." The white dew is symbolic of clear, cool qi, a qi which can disperse pernicious clouds and fogs, and, in long summer, damp heat prevails, but, when autumn comes, the clear, depurating qi does away with stuffy heat and dampness as if giving vent to something malign or ill.

The above teaching explains that if people do not try to avoid great cold which damages the form, great heat which damages the qi, or the abnormal vicissitude of qi in the four seasons, terms, and signposts, or if people are not disciplined in drinking and eating, tax themselves unwisely, and let their hearts be governed by good and bad [or what they like and do not like], their original qi will not move. [Instead,] qi will transform to make fire. According to the Chinese lunar calendar, five days form what is technically called a signpost. Three such signposts form a term and six terms form a season. This is the cause of premature loss of life.

Endnote
[1] *Su Wen*, Ch. 2

10

Treatment Experiences in Regulating & Rectifying the Spleen & Stomach:

Treatise on Inadvertent Detriment Due to Mistakes Out of Ignorance in the Use of Upbearing & Downbearing, Floating & Sinking Treatment Methods in Medication

I myself suffered from a disease of enduring spleen-stomach debility, losing half [my] vision and hearing. This would explain Li's recurrent discussion of the nine orifices. This was [a disease of] yin exuberance overwhelming yang. In other words, of dampness and turbidity overwhelming the yang qi. In addition, [I had] shortness of breath, essence spirit insufficiency, and bowstring pulse due to vacuity [in turn due] to speaking too much. Note the bowstring pulse. This pulse image is not generally thought of as a sign of vacuity. However, when the spleen is damaged by damp evils, it no longer engenders and transforms sufficient blood to nourish the liver. In this case, the liver qi can no longer function properly, *i.e.*, govern coursing and discharge. Thus the liver becomes depressed, the qi becomes stagnant, and the pulse becomes bowstring. Readers should also note how deleterious Li thinks too much speaking is. In fact, speaking, including singing and chanting, consumes large quantities of heart and lung qi which are both derived from the spleen. Li regards damage to the qi due to speaking excessively so important, that the last lines of this, his last book, end with yet another admonishment against speaking unnecessarily. All these [symptoms indicated] yang qi debility and weakness. [Since the yang qi] was deeply lying within yin, it could not obtain soothing and extension. This means that, because of encumbrance by damp, heavy, turbid yin evils, the clear yang qi was not able to upbear and effuse.

Between the sixth and the seventh months in the *gui mao* year, licentious [*i.e.*, excessive] rain and yin cold did not stop for over a month. The 60 year Chinese lunar calendar is arranged by matching one heavenly stem to one earthly branch. Therefore, the *gui mao* year Li Dong-yuan is referring to was 1245 CE when the author was 65 years old. At this time, many people became diseased with diar-

rhea and dysentery since profuse dampness is liable to result in the five diar-
rheas. These are stomach diarrhea (swill), spleen diarrhea (soft stool), large intestine diarrhea (throughflux), small intestine diarrhea (blood), and major
conglomeration diarrhea (intestinal afflux). One day, I felt a generalized heaviness and aching pain in the joints of my limbs and had swill diarrhea three times
along with urinary blockage and obstruction. In terms of the treatment, the *Biao
Ben Lun (Treatise on Tip [or Branch] & Root)* [in] the *Nei Jing (Inner Classic)*
[says,] "[In case of] inhibited defecation or urination, do not ask [whether this
is] root or tip. First [simply] disinhibit defecation or urination."[1] It also says,
"Exhaust it by abducting it out if [the evils] are in the lower."[2] This also means
[that one should] first disinhibit urination [in such cases]. It also says [that one
should] first separate and distinguish between the various types of diarrhea and
dysentery and inhibited urination. Yet again it states that this is never an appropriate treatment for dampness except with inhibition of urination. In all such
cases, the only method seems to be to disinhibit urination and, to do this, there
is no other choice but to use percolating, draining formulas with bland flavors.
Although the methods of the sages are published in their books, there may be
some shortcomings, and [we] should carry out investigation and make correc-
tions. Here Li is alluding to the authors of the *Nei Jing*.

Now, [in my case,] the intruding evils of excessive cold and dampness [were mov-
ing] from external to internal in a violent way. If bland, percolating formulas
were used to eliminate this according to the above methods and parameters, the
disease might have been cured promptly, but it would have been downbearing
what was also downborne. Without simultaneously fortifying the spleen and
upbearing yang, simply seeping water downward would have further led to the
downward falling of the central qi. This is because, it is qi which moves fluids in
the body. Wherever fluids flow, qi follows. Therefore, by promoting urination,
one runs the risk of draining the righteous qi along with damp evils. This would
be [the same as] repeatedly boosting yin and doubly exhausting the yang qi. Since
this would worsen spleen vacuity and the spleen governs the movement and
transformation of water fluids in the body, weakening the spleen is tantamount
to engendering damp evils. The yang qi would be whittled away all the more,
and the essence spirit would become shorter. Yin would be doubly strengthened,
and yang would be doubly debilitated. [In other words, this method] would contrarily strengthen the evils. Therefore, [in such cases,] it is necessary to use yang-
upbearing, windy medicinals. This implies that, with invasion of external (guest)
evils, the yang qi is depressed and, therefore, this should be overcome by effusing and dissipating. [Then true or complete] recovery will be affected. [Such
medicinals] include *Qiang Huo* (Radix Et Rhizoma Notopterygii), *Du Huo* (Radix
Angelicae Pubescentis), *Chai Hu* (Radix Bupleuri), *Sheng Ma* (Rhizoma

Cimicifugae), one *qian* for each of the above, *Fang Feng* (Radix Ledebouriellae Divaricatae) cut to pieces, 0.5 *qian*, mix-fried *Gan Cao* (Radix Glycyrrhizae Uralensis) cut to pieces, 0.5 *qian*, all to be sliced. These should be boiled in four medium-sized cups of water down to one cupful and taken slightly hot after removing the dregs. The general principle says that overwhelming cold dampness can be leveled [or calmed] with the assistance of windy [medicinals]. It also says that that which has descended should be lifted. When the yang qi obtains upbearing and soaring, [the evils] will be removed.In other words, dampness will be downborne if the clear yang is upborne. This is such an important principle in clinical practice which is, in my opinion, far too often overlooked or insufficiently appreciated. Another principle says that the guest should [be treated] by eliminating.Guest here means the externally contracted evils. While normally these should be eliminated from the body, because of concomitant righteous vacuity, Li thinks it is more important to upbear the clear and restore the health of the yang qi. Then the yang qi will automatically move and transform the yin evils. This is [a way of] helping the curved by means of straightening. The method of the sage can be applied based on this analogy. From this one instance, inference can be drawn about hundreds of diseases. One who is unacquainted with the mechanisms of upbearing and downbearing, floating and sinking is lucky if they have ever achieved a cure by applying an indiscriminate treatment.

Early in the early sixth month of the *wu shen* year [1240 CE], Secretary of the Ministry of Defense, Bai Wen-ju, aged 62, who habitually had a spleen-stomach vacuity detriment disease, suffered from an intermittent eye disease with generalized yellowing of the face and eyes, sometimes yellow, sometimes whitish urine, irregular defecation, reduced drinking and eating, shortness of breath with qi ascent, fatigue and somnolence, and uncontrollable [*i.e.*, debilitated] limbs. In the middle of the sixth month, his eye disease recurred and the [attending] physician administered *Xie Gan San* (Drain the Liver Powder)[3] which caused diarrhea and made his disease even worse than before. I concluded that *Da Huang* (Radix Et Rhizoma Rhei) and *Qian Niu Zi* (Semen Pharbiditis), though able to eliminate dampness and heat, had not been able to penetrate the channels and network vessels and, after being swallowed, did not enter the liver channel but entered the stomach first. *Da Huang* (Radix Et Rhizoma Rhei), bitter and cold, made the stomach doubly vacuous, while *Qian Niu Zi* (Semen Pharbiditis), whose flavor is extremely acrid, was capable of draining qi, making the root of the lungs more vacuous and resulting in severe cough. While the tip [or branch] repletion was not relieved, the root vacuity was made [all] the more serious. [Even worse,] this happened in a time of rainy summerheat. This could not but worsen [the condition of] a patient who formerly had jaundice. What was appropriate [in this case] was to attend to the viscera proper of the spleen, stomach, and lungs and to drain damp heat from the exterior channels. [Therefore, I] composed *Qing Shen Yi Qi Tang* (Clear the Spirit & Boost the Qi Decoction) to treat [this patient's condition] and cure was affected.

Qing Shen Yi Qi Tang (Clear the Spirit & Boost the Qi Decoction)

Fu Ling (Sclerotium Poriae Cocos)
Sheng Ma (Rhizoma Cimicifugae), 2 *fen* each
Ze Xie (Rhizoma Alismatis Orientalis)
Cang Zhu (Rhizoma Atractylodis)
Fang Feng (Radix Ledebouriellae Divaricatae), 3 *fen* [for each of] the above
Sheng Jiang (uncooked Rhizoma Zingiberis Officinalis), 5 *fen*

These medicinals are able to penetrate the channels and eliminate damp heat without settling. Therefore, they do not drain the viscera proper. [Instead,] they supplement the vacuity and weakness of the qi proper of the lungs as well as of the spleen and the stomach.

Qing Pi (Pericarpium Citri Reticulatae Viride), 1 *fen*
Chen Pi (Pericarpium Citri Reticulatae)
uncooked *Gan Cao* (Radix Glycyrrhizae Uralensis)
Bai Shao (Radix Albus Paeoniae Lactiflorae)
Bai Zhu (Rhizoma Atractylodis Macrocephalae), 2 *fen* [for each of]
     the above
Ren Shen (Radix Panacis Ginseng), 5 *fen*

These medicinals are able to settle in the root and do not penetrate the channels. Those that do not penetrate the channels will not enrich the evils within those channels, and those that settle are able to supplement the original qi of the viscera. This is an interesting explanation for why supplementing medicinals do not necessarily supplement evils when administered at the same time as draining medicinals.

Huang Bai (Cortex Phellodendri), 1 *fen*
Mai Men Dong (Tuber Ophiopogonis Japonici)
Ren Shen (Radix Panacis Ginseng), 2 *fen* each
Wu Wei Zi (Fructus Schisandrae Chinensis), 3 *fen*

These medicinals remove seasonal floating heat and steaming dampness. Slice the above ingredients the size of cannabis seeds. [Take] all as one dose, boiled in two cups of water down to one cupful and taken while moderately warm on an empty stomach after removing the dregs.

When fire blazes extremely at the time of metal hiding, cold water is defunct. Fire blazing implies extremely hot summer weather. The three hidings are the period of the hottest weather in the year, each consisting of 10 days. The last hiding begins on the first *geng* (S7) day (lung metal is represented by *geng*) after the Beginning of Autumn. Because of this, metal hiding still sees very hot days. This period necessitates speedy emergency [treatment] with *Sheng Mai San* (Engender the Pulse Powder)[4] to eliminate damp heat since very severe [damp heat must be] repelled. Note that the ingredients of *Sheng Mai San* are included in the above formula. The lungs desire restraint, and the heart is bitter about relaxation. For both of them, sour [medicinals] can accomplish restraint, [while] heart fire exuberance leads to draining by the sweet. Therefore, the sweetness of *Ren Shen* is assisted by the sourness of *Wu Wei Zi*. Sun Si-miao said that, in the summer months, [one should] commonly [or regularly] administer *Wi Wei Zi* in order to supplement the qi of the five viscera. *Mai Men Dong*, which is slightly bitter and cold, is able to enrich the source of water in the metal phase and to clear and depurate the lung qi. This implies that the lungs should be enriched since they are metal, the engenderer of kidney water. It is also able to eliminate coughing due to fire tormenting metal and to constrain phlegm evils. Then, a tiny [amount] of *Huang Bai*, which is bitter and cold, is added to protect and enrich the flow of water and settle and harden the floating qi so as to eliminate wilting and weakness of both feet. Water flow or the flow of water here means the kidneys. Settle and harden is a reference to the upwardly counterflowing ministerial/life-gate fire which should be rooted in the lower burner. Today, we primarily talk about hardening the kidneys. However, functionally, this means the same thing, *i.e.*, to make the kidneys strong and healthy by clearing and settling upwardly stirring ministerial/life-gate fire.

The wife of Fan Tian-song, who habitually had had a spleen-stomach disease, suffered from vexation and agitation from time to time with inhibition within the chest and non-freely flowing stools. In early winter, she went out and returned late [in the evening] having been assailed and depressed by cold qi. Oppression and chaos [*i.e.*, fidgeting] attacked violently. This was due to fire not obtaining extension. In other words, external contraction of cold on top of a defensive qi vacuity due to habitual spleen vacuity had resulted in the depression of yang qi internally. Because the yang qi could not upbear and effuse, it had transformed into depressive heat. Such liver depression qi stagnation would aggravate any pre-existing tendency to chest oppression, and depressive heat ascending to harass the heart spirit would result in aggravation of any tendency to vexation, agitation, and restlessness. Suspecting of the existence of heat, the [attending] physician treated her with *Shu Feng Wan* (Coursing Wind Pills).[5] [As a result of these,] her stools were moved but the disease [as a whole] was not decreased. This time, suspecting that the medicinals had not been strong enough, [the physician] prescribed 70-80 more pills. Two [times more stools]were moved downward, but the former condition still did not diminish. Instead, a new problem, counterflow retching [cropped up]. Food was not able to collect [*i.e.*, there was diarrhea], and thick, sticky phlegm and spittle gushed out incessantly. [The woman suffered from] black eyes [or dim vision], spinning head, nausea, vexation, oppression, shortness of breath, distressed rapid breathing and panting, lack of strength, no desire to speak, perverted heart spirit, incessant daze, not daring to open the eyes, [feeling] as if in wind and clouds, tormenting headache as if the head were about to split, generalized heaviness like a mountain, reversal chilling of the four limbs, and inability to obtain quiet sleep. [Therefore,] I concluded that the earlier condition had been stomach qi detriment, and that, after precipitation twice, the stomach was made the more vacuous with attack of phlegm reversal headache as a result. [Thus, I] composed *Ban Xia Bai Zhu Tian Ma Tang* (Pinellia, Atractylodes & Gastrodia Decoction) to treat [this woman's condition] and [she] was cured.

Ban Xia Bai Zhu Tian Ma Tang (Pinellia, Atractylodes & Gastrodia Decoction)

Huang Bai (Cortex Phellodendri), 2 *fen*
Gan Jiang (dry Rhizoma Zingiberis Officinalis), 2 *fen*
Tian Ma (Rhizoma Gastrodiae Elatae)
Cang Zhu (Rhizoma Atractylodis)
Fu Ling (Sclerotium Poriae Cocos)
Huang Qi (Radix Astragali Membranacei)
Ze Xie (Rhizoma Alismatis Orientalis)
Ren Shen (Radix Panacis Ginseng), 5 *fen* [for each of] the above
Bai Zhu (Rhizoma Atractylodis Macrocephalae)
Shen Qu (Massa Medica Fermentata), stir-fried, 1 *qian* each
Ban Xia (Rhizoma Pinelliae Ternatae), washed with boiled water 7 times
powdered *Mai Ya* (Fructus Germinatus Hordei Vulgaris)
Chen Pi (Pericarpium Citri Reticulatae), 1.5 *qian*

This is not the *Ban Xia Bai Zhu Tian Ma Tang* which is commonly thought of today under this name. That formula was orginally found in Cheng Guo-peng's Qing dynasty *Yi Xue Xin Wu (New Materials in the Study of Medicine)*.

Slice the above ingredients [and take] 0.5 *liang* per dose, boiled in two cups of water down to one cupful. Take while warm before meals after removing the dregs. This kind of tormenting headache is referred to as a foot tai yin phlegm reversal headache. Nothing but *Ban Xia* can cure it. Black eyes [or dim vision] with spinning head is due to wind vacuity attacking internally. Nothing but *Tian Ma* is able to eliminate it. [*Tian Ma*] sprouts make [are called] stable [in the] wind herb, the only herb that is not stirred by the wind. *Huang Qi*, sweet and warm, drains fire and supplements the original qi. Huang Qi drains depressive fire by upbearing and effusing yang qi and thus resolving depression. *Ren Shen*, sweet and warm, drains fire, supplements the center, and boosts the qi. *Cang Zhu* and *Bai Zhu*, both sweet, bitter, and warm—sweetness being able to eliminate dampness—supplement the center and boost the qi. *Ze Xie* disinhibits urination and abducts dampness. *Chen Pi*, bitter and warm, boosts the qi, regulates the center, and upbears yang. *Shen Qu* disperses food and sweeps away stagnant qi in the stomach. Powdered *Mai Ya* loosens the center and assists the stomach qi. *Gan Jiang*, acrid and hot, is used to clear center cold. *Huang Bai*, bitter and intensely cold, can, after being washed with wine, prevent the small fire existing in the spring from developing dryness. The fire that engenders the original qi. It is located in the lower abdomen (spring) and is associated with the kidneys (winter).

This is a very interesting formula. It is a typical Li prescription although it is no longer commonly used. It is for the treatment of migraine headaches and Meniere's disease in patients with a liver-spleen disharmony, profuse phlegm dampness, depressive heat, and an element of wind. Because it supplements the spleen more forcefully as well as rectifies the qi more forcefully than Cheng Guo-peng's formula of the same name, I think it is more useful in many contemporary patients than Cheng's formula. Obviously, it can be further modified from here.

In the *wu shen* year, in the middle of the seventh month, [I received] a poor person who had contracted a spleen-stomach vacuity weakness disease with distressed rapid breathing and emaciation. [I] accordingly prescribed *Ren Shen Shao Yao Tang* (Ginseng & Peony Decoction).

Ren Shen Shao Yao Tang
(Ginseng & Peony Decoction)

Mai Men Dong (Tuber Ophiopogonis Japonici), 2 *fen*
Dang Gui (Radix Angelicae Sinensis)
Ren Shen (Radix Panacis Ginseng), 3 *fen* [for each of] the above
mix-fried *Gan Cao* (Radix Glycyrrhizae Uralensis)
Bai Shao (Radix Albus Paeoniae Lactiflorae)

Huang Qi (Radix Astragali Membranacei), 1 *qian* [for each of] the above
Wu Wei Zi (Fructus Schisandrae Chinensis), 5 pieces

This formula supplements the qi, blood, and yin at the same time as it supplements the spleen and lungs in terms of the viscera.

Slice the above ingredients and divide into two doses. Boil each dose in two cups of water down to one cupful and take while moderately hot after removing the dregs. After recuperating, living in an empty room in winter and sleeping on a heated *kang* led [the patient] to vomit blood several times. To this day in north China, many people prefer to sleep on a *kang* which is a raised platform built of clay bricks connected as part of the flue to the stove. Therefore it is comfortably warm to sleep on. I concluded that this patient had been vacuous and weak for a long [time] with something tangible attaching to the umbilicus, great internal heat, qi insufficiency in the upper, and external vacuity of the yang qi. [Therefore,] it was necessary to supplement the yang qi externally and drain vacuity heat internally. Living in an empty room with thin clothes doubly evacuated [this woman's] yang. Since great cold in the exterior confines heat in the interior, fire evils could not [in this case] be soothed or spread. Hence blood exited through the mouth. In other words, because they were depressed internally by cold, heat evils could not find a way out of the body by normal effusion and dissipation. This resulted in driving these disease evils deeper into the blood aspect. Heat then stirred the blood causing it to move frenetically outside its pathways. Thus there was blood exiting from the mouth. I was reminded of [Zhang] Zhong-jing's treatment of tai yang cold damage requiring sweating with *Ma Huang Tang* (Ephedra Decoction).[6] If treated with some other [method], nose-bleeding may occur, but, when this decoction is administered, [epistaxis] may be cured immediately after taking. [Since that formula] is quite similar to the present case, I prescribed *Ma Huang Ren Shen Shao Yao Tang* (Ephedra, Ginseng & Peony Decoction).

Ma Huang Ren Shen Shao Yao Tang (Ephedra, Ginseng & Peony Decoction)

Ren Shen (Radix Panacis Ginseng), to boost insufficient original qi of the
    triple burner and replenish the exterior
Mai Men Dong (Tuber Ophiopogonis Japonici), 3 *fen* each
Gui Zhi (Ramulus Cinnamomi Cassiae), to supplement exterior vacuity
Dang Gui (Radix Angelicae Sinensis), to harmonize and nourish the
    blood, 5 *fen* each
Ma Huang (Herba Ephedrae), to remove external cold
mix-fried *Gan Cao* (Radix Glycyrrhizae Uralensis), to supplement the spleen

Bai Shao (Radix Albus Paeoniae Lactiflorae)
Huang Qi (Radix Astragali Membranacei), 1 *qian* [for each of] the above
Wu Wei Zi (Fructus Schisandrae Chinensis), 2 pieces, to quiet the lung qi

Slice the above ingredients and [take] all as one dose. *Ma Huang* should be boiled alone in three cups of water. Continue to boil, remove the scum, and put in the other ingredients when the solution is boiled down to two cupfuls. [Then] boil it down to one cupful and take while hot before sleep after removing the dregs.

This prescription shows just how one can supplement and drain at the same time. It also shows how one can clear heat through upbearing and effusing without using any bitter, cold medicinals. It is an extremely masterful demonstration of virtuosity.

Sheng Yang San Huo Tang
(Upbear Yang & Dissipate Fire Decoction)

[This formula] is indicated in males and females for heat in the four limbs, heat of the muscles, sinew impediment heat, heat in the bone marrow, drowsiness, and heat in the hands which feels like being burnt with fire. In most cases, this [kind of] disease is due to blood vacuity. Or it may [come from] suppression and confinement of yang qi within spleen earth due to stomach vacuity and eating too many chilled things. Clinically, it is important to understand that overeating chilled foods does not just damage the spleen and lead to vacuity. It also causes stomach heat. Li's explanation for this is that the cold of the chilled foods causes depression of stomach yang with transformative heat. Fire depression [or depressed fire] requires effusing.

uncooked *Gan Cao* (Radix Glycyrrhizae Uralensis), 2 *qian*
Fang Feng (Radix Ledebouriellae Divaricatae), 2.5 *qian*
mix-fried *Gan Cao* (Radix Glycyrrhizae Uralensis), 3 *qian*
Sheng Ma (Rhizoma Cimicifugae)
Ge Gen (Radix Puerariae)
Du Huo (Radix Angelicae Pubescentis)
Bai Shao (Radix Albus Paeoniae Lactiflorae)
Qiang Huo (Radix Et Rhizoma Notopterygii)
Ren Shen (Radix Panacis Ginseng), 5 *qian* [for each of] the above
Chai Hu (Radix Bupleuri), 8 *qian*

Slice the above [and take] 0.5 *liang* per dose, boiled in three large cups of water down to one cupful and taken while moderately hot after removing the dregs.

[In this case,] cool or cold things and chilled [or iced] water are prohibited for a month or more.

From "An Examination of Li Dong-yuan's Method of 'Upbearing Clear Yang & Scattering Yin Fire'" by Wang Mao-song, *Shan Xi Zhong Yi (Shanxi Chinese Medicine)*, #5, 2001, p. 60-61

CASE 1: Sjögren's syndrome

The patient was a 56 year-old female who was first examined on Aug. 21, 1997. The woman had suffered from dry mouth and dry eyes for 10 years. Two years ago, tears, saliva, and sweat had become even more scanty. This was accompanied by bodily fatigue, lack of strength, tidal heat, red cheeks, and hot flashes. When these hot flashes occurred, she felt a general malaise and had to eat or drink chilled things or apply cool compresses. For a number of years she had seen both Western and Chinese doctors for treatment and had been diagnosed as suffering from Sjögren's syndrome. However, neither Chinese nor Western medicines had had any effect. These previous doctors had discriminated her pattern as yin vacuity with internal heat and had treated her with yin-nourishing, heat-clearing medicinals to no effect. Dr. Wang, however, thought the patient suffered from central qi insufficiency with yin fire flaming upward. Therefore, he prescribed the following medicinals based on the above-discussed principles for yin fire: *Tai Zi Shen* (Radix Pseudostellariae Heterophyllae), 15g, *Mai Men Dong* (Tuber Ophiopogonis Japonici), 10g, *Sheng Di* (uncooked Radix Rehmanniae Glutinosae), 20g, *Ge Gen* (Radix Puerariae), 10g, *Sheng Ma* (Rhizoma Cimicifugae), 8g, *Zhi Mu* (Rhizoma Anemarrhenae Aspheloidis), 10g, *Huang Bai* (Cortex Phellodendri), 10g, *Xuan Shen* (Radix Scrophulariae Ningpoensis), 10g, *Shi Hu* (Herba Dendrobii), 15g, and *Gan Cao* (Radix Glycyrrhizae Uralensis), 5g. After taking 10 packets of these medicinals, the patient reported that she felt psychologically much better and that her dry mouth, eyes, sweating, and tidal heat were all improved. After another 30 packets of the above formula, all her symptoms had disappeared.

It is not that Dr. Wang did not nourish yin or did not clear heat as had the previous physicians. However, on top of those methods, Dr. Wang added fortifying the spleen and upbearing the clear. This upbearing of the clear and scattering of yin fire was accomplished not only by *Sheng Ma* but also by *Ge Gen*. By choosing medicinals that accomplish more than a single function, Dr. Wang was able to craft a very elegant and compact formula for this patient's otherwise recalcitrant condition.

The following two case histories do not use *Sheng Yang San Huo Tang* but are based on the treatment principles of upbearing yang and scattering fire. This is actually how I suggest readers use the information presented in this book —not the rote prescription of formulas created by Li but rather the crafting of formulas based on Li's principles and models.

CASE 2: Neurologic tinnitus

The patient was a 48 year-old female who was first examined on May 14, 1998. The woman had had tinnitus for one year. This had started in one ear but had gradually gotten worse until it occurred in both ears and sounded like cicadas. In addition, her hearing had gotten worse. This was accompanied by dizziness, headache, chest oppression and discomfort. The patient had been diagnosed as suffering from neurologic tinnitus and was treated with a multivitamin, adenosine triphosphate, and blood vessel dilating medicines, however, without result. Initially, Dr. Wang tried treating the patient based on the principles of enriching the kidneys and boosting the essence, assisted by leveling (the liver) and subduing (yang), but this also failed to achieve any positive effect. Therefore, based on the line from the *Nei Jing (Inner Classic)*, "Clear yang issues from the upper orifices," Dr. Wang decided to try Li Dong-yuan's method of upbearing yang and scattering fire. Therefore, he prescribed *Yi Qi Cong Ming Tang Jia Jian* (Boost the Qi & Brighten the Hearing Decoction with Additions & Subtractions). Unfortunately, Dr. Wang does not describe the specific medicinals he employed. However, Li Dong-yuan's basic formula consists of: *Huang Qi* (Radix Astragali Membranacei), *Gan Cao* (Radix Glycyrrhizae Uralensis), *Bai Shao* (Radix Albus Paeoniae Lactiflorae), *Huang Bai* (Cortex Phellodendri), *Ren Shen* (Radix Panacis Ginseng), *Sheng Ma* (Rhizoma Cimicifugae), *Ge Gen* (Radix Puerariae), and *Jing Jie Sui* (Herba Seu Flos Schizonepetae Tenuifoliae). After taking these medicinals, Dr. Wang says the patient's tinnitus markedly decreased and that regulating therapy for a month was able to basically cure the woman.

CASE 3: Hypertension

The patient was a man of undisclosed age who was first seen on Sept. 22, 1998. The man had had hypertension for 30 years and commonly had headache, dizziness, chest oppression, heart palpitations, insomnia, and impaired memory. He had been treated with Western hypotensive medicines for a long time and his blood pressure had stabilized and would not go below 22-23/12kPa. At the time Dr. Wang examined this patient, all the above symptoms were worse and were accompanied by shortness of breath, chest noises, and nocturnal profuse urination. ECG showed myocardial damage. Physical examination revealed that the man was obese, his tongue tended towards red, the fur was thin and white, and both pulses were bowstring, small, and slippery. Based on these signs and symptoms, Dr. Wang concluded that the clear yang was not being upborne but that vacuity wind was harassing above. Based on that assessment, Dr. Wang prescribed the following medicinals: *Tai Zi Shen* (Radix Pseudostellariae Heterophyllae), 15g, *Huang Qi* (Radix Astragali Membranacei), 10g, *Ge Gen* (Radix Puerariae), 10g, *Bai Ji Li* (Fructus Tribuli Terrestris), 10g, *Tian Ma* (Rhizoma Gastrodiae Elatae), 10g, *Gou Teng* (Ramulus Uncariae Cum Uncis), 15g, *Ling Yang Jiao* (Cornu Antelopis Saiga-tatarici), 0.3g swallowed with the decoction, *Dan Shen* (Radix Salviae Miltiorrhizae), 12g, *Fu Ling* (Sclerotium Poriae Cocos), 10g, *Ju Hua* (Flos Chrysanthemi Morifolii), 10g, and *Bai Shao* (Radix Albus Paeoniae Lactiflorae), 10g. After 10 packets of these medicinals, the headache markedly decreased and the blood pressure went down to 20/11kPa. After another 10 packets, the man was able to reduce the dose of his Western hypotensive medicines. On follow-up after an unspecified period of time, his blood pressure was still 20/11kPa. On follow-up in 2001, the man's blood pressure had still not risen. As Dr. Wang notes, based on yin fire theory, a person can have ascendant liver yang hyperactivity at the same time as clear yang not being upborne. In that case, simply leveling the liver and subduing yang will not result in lowering of the blood pressure.

An Wei Tang
(Quiet the Stomach Decoction)

[This formula] treats hemiplegia with hemilateral wind, wilting, and impediment due to sweating while drinking and eating. [If this] goes on for days, [it leads to] vacuity within the heart. [Hence] wind vacuity evils [invade, resulting in this disease. In other words, wind evils invade by taking advantage of this vacuity. In this case, one] must first eliminate the sweating. [Then] the swift and impetuous qi [*i.e.*, wind evils] can be restrained by suppression.

Huang Lian (Rhizoma Coptidis Chinensis), sorted and stripped of hair
Wu Wei Zi (Fructus Schisandrae Chinensis), with seed removed
Wu Mei (Fructus Pruni Mume), cored
uncooked *Gan Cao* (Radix Glycyrrhizae Uralensis), 5 *fen* [for each of]
    the above
mix-fried *Gan Cao* (Radix Glycyrrhizae Uralensis), 3 *fen*
Sheng Ma (Rhizoma Cimicifugae), 2 *fen*

Slice all the above and separate into two doses. Boil [each dose] in two cups of water down to one cupful and take while warm between meals after removing the dregs. Sodden wheat food, wine, the five acrids, and spices are prohibited. The five acrids consist of garlic, scallion, ginger, onion, and hot pepper.

Qing Wei San
(Clear the Stomach Powder)

[This formula] treats unbearable pain in the upper and lower teeth leading to heat and severe pain all over the head and brains as a result of administering hot, stomach-supplementing medicinals. The divergent network vessel of the foot yang ming enters the brains. [The stomach] is fond of cold but is averse to heat. [Therefore,] exuberant heat in the yang ming channel brings on [this disease]. This is the same disease mechanism which causes the vast majority of pediatric earache. Due to food stagnation, stomach heat follows the network vessels and/or divergent channels upward to the head. Because the inner ear is enclosed in a bony box, once heat arrives there, it has no way to be out-thrust and effused. Therefore, it steams and brews, transforming toxins and causing purulence.

Sheng Di (uncooked Radix Rehmanniae Glutinosae)
Dang Gui (Radix Angelicae Sinensis), 3 *fen* each
Dan Pi (Cortex Radicis Moutan), 0.5 *qian*
Huang Lian (Rhizoma Coptidis Chinensis), sorted, 6 *fen*; add [an extra] 2
    fen if bad quality; double the amount in summer months. On the
    whole, quantities should vary depending on the seasons.
Sheng Ma (Rhizoma Cimicifugae), 1 *qian*

Powder the above [and take] all as one dose, boiled in 1 1/2 cups of water down to 7/10 [of one cupful] taken when cooled after removing the dregs.

Qing Yang Tang
(Clear Yang Decoction)

[This formula] treats deviated mouth with spasmed, hard cheek. [If there is] exuberant fire in the stomach, there must [also] be incessant sweating and frequent urination. Once again Li says that stomach heat may result in frequent, excessive urination.

Hong Hua (Flos Carthami Tinctorii)
wine-processed *Huang Bai* (Cortex Phellodendri)
Gui Zhi (Ramulus Cinnamomi Cassiae), 1 *fen* [for each of] the above
uncooked *Gan Cao* (Radix Glycyrrhizae Uralensis)
Su Mu (Lignum Sappan), 5 *fen* each
mix-fried *Gan Cao* (Radix Glycyrrhizae Uralensis), 1 *qian*
Ge Gen (Radix Puerariae), 1.5 *qian*

Dang Gui (Radix Angelicae Sinensis)
Sheng Ma (Rhizoma Cimicifugae)
Huang Qi (Radix Astragali Membranacei), 2 *qian* [for each of] the above

Slice the above ingredients [and take] all as one dose. Boiled in three large cups of wine down to 1 2/10 cupfuls and take while moderately warm before a meal after removing the dregs. After taking this, iron and massage the rigid place and cure will be affected. Deviated mouth with hypertonicity of the sinews is attributed to great cold in the sinews and blood network vessels. As a substitute for fire needling, this formula breaks the blood, thus removing congelation and binding and, [at the same time,] draining the raging fire of the penetrating vessel internally.

Wei Feng Tang
(Stomach Wind Decoction)

[This formula] treats vacuity [plus] wind condition with ability to eat, numbness, spasmed, clenched jaws, twitching in the eyes, wind existing in the stomach, and swelling only in the face. Given the signs and symptoms, it appears that Li is referring to a qi vacuity allowing entrance to externally contracted wind evils.

Man Jing Zi (Fructus Viticis), 1 *fen*
Gan Jiang (dry Rhizoma Zingiberis Officinalis), 2 *fen*
Cao Dou Kou (Semen Alpiniae Katsumadai)
Huang Bai (Cortex Phellodendri)
Qiang Huo (Radix Et Rhizoma Notopterygii)
Chai Hu (Radix Bupleuri)
Gao Ben (Radix Et Rhizoma Ligustici Sinensis), 3 *fen* [for each of]
    the above
Ma Huang (Herba Ephedrae), 5 *fen*, with the joints preserved
Dang Gui (Radix Angelicae Sinensis)
Cang Zhu (Rhizoma Atractylodis)
Ge Gen (Radix Puerariae), 1 *qian* [for each of] the above
fresh *Bai Zhi* (Radix Angelicae Dahuricae), 1.2 *qian*
mix-fried *Gan Cao* (Radix Glycyrrhizae Uralensis), 1.5 *qian*
Sheng Ma (Rhizoma Cimicifugae), 2 *qian*
Da Zao (Fructus Zizyphi Jujubae), 4 pieces

Slice the above the size of cannabis seeds and separate into two doses, each boiled in two cups of water down to one cupful. Take while hot after meals after removing the dregs.

It has always seemed like overkill to me to treat twitching eyelids due to transient stress with wind-extinguishing formulas. The severity of the symptom never seemed to match the treatment principles of settling the liver and extinguishing wind. This formula suggests another approach: coursing of the liver and rectifying the qi, fortifying of the spleen and supplementing the blood, resolving the exterior and coursing wind, and eliminating dampness and clearing heat. In this case, a chronic spleen qi vacuity has made it easy for wind evils to enter the body from outside due to a defensive qi vacuity. I have seen many patients over the last two or more decades with twitching eyelids presenting a pattern of liver-spleen disharmony with dampness and depressive or damp heat. I must honestly say that, till now, it did not occur to me that the twitching eyelids may have been due to externally contracted wind.

Endnotes

1 *Su Wen,* Ch. 65

2 *Ibid.*

3 There are various *Xie Gan San* (Drain the Liver Powders), but there are none found by the translator that are composed of *Qian Niu Zi* (Semen Pharbiditis). For reference, a typical *Xie Gan San* formula is composed of: *Jie Geng* (Radix Platycodi Grandifori), *Huang Qin* (Radix Scutellariae Baicalensis), *Da Huang* (Radix Et Rhizoma Rhei), *Zhi Zi* (Fructus Gardeniae Jasminoidis), *Che Qian Zi* (Semen Plantaginis), and *Mang Xiao* (Mirabilitum).

4 This is composed of: *Ren Shen* (Radix Panacis Ginseng), 5 *qian,* *Mai Men Dong* (Tuber Ophiopogonis Japonici), and *Wu Wei Zi* (Fructus Schisandrae Chinensis), 3 *qian* each.

5 This formula may be composed of: processed *Zhi Ke* (Fructus Citri Aurantii), *Fang Feng* (Radix Ledebouriellae Divaricatae), *Qiang Huo* (Radix Et Rhizoma Notopterygii), *Du Huo* (Radix Angelicae Pubescentis), *Bin Lan* (Semen Arecae Catechu), *Bai Zhi* (Radix Angelicae Dahuricae), *Wei Ling Xian* (Radix Clematidis Chinensis), stir-fried *Bai Ji Li* (Fructus Tribuli Terrestris), stir-fried *Huo Ma Ren* (Semen Cannabis Sativae), *Xing Ren* (Semen Pruni Armeniacae), *Gan Cao* (Radix Glycyrrhizae Uralensis), and honey (*Mi Tang*).

11

Treatise on the Yang Ming Disease of Overwhelming Dampness & Spontaneous Perspiration

Some people may ask, between dampness and sweating, which is yin and which is yang? It is said [they both correspond to] *kun* earth of the southwest [as do] the spleen and stomach. This suggests that dampness and sweating are both related to earth, *i.e.,* the spleen and stomach. *Kun* is one of the eight trigrams. It corresponds to the southwest in space and earth in the five phases. Sweating is to humans what rain is to heaven and earth. Enriched by yin, dampness turns into mist, dew, and rain. Yin dampness is the cold, downward movement of the earth qi. This relates dampness to yin and also connotes something excessive or chilling. Profuse sweating leads to collapse of yang. When yang is gone, yin overwhelms, and, in serious [cases,] center cold [ensues]. With dampness overwhelming, the voice is heard as if issuing from a jar. This shows that, [in this case,] the dampness is [as serious] as water stroke. Some people pronounce the word earth as from a deep jar. The Chinese pronunciation of the word earth is *tu*. The issue of the pronunciation of the word *tu* is apparently raised to describe a property of earth or the spleen and stomach and to relate dampness to earth. This is descriptive of a muffled sound as if coming from a distance, [a voice] not issuing [or articulated with difficulty]. From this, it is evident that [there is] dampness. [From this,] it is also known that both of these [*i.e.,* profuse sweating and dampness] are [ascribed to] yin cold. The *Nei Jing (Inner Classic)* says, "Qi vacuity leads to exterior cold."[1] For instance, center heat with steaming perspiration, however intense, will be transmuted into great cold in the end. It is known that, because of exterior vacuity and yang collapse, center heat cannot resist external cold and will be transmuted into center cold eventually, giving rise to impediment cold in most cases. This describes the progression of diabetes mellitus where first there is internal heat mixed with spleen vacuity. Eventually, the spleen and kidneys become so vacuous and weak that vacuity cold is engendered. Because of this vacuity cold and lack of qi to propel the blood, there is blood stasis causing chest impediment associated with cardiovascular disease. Sweating abnormalities, including spontaneous perspiration, are one of the neuropathic complications of diabetes. The [facial] color [or complexion] reflects heaven, while the pulse reflects the earthly form. Heaven here may mean the exterior, while the earth may mean the interior. Because of the ambiguity of this phrase, the sentence may also be rendered: "Examine the face regarding the complexion; examine the inch opening regarding the pulse." That is, the yin and yang of earth. Therefore, via the signs of the pulse and qi, one can see [both] the form and the formless. Qi here most likely means the complexion. Even to this day in colloquial Chinese, *qi se* or qi color is often used to denote the complexion.

Tiao Wei Tang
(Regulating the Defensive Decoction)

[This formula] treats overwhelming dampness and spontaneous perspiration. It supplements defensive qi vacuity weakness with exterior vacuity not resisting external cold.

Su Mu (Lignum Sappan)
Hong Hua (Flos Carthami Tinctorii), 1 *fen* each
Zhu Ling (Sclerotium Polypori Umbellati), 2 *fen*
Mai Men Dong (Tuber Ophiopogonis Japonici)
Sheng Di (uncooked Radix Rehmanniae Glutinosae), 3 *fen* [for each of] the above
Ban Xia (Rhizoma Pinelliae Ternatae), washed with boiled water 7 times
uncooked *Huang Qin* (Radix Scutellariae Baicalensis)
uncooked *Gan Cao* (Radix Glycyrrhizae Uralensis)
Dang Gui Shao (Extremitas Radicis Angelicae Sinensis), 5 *fen* [for each of] the above
Qiang Huo (Radix Et Rhizoma Notopterygii), 7 *fen*
Ma Huang Gen (Radix Ephedrae)
Huang Qi (Radix Astragali Membranacei), 1 *qian* each
Wu Wei Zi (Fructus Schisandrae Chinensis), 7 pieces

Slice the above the size of cannabis seeds and [take] all in one dose. Boiled in two cups of water down to one cupful and take while moderately hot after removing the dregs. Wind stroke condition is invariably accompanied by spontaneous perspiration. Since the promotion of perspiration is not allowed in case of profuse sweating, *Ma Huang* (Herba Ephedrae) is prohibited and its root nodes are used [instead].

Endnotes

[1] *Su Wen*, Ch. 53

12

Treatise on Damp Heat Producing Wilting & Lung Metal Suffering Evils

In the sixth and seventh months, the governance of dampness is exercised vigorously. Because the child is capable of causing repletion in the mother, heat becomes effulgent. Dampness corresponds to the spleen which is earth. According to five phase theory, earth (dampness) is engendered by fire (*i.e.*, the heart). Based on this idea, this sentence implies that dampness (the child) makes heart fire (the mother) effulgent. Dampness and heat conspire to torment *geng* (S7), the large intestine. Therefore cold and cool [medicinals] should be used to rescue it. Since dry metal suffers from evil damp heat, the source of engenderment and transformation of cold water is exhausted. As a result of this source exhaustion, the kidneys become depleted. Hence the disease of wilting and reversal occurs with wilting, limpness, paralysis, and inability to stir [or move] the low back and below. Movement and standing are not correct [or healthy] and both feet step awry. [For this,] *Qing Zao Tang* (Clear Dryness Decoction) is indicated.

Li clearly appreciated the clinical fact that most patients with what we now refer to as autoimmune diseases accompanied by paralysis and atrophy present a liver-spleen disharmony, damp heat, and liver-kidney vacuity. Whether Li's five phase explanation of the disease mechanisms is germane or not, his treatment strategy exactly matches these disease mechanisms.

Qing Zao Tang (Clear Dryness Decoction)

Huang Lian (Rhizoma Coptidis Chinensis), stripped of hair
wine-processed *Huang Bai* (Cortex Phellodendri)
Chai Hu (Radix Bupleuri), 1 *fen* [for each of] the above
Mai Men Dong (Tuber Ophiopogonis Japonici)
Dang Gui (Radix Angelicae Sinensis)
Sheng Di (uncooked Radix Rehmanniae Glutinosae)
mix-fried *Gan Cao* (Radix Glycyrrhizae Uralensis)

Zhu Ling (Sclerotium Polypori Umbellati)
Shen Qu (Massa Medica Fermentata), 2 *fen* [for each of] the above
Ren Shen (Radix Panacis Ginseng)
Fu Ling (Sclerotium Poriae Cocos)
Sheng Ma (Rhizoma Cimicifugae), 3 *fen* [for each of] the above
Chen Pi (Pericarpium Citri Reticulatae)
Bai Zhu (Rhizoma Atractylodis Macrocephalae)
Ze Xie (Rhizoma Alismatis Orientalis), 5 *fen* [for each of] the above
Cang Zhu (Rhizoma Atractylodis), 1 *qian*
Huang Qi (Radix Astragali Membranacei), 1.5 *qian*
Wu Wei Zi (Fructus Schisandrae Chinensis), 9 pieces

Within this formula, *Huang Qi, Ren Shen, Bai Zhu, Fu Ling, Cang Zhu, and* mix-fried *Gan Cao* all fortify the spleen and supplement the qi. *Chai Hu, Sheng Ma,* and *Chen Pi* course the liver and resolve depression, upbear the clear and disin-hibit the qi mechanism. *Huang Lian* and *Huang Bai* clear heat and eliminate damp-ness. *Zhu Ling, Fu Ling,* and *Ze Xie* seep dampness, while *Bai Zhu* and *Cang Zhu* dry dampness. *Mai Men Dong* and *Wu Wei Zi* enrich yin and engender fluids which have been damaged by enduring heat. *Dang Gui* and *Sheng Di* nourish, cool, and quicken the blood. *Shen Qu* transforms food and abducts stagnation in case spleen qi vacuity, liver depression, and damp obstruction have resulted in food stagnation. This is still an excellent formula for use in contemporary clin-ical practice with conditions such as MS and SLE.

Slice the above the size of cannabis seeds and [take] 0.5 *liang* per dose. Boil in two and a half cups of water down to one cupful and take while moderately hot on an empty stomach after removing the dregs.

Zhu Yang He Xue Bu Qi Tang (Assist Yang, Harmonize the Blood & Supplement the Qi Decoction)

[This formula] treats the sequelae of eye [diseases] with congestion of heat in the upper [body] reddening of the whites of the eyes, profuse eye discharge and tears, and painless, itching eyes which are difficult to open. This [is due to] exces-sive administration of bitter, cold medicinals which have disabled the true qi from freely flowing to the nine orifices. Therefore, [there is] clouded, flowery, unclear vision. [In this case,] one should assist yang, harmonize the blood, and supplement the qi. Overdosage of bitter, cold medicinals has caused damage to the spleen yang. Because it cannot upbear and out-thrust, it has become depressed and transformed into heat. This heat has then followed the stomach channel upward to the eye, thus resulting in the above signs and symptoms. This is, yet again, a depressive heat scenario, where there is a concomitant spleen qi vacuity. Therefore, when Li says one should assist yang, he does not mean in the contemporary sense of invigorating yang but rather promoting the upbearing and effusing of the clear yang of the middle burner. In addition, a spleen qi vacuity has resulted in a qi and blood dual vacuity. Therefore, the eyes are also not being nourished and empowered at the same time as they are being harassed by ascending heat.

> fresh *Bai Zhi* (Radix Angelicae Dahuricae), 2 *fen*
> *Man Jing Zi* (Fructus Viticis), 3 *fen*
> mix-fried *Gan Cao* (Radix Glycyrrhizae Uralensis)
> *Dang Gui* (Radix Angelicae Sinensis), wine-washed
> *Chai Hu* (Radix Bupleuri), 5 *fen* [for each of] the above
> *Sheng Ma* (Rhizoma Cimicifugae)
> *Fang Feng* (Radix Ledebouriellae Divaricatae), 7 *fen* each
> *Huang Qi* (Radix Astragali Membranacei), 1 *qian*

Slice the above [and take] all in one dose. Boil in 1 1/2 cups of water down to one cupful and take while hot before going to bed after removing the dregs. Sleep under protection from the wind, guard against wind and cold, and refrain from cold food.

Although this is not a hugely useful formula in contemporary clinical practice, it still exemplifies Li's basic prescriptive methodology.

Sheng Yang Tang (Upbear Yang Decoction)

[This formula] treats 3-4 bowel movements per day with loose but not profuse stools, occasional diarrhea, rumbling in the abdomen, and yellow urine.

> *Chai Hu* (Radix Bupleuri)
> *Yi Zhi Ren* (Fructus Alpiniae Oxyphyllae)
> *Dang Gui* (Radix Angelicae Sinensis)
> *Chen Pi* (Pericarpium Citri Reticulatae), 3 *fen* [for each of] the above
> *Sheng Ma* (Rhizoma Cimicifugae), 6 *fen*
> *Gan Cao* (Radix Glycyrrhizae Uralensis), 2 *qian*
> *Huang Qi* (Radix Astragali Membranacei), 3 *qian*
> *Hong Hua* (Flos Carthami Tinctorii), a small amount

Separate the above into two doses. Boil each in two large cups of water down to one cupful and take while moderately hot after removing the dregs.

This is another potential base formula for the treatment of irritable bowel syndrome due to a liver-spleen disahrmony.

Sheng Yang Chu Shi Tang
(Upbear Yang & Eliminate Dampness Decoction)

[This formula] treats spleen-stomach vacuity weakness [with] no thought for food, borborygmus, abdominal pain, unchecked diarrhea, yellow urine, and encumbrance and weakness of the four limbs.

> Gan Cao (Radix Glycyrrhizae Uralensis)
> powdered Mai Ya (Fructus Germinatus Hordei Vulgaris), introduced in
>   case of cold stomach and rumbling in the abdomen
> Chen Pi (Pericarpium Citri Reticulatae)
> Zhu Ling (Sclerotium Polypori Umbellati), 3 fen [for each of] the above
> Ze Xie (Rhizoma Alismatis Orientalis)
> Yi Zhi Ren (Fructus Alpiniae Oxyphyllae)
> Ban Xia (Rhizoma Pinelliae Ternatae)
> Fang Feng (Radix Ledebouriellae Divaricatae)
> Shen Qu (Massa Medica Fermentata)
> Sheng Ma (Rhizoma Cimicifugae)
> Chai Hu (Radix Bupleuri)
> Qiang Huo (Radix Et Rhizoma Notopterygii), 5 fen [for each of] the above
> Cang Zhu (Rhizoma Atractylodis), 1 qian

Slice the above [and take] all in one dose. Boil in three large cups of water together with three slices of ginger and two dates down to one cupful. Take on an empty stomach after removing the dregs.

This is another potential formula for the treatment of irritable bowel syndrome with a liver-spleen disharmony and lots of dampness but no or not much heat. The patient may also suffer from damp impediment pain or bodily heaviness.

Yi Wei Tang
(Boost the Stomach Decoction)

[This formula] treats head oppression, slight headache following taxation and stirring, no liking for food or drink, fatigue of the four limbs, agitating heat, shortness of breath, inability of the mouth to know flavor [or taste the flavor of food], borborygmus, slightly loose, yellow-colored stools, bodily languor, and a dry mouth with no liking for chilled foods. Slightly loose, possibly ribbon-like, yellow-colored stools typically indicate a spleen vacuity with damp heat in which dampness is more than heat. It is a commonly seen presentation with patients with such intestinal dysbioses as candidiasis.

> *Huang Qi* (Radix Astragali Membranacei)
> *Gan Cao* (Radix Glycyrrhizae Uralensis)
> *Ban Xia* (Rhizoma Pinelliae Ternatae), 2 *fen* [for each of] the above
> *Huang Qin* (Radix Scutellariae Baicalensis)
> *Chai Hu* (Radix Bupleuri)
> *Ren Shen* (Radix Panacis Ginseng)
> *Yi Zhi Ren* (Fructus Alpiniae Oxyphyllae)
> *Bai Zhu* (Rhizoma Atractylodis Macrocephalae), 3 *fen* [for each of] the above
> *Dang Gui Wei* (Extremitas Radicis Angelicae Sinensis)
> *Chen Pi* (Pericarpium Citri Reticulatae)
> *Sheng Ma* (Rhizoma Cimicifugae), 5 *fen* [for each of] the above
> *Cang Zhu* (Rhizoma Atractylodis), 1.5 *qian*

Slice the above (and take) in one dose, boiled in 2 large cups of water down to 1 cupful while moderately hot before a meal after removing the dregs. Refrain from dietary irregularity, raw, cold, and hard foods, wine, and sodden wheat food.

This is yet another good formula for the treatment of IBS due to a liver-spleen disharmony with dampness and heat. In this case, dampness is more and heat is less. When heat is more, the stools typically turn dark in color and become foul-smelling. This formula is basically a modification of *Bu Zhong Yi Qi Tang* (Supplement the Center & Boost the Qi Decoction). *Ban Xia, Cang Zhu,* and *Yi Zhi Ren* have been added to further eliminate dampness and stop diarrhea, while *Huang Qin* has been added to gently clear heat from the stomach and intestines.

Sheng Jiang He Zhong Tang (Fresh Ginger Harmonize the Center Decoction)

[This formula] treats inability to descend food [*i.e.,* eat], a dry mouth, vacuity thirst, and encumbrance and fatigue of the four limbs.

> uncooked *Gan Cao* (Radix Glycyrrhizae Uralensis)

mix-fried *Gan Cao* (Radix Glycyrrhizae Uralensis), 1 *fen* each
wine-processed *Huang Qin* (Radix Scutellariae Baicalensis)
Chai Hu (Radix Bupleuri)
Chen Pi (Pericarpium Citri Reticulatae), 2 *fen* [for each of] the above
Sheng Ma (Rhizoma Cimicifugae), 3 *fen*
Ren Shen (Radix Panacis Ginseng)
Ge Gen (Radix Puerariae)
Gao Ben (Radix Et Rhizoma Ligustici Sinensis)
Bai Zhu (Rhizoma Atractylodis Macrocephalae), 5 *fen* [for each of]
    the above
Qiang Huo (Radix Et Rhizoma Notopterygii), 7 *fen*
Cang Zhu (Rhizoma Atractylodis), 1 *qian*
uncooked *Huang Qin* (Radix Scutellariae Baicalensis), 2 *qian*

Slice the above [and take] in one dose. Boil in one cup of water together with five slices of ginger and two broken dates down to one cupful. Take while moderately hot before a meal after removing the dregs.

Qiang Wei Tang
(Invigorate the Stomach Decoction)

[This formula] treats the results of damage by drinking and food, and taxation and overwork, abdominal and rib-side fullness and oppression, shortness of breath, a bland, flavorless taste in the mouth in spring, aversion to cold despite heat in summer, constant satiation, and no liking for eating chilled things.

Huang Bai (Cortex Phellodendri)
Gan Cao (Radix Glycyrrhizae Uralensis), 5 *fen* each
Sheng Ma (Rhizoma Cimicifugae)
Chai Hu (Radix Bupleuri)
Dang Gui (Radix Angelicae Sinensis)
Chen Pi (Pericarpium Citri Reticulatae), 1 *qian* [for each of] the above
Sheng Jiang (uncooked Rhizoma Zingiberis Officinalis)
Shen Qu (Massa Medica Fermentata), 1.5 *qian*
Cao Dou Kou (Semen Alpiniae Katsumadai), 2 *qian*
Ban Xia (Rhizoma Pinelliae Ternatae)
Ren Shen (Radix Panacis Ginseng), 3 *qian* each
Huang Qi (Radix Astragali Membranacei), 1 *liang*

Slice the above and [take] three *qian* per dose, boiled in two large cups of water down to one cupful. Take while warm before meals after removing the dregs.

Still another liver-spleen disharmony formula with dampness and heat, but mostly dampness. This formula is also appropriate for a liver-spleen disharmony with summerheat dampness as opposed to summerheat heat.

Wen Wei Tang
(Warm the Stomach Decoction)

[This formula] particularly treats spleen-stomach vacuity weakness with stomach duct pain [as a result of] administering too many cold medicinals.

Ren Shen (Radix Panacis Ginseng)
Gan Cao (Radix Glycyrrhizae)
Yi Zhi Ren (Fructus Alpiniae Oxyphyllae)
Sha Ren (Fructus Amomi)
Hou Po (Cortex Magnoliae Officinalis), 2 *fen* [for each of] the above
Bai Dou Kou (Fructus Cardamomi)
Sheng [*Jiang* and] *Gan Jiang* (uncooked and dry Rhizoma Zingiberis Officinalis)
Ze Xie (Rhizoma Alismatis Orientalis)
Jiang Huang (Rhizoma Curcumae Longae), 3 *fen* [for each of] the above
Huang Qi (Radix Astragali Membranacei)
Chen Pi (Pericarpium Citri Reticulatae), 7 *fen* each

Powder the above ingredients very finely. (Then take) three *qian* per dose, boiled in one cup of water down to half a cupful. Take while warm before meals.

He Zhong Wan
(Harmonize the Center Pills)

Ren Shen (Radix Panacis Ginseng)
Sheng [*Jiang* and] *Gan Jiang* (uncooked and dry Rhizoma Zingiberis Officinalis)
Ju Hong (Pericarpium Citri Erythrocarpae), 1 *qian* [for each of] the above
dry *Mu Gua* (Fructus Chaenomelis Lagenariae), 2 *qian*
mix-fried *Gan Cao* (Radix Glycyrrhizae Uralensis), 3 *qian*

Powder the above and make the steamed cake into pills the size of Chinese parasol tree seeds. Take 30-50 pills per dose with warm water before meals. Steamed cake refers to fermented wheat flour which is shaped into pancake form and then steamed to cook.

Huo Xiang An Wei San
(Agastaches Calm the Stomach Powder)

[This formula] treats spleen-stomach vacuity weakness with inability to ingest food and drink, and spitting and vomiting [before the food has time] to obtain rottening and ripening.

Huo Xiang (Herba Agastachis Seu Pogostemi)
Ding Xiang (Flos Caryophylli)
Ren Shen (Radix Panacis Ginseng), 2.5 qian
Ju Hong (Exocarpium Citri Erythrocarpae), 5 qian

Powder the above four ingredients (and take) two qian per dose. Boil in one large cup of water together with one slice of ginger down to 7/10 and take while cold before a meal without the dregs removed.

Yi Gong San
(Wonder-working Powder)

[This formula] treats spleen-stomach vacuity cold [with] borborygmus and pain, self-disinhibited [stools, i.e., loose stools], and no thought for drinking and eating.

Ren Shen (Radix Panacis Ginseng)
Fu Ling (Sclerotium Poriae Cocos)
Bai Zhu (Rhizoma Atractylodis Macrocephalae)
Gan Cao (Radix Glycyrrhizae Uralensis)
Chen Pi (Pericarpium Citri Reticulatae), 5 fen [for each of] the above

Powder the above coarsely [and take] five qian per dose. Boil in two large cups of water together with three slices of ginger and two dates down to one cupful. Take while warm before meals after removing the dregs. First administer several doses [of the above prescription] to rectify the [stomach] qi.

This formula is only one medicinal shy of being Liu Jun Zi Tang (Six Gentlemen Decoction).

13

Treatise on Drinking & Eating Damaging the Spleen

The *Si Shi Jiu Nan (49th Difficulty)* states, "Food and drink and taxation fatigue may lead to damage of the spleen."[1] It is also stated that [if one eats] twice the ordinary food intake, this will damage the stomach and intestines and intestinal afflux may thus cause piles. Intestinal afflux refers to noisy diarrhea and dysentery. The spleen moves the stomach fluids and humors, grinds grain within the stomach, and governs the five flavors. [If] the stomach is damaged, this leads to food and drink not being transformed, no knowledge of flavor in the mouth [*i.e.*, inability to taste food], fatigue and encumbrance of the four limbs, heart and abdominal glomus and fullness, daze, a desire to vomit, aversion to food, and swill diarrhea or intestinal afflux. [In this case,] it is clear that the spleen as well as the stomach has been damaged. Generally speaking, damage [due to] drinking and damage [due to] eating are not treated the same. Damage [due to] drinking is a damage done by formless qi. [Therefore,] it should [be treated] by effusing sweat and disinhibiting urination in order to abduct dampness. Damage [due to] eating is a damage [due to] a substance that has form. A mild [case] calls for dispersion and transformation, though reducing grains is the wondrous [or best way]. Only a serious [case] allows for ejection and precipitation. This is a direct rebuttal of suggestions by Zhang Zi-he. Several formulas have been composed and are listed below with classification and analysis [for this condition]. In fact, there is only one formula given in this chapter. It is believed that the last seven formulas in the preceding chapter and several formulas in the next chapter should have been placed in the present chapter.

Because of the interrelationship and interdependence between the spleen and stomach, Li is extremely concerned about the effect of and treatments for food stagnation. Food stagnation complicates many patients' conditions when there is a liver-spleen disharmony and a superabundance of rich, flavorful food as in the developed world.

Wu Ling San
(Five [Ingredients] Poria Powder)

[This formula] treats vexatious thirst with excessive drinking or vomiting immediately upon entry of water, a rippling [*i.e.*, sloshing] sensation within [or below]
the heart, dampness collected internally, and inhibited urination.

Gui Zhi (Ramulus Cinnamomi Cassiae), 1 *liang*
Fu Ling (Sclerotium Poriae Cocos)
Zhu Ling (Sclerotium Polypori Umbellati)
Bai Zhu (Rhizoma Atractylodis Macrocephalae), 1.5 *liang*
Ze Xie (Rhizoma Alismatis Orientalis), 2.5 *liang*

Powder the above [medicinals and take] two *qian* per dose with hot, boiled water
at any time. After taking [this prescription], drink plenty of hot soup. When
sweat exists, there will be a cure. For heat stasis in the interior with jaundice, take
[the above] mixed with thickly boiled *Yin Chen Tang* (Artemisia Capillaris
Decoction)[2] before meals. In case of jaundice with thirst or summerheat stroke
leading to drinking, it can also be taken mixed with water.

This formula is for the treatment of water stagnating in the stomach below the
heart. This is what Li refers to as damage (due to) drinking or drink damage.
While modern Western medicine recommends drinking at least eight large glasses
of water per day, this is not always a good idea. In clinical practice, every once
and a while one will come across a patient with stagnant water in his or her stomach. This patient may be thirsty and complain of a dry mouth. This is because
the water they drink is not being transformed and dispersed to the rest of the
body. Instead, it has collected and is stagnant in the stomach. Therefore, the rest
of the body registers dehydration and thirst. If one suspects that such is the case,
one should have the patient lie down on their back. Then lightly jiggle their epigastrium with one or both hands. If there is stagnant water in the stomach, one
will literally hear it sloshing around. One can also ask the patient if they hear
water sloshing in their stomach when they roll from side to side. The elimina-
tion of this stagnant water by such a formula as Li suggests usually achieves a
remarkably speedy reduction in signs and symptoms. However, the patient must
be cautioned not to drink water during this process, even if they are very thirsty.
To do so defeats the purpose of this treatment.

Endnotes

[1] *Nan Jing*, 49th Difficulty

[2] This formula is composed of: *Yin Chen Hao* (Herba Artemisiae Capillaris) and *Bai Xian Pi*
(Cortex Radicis Dictamni Dasycarpi).

14

Treatise on Damage Due to Excessive Drinking of Alcohol

This chapter is a collection of relatively simple formulas for the treatment of acute food stagnation. As such, it does not specifically deal with yin fire except parenthetically in the first paragraph. In my opinion, it is not one of the more important chapters in this book. Since Li's time, the insights and combinations suggested in this chapter have been incorporated as standard into professional Chinese medicine. However, this chapter does also provide a model of how to start with a simple two medicinal combination and then create more and more complex formulas for more complex presentations.

Wine [*i.e.*, alcohol] is greatly hot and has toxins. [Its] qi and flavor are both yang. It is a formless substance. This implies that, due to its volatility, the qi of wine is insubstantial. If damaged by it, stop drinking and one must effuse and dissipate. [As soon as] sweat exists, this will lead to cure. The second best choice is to disinhibit urination. These two [methods] separate and disperse dampness below and above [respectively]. These days, alcoholics are usually [made] to take the greatly hot medicinals of *Jiu Zhen Wan* (Wine Relieving Pills)[1] to precipitate. In addition, [some] use *Qian Niu Zi* (Semen Pharbiditis) and *Da Huang* (Radix Et Rhizoma Rhei) to precipitate. [However,] this is [tantamount to] erroneously precipitating formal yin blood when the formless original qi is suffering from disease. It is a colossal mistake. Already damaged by alcohol whose nature is intensely hot, the original qi now suffers from further drainage. Even worse, kidney water also [suffers] detriment. True yin [*i.e.*, kidney yin] and formal yin blood [thus] both become insufficient. [In this case,] yin blood is made [all] the more vacuous and true water [all] the weaker. [Hence] heat from yang toxins becomes greatly effulgent and yin fire increases contrarily, [*i.e.*, undesirably]. This is [none other than] dispersing and consuming the original qi, thus shortening the person's length of life. Even if [that does] not [happen], vacuity detriment disease will develop. [If] wine jaundice [is treated by] precipitation, eventually it will develop into black jaundice. Wine jaundice refers to jaundice induced by dissipation in wine and manifested by fever with vexation, inability to take in food, and vomiting. Black jaundice develops from wine jaundice as a result of inappropriate precipitating treatment. Black jaundice is manifested by blue-green eyes, a black facial complexion, and blackish stool with a sensation in the cardiac region of biting or burning as if having eaten a lot of garlic. Caution must be taken not to commit this blunder. *Ge Hua Jie Cheng Tang* (Pueraria Flower Resolve Hangover Decoction) is indicated [for this].

Ge Hua Jie Cheng Tang (Pueraria Flower Resolve Hangover Decoction)

[This formula] treats excessive drinking of alcohol [with] retching, vomiting, phlegm counterflow, heart spirit vexation and chaos, chest and diaphragmatic glomus and obstruction, trembling, rocking hands and feet, reduced eating and drinking, and inhibited urination.

Qing Pi (Pericarpium Citri Reticulatae Viride) with the pulp removed, 3 *fen*
Mu Xiang (Radix Auklandiae Lappae), 5 *fen*
Chen Pi (Pericarpium Citri Reticulatae), with the white inner skin removed
Ren Shen (Radix Panacis Ginseng), stemmed
Zhu Ling (Sclerotium Polypori Umbellati), stripped of the black skin
Fu Ling (Sclerotium Poriae Cocos), 1.5 *qian* [for each of] the above
Shen Qu (Massa Medica Fermentata), stir-fried to yellow
Ze Xie (Rhizoma Alismatis Orientalis)
Sheng [*Jiang*] (uncooked Rhizoma Zingiberis Officinalis) [&] *Gan Jiang* (dry Rhizoma Zingiberis Officinalis)
Bai Zhu (Rhizoma Atractylodis Macrocephalae), 2 *qian*
Bai Dou Kou (Fructus Cardamomi)
Ge Hua (Flos Puerariae)
Sha Ren (Fructus Amomi), 5 *qian* [for each of] the above

Powder the above medicinals finely, weigh, and mix evenly. [Take] three coins per dose brewed with boiled water. "Three coins" refers to a coin minted in the Han dynasty and used both as a unit of and an instrument for measurement. It was almost two grams in weight. If [one] only sweats slightly, the alcohol disease is gone. This [remedy should be] used only when necessary, [*i.e.*, as a last resort]. No one should think that they can drink alcohol day after day once in possession of this formula. This formula is acrid in qi and hot in flavor, and, only if taken to cure hangover once in a long while, will there not be detriment to the original qi. There is no [completely safe] remedy for [drinking] alcohol [to the point of drunkenness].

Zhi Zhu Wan
(Immature Citrus Aurantium & Atractylodes Pills)

[This formula] treats glomus. It disperses food and strengthens the stomach.

Zhi Shi (Fructus Immaturus Citri Aurantii), stir-fried to yellow with wheat
　bran and stripped of the pulp, 1 liang
Bai Zhu (Rhizoma Atractylodis Macrocephalae), 2 liang

Powder the above [medicinals] finely and make into pills the size of Chinese
parasol tree seeds with rice cooked with lotus leaves as a wrapping. Each time
take 50 pills with plenty of boiled water at no [particular] time. Bai Zhu is not
chosen specifically to transform food quickly but to strengthen stomach qi [so
that] there is no repeat damage.

Ju Pi Zhi Zhu Wan
(Orange Peel, Immature Citrus Aurantium
& Atractylodes Pills)

[This formula] treats [both] old and young with original qi vacuity weakness,
nondispersion of food and drink, lack of regulation of the viscera and bowels,
and glomus and fullness below the heart.

Zhi Shi (Fructus Immaturus Citri Aurantii), stir-fried with wheat bran and
　stripped of the pulp
Chen Pi (Pericarpium Citri Reticulatae), 1 liang each
Bai Zhu (Rhizoma Atractylodis Macrocephalae), 2 liang

Powder the above ingredients and make into pills the size of Chinese parasol tree
seeds with rice cooked with lotus leaves as a wrapping. Each time take 50 pills
between meals with warm water. The general principle for using these medicinals
is to value [i.e., lay great store in] strengthening the patient's stomach qi. If the
stomach qi is boosted and made thick, even [eating] ravenously, overeating, or eating double [as often] cannot damage it. This [requires] ability [or proficiency] in
using food [intake increasing] medicinals. These medicinals boost the stomach qi
if administered for a long [time]. Thus there is no recurrence of damage.

This formula is for the treatment of food damage with a spleen qi vacuity. Li theoretically might have suggested the combination of Zhi Shi and Chen Pi with
Ren Shen (Radix Panacis Ginseng) or Dang Shen (Radix Codonopsitis Pilosulae),

both qi-supplementing medicinals. However, both these medicinals tend to engender fluids, and food depression tends to become complicated by damp depression because both food and fluids are moved and dissipated by the qi. Therefore, Li has chosen the acrid and drying *Bai Zhu* in order to supplement the qi. This medicinal transforms dampness rather than engenders fluids. Hence it is a better choice for the treatment of spleen qi vacuity concomitant with food stagnation, at least when one is using such a small, little formula.

Ban Xia Zhi Zhu Wan
(Pinellia, Immature Citrus Aurantium & Atractylodes Pills)

[This formula] treats internal damage due to chilled foods.

> *Ban Xia* (Rhizoma Pinelliae Ternatae), washed with ginger juice 7 times & baked dry
> *Zhi Shi* (Fructus Immaturus Citri Aurantii), stir-fried to yellow with wheat bran
> *Bai Zhu* (Rhizoma Atractylodis Macrocephalae), 2 *liang* [for each of] the above

Powder the above together finely and make into pills the size of Chinese parasol tree seeds with rice cooked with lotus leaves as a wrapping. Take 50 pills each time. The dosage can be larger. [These pills] can be made in other ways, for example, with steamed cake soaked in boiled water.

In case of food damage [from] unregulated [eating] of cold and hot [foods], add 10 pills of *San Huang Wan* (Three Yellows Pills)[2] to each dose and take with boiled water. Another formula is composed of *Ze Xie* (Rhizoma Alismatis Orientalis), 1 *liang*, added [to the formula] and made into pills. It is used for patients with [accompanying] strangury.

Mu Xiang Gan Jiang Zhi Zhu Wan
(Auklandia, Dry Ginger, Immature Citrus Aurantium
& Atractylodes Pills)

[This formula] breaks and eliminates cold, stagnant qi and disperses cold food and drink.

> *Mu Xiang* (Radix Auklandiae Lappae), 3 *qian*
> blast-fried *Gan Jiang* (dry Rhizoma Zingiberis Officinalis), 5 *qian*

Zhi Shi (Fructus Immaturus Citri Aurantii), stir-fried, 1 *liang*
Bai Zhu (Rhizoma Atractylodis Macrocephalae), 1.5 *liang*

Powder the above finely and make into pills the size of Chinese parasol tree seeds with rice cooked with lotus leaves as a wrapping. Take 30-50 pills each time with warm water before meals.

Mu Xiang Ren Shen Sheng Jiang Zhi Zhu Wan
(Auklandia, Ginseng, Fresh Ginger, Immature Citrus Aurantium & Atractylodes Pills)

[This formula] opens the stomach and increases food intake.

Gan Sheng Jiang (dry & uncooked Rhizoma Zingiberis Officinalis), 2.5 *qian*
Mu Xiang (Radix Auklandia Lappae), 3 *qian*
Ren Shen (Radix Panacis Ginseng), 3.5 *qian*
Chen Pi (Pericarpium Citri Reticulatae), 4 *qian*
Zhi Shi (Fructus Immaturus Citri Aurantii, stir-fried to yellow,
    1 *liang*
Bai Zhu (Rhizoma Atractylodis Macrocephalae), 1.5 *liang*

Powder the above and make pills the size of Chinese parasol tree seeds with rice cooked with lotus leaves as a wrapping. Take 30-50 pills each time with warm water before meals. Overeating is prohibited.

He Zhong Wan
(Harmonize the Center Pills)

[This formula] treats enduring diseases of vacuity weakness [with a constant] satiated sensation, inability to eat, and constipation or diarrhea with thin stool. This is [a case of] stomach qi vacuity weakness. Constant administration [of this formula] harmonizes the center and rectifies the qi, disperses phlegm and eliminates dampness, thickens the stomach and intestines, and promotes drinking and eating.

Mu Xiang (Radix Auklandiae Lappae), 2.5 *qian*
Zhi Shi (Fructus Immaturus Citri Aurantii), stir-fried with wheat bran
mix-fried *Gan Cao* (Radix Glycyrrhizae Uralensis), 3.5 *qian* each
Bin Lan (Semen Arecae Catechu), 4.5 *qian*
Chen Pi (Pericarpium Citri Reticulatae), stripped of the inner white
    skin, 8 *qian*

Ban Xia (Rhizoma Pinelliae Ternatae), washed with boiled water 7 times
Hou Po (Cortex Magnoliae Officinalis), processed with ginger, 1 *liang* each
Bai Zhu (Rhizoma Atractylodis Macrocephalae), 1.2 *liang*

Powder the above, soak thoroughly with ginger juice, steam like bread, and make into pills the size of Chinese parasol tree seeds. Take 30-50 pills each time with warm water before or between meals.

Jiao Tai Wan
(Crossing Prosperity Pills)

The ascent of earthly qi and the descent of heavenly qi is called crossing prosperity. This describes the normal, healthful, natural condition of yin and yang in the phenomenal world according to the *Yi Jing (Classic of Change)*.

[This formula] upbears the yang qi, drains yin fire, regulates the constructive qi, promotes drinking and eating, assists the essence spirit, loosens the abdomen and center, and eliminates fatigue and somnolence, lack of control of the four limbs [*i.e.*, debilitation of the limbs], drowsiness, and languor.

blast-fried *Gan Jiang* (dry Rhizoma Zingiberis Officinalis), 3 *fen*
Ba Dou Shuang (Pulvis Semenis Praeparati Crotonis Tiglii)
Ren Shen (Radix Panacis Ginseng), stemmed
Rou Gui (Cortex Cinnamomi Cassiae), debarked, 1 *qian* each
Chai Hu (Radix Bupleuri), with sprouts sorted out
Xiao Jiao (Fructus Zanthoxyli Bungeani), deoiled by stir-frying. Pick out
    the uncracked fruit, and remove the seeds.
Bai Zhu (Rhizoma Atractylodis Macrocephalae), 1.5 *qian* [for each of]
    the above
Hou Po (Cortex Magnoliae Officinalis), skinned, grated & stir-fried,
    increase by 4 *qian* in autumn and winter
wine-boiled *Chuan Lian Zi* (Fructus Meliae Toosendanis)
Fu Ling (Sclerotium Poriae Cocos)
Sha Ren (Fructus Amomi), 3 *qian* [for each of] the above
Chuan Wu Tou (Radix Aconiti Carmichaeli), with skin and navel removed
    by blast-frying, 4.5 *qian*
Zhi Mu (Rhizoma Anemarrhenae Aspheloidis), 4 *qian*, half stir-fried, half
    washed with wine. This ingredient is appropriate in spring and summer
    but deleted in autumn and winter.
Wu Zhu Yu (Fructus Evodiae Rutecarpae), washed with boiled water 7
    times, 5 *qian*

Huang Lian (Rhizoma Coptidis Chinensis), stripped of hair, reduced by 1.5
   qian in autumn and winter
Zao Jiao (Fructus Gleditschiae Sinensis), washed with water, remove the
   pod by roasting
Zi Wan (Radix Asteris Tatarici), with sprouts sorted out, 6 *qian* [for each
   of]the above

Except for *Ba Dou Shuang* which should be taken separately, powder the
above finely and make into pills the size of Chinese parasol tree seeds with
heated honey. Take 10 pills each time with warm water. Add and subtract
[dosages or medicinals depending] on vacuity or repletion.

San Leng Xiao Ji Wan
(Sparganium Disperse Accumulation Pills)

[This formula] is for damage [caused by] uncooked, chilled, and hard things
[which are] unable to be dispersed and transformed [or digested] with heart and
abdominal fullness and oppression.

Ding Pi (Cortex Caryophylli)
Yi Zhi Ren (Fructus Alpiniae Oxyphyllae), 3 *qian* each
Ba Dou (Semen Crotonis Tiglii), char-fried with rice which is
   removed afterwards
Xiao Hui Xiang (Fructus Foeniculi Vulgaris)
Chen Pi (Pericarpium Citri Reticulatae)
Qing Pi (Pericarpium Citri Reticulatae Viride), 5 *qian* [for each of] the above
San Leng (Rhizoma Sparganii Stoloniferi), blast-fried
E Zhu (Rhizoma Curcumae Zedoariae), blast-fried
stir-fried *Shen Qu* (Massa Medica Fermentata), 7 *qian* [for each of] the above

Powder the above ingredients and make into pills the size of Chinese parasol tree
seeds with a paste of vinegar and flour. Take 10-20 pills each time with warm
fresh ginger soup before meals. Depending on vacuity or repletion, add and subtract [dosages and/or medicinals]. Once the bowels become relaxed, stop [fur-
ther] administration.

Bei Ji Wan
(Contingency Pills)

[This formula] treats sudden piercing pain in hundreds of heart and abdominal
diseases. They are also [indicated for] distention, fullness, lack of happiness, and
distressed rapid breathing.

striped Sichuan *Da Huang* (Radix Et Rhizoma Rhei)
Gan Jiang (dry Rhizoma Zingiberis Officinalis), powdered by blast-frying
Ba Dou (Semen Crotonis Tiglii), with the skin and core washed off, ground
    into paste, deoiled, used in the form of powder

Grind equal amounts of the above three ingredients and prepare with heated honey. Pound in a mortar hundreds of times and make into pills the size of a big pea. Take one pill with warm water before going to bed in the evening. In case of qi repletion, add one pill. [In case of] sudden attack of disease, take this any time. Administration [of this formula] is not ok for pregnant women. If the food that causes the damage stays somewhere in the chest and diaphragm with the stomach turning, desire to vomit, and repeated oppression and agitation, remove this by probing [the throat] with something [to cause vomiting].

Shen Bao Wan
(Spirit-protecting Pills)

[This formula] treats heart and diaphragmatic pain, abdominal pain, blood pain, kidney qi pain [*i.e.*, low back pain with weak feet and knees], rib-side pain, non-freely flowing stools, qi choking, and food retention without dispersion.

Mu Xiang (Radix Auklandiae Lappae
Hu Jiao (Fructus Piperis Nigri), 2.5 *qian* each
Ba Dou (Semen Crotonis Tiglii), 10 pieces, skinned, deoiled, cored
    & ground
dried *Quan Xie* (Buthus Martensis), 7 pieces

Powder the above four flavors [or ingredients] and make into pills the size of cannabis seeds with boiled water soaked steamed cake coated with three *qian* of *Zhu Sha* (Cinnabaris). Take five pills each time.

In case of heart and diaphragmatic pain, take these with *Shi Di* (Calyx Diospyri Khaki) and *Deng Xin Cao* (Medulla Junci Effusi) soup. In case of abdominal pain, take these with *Shi Di* (Calyx Diospyri Khaki) and roasted ginger soup. In case of blood pain, take these with stir-fried ginger and vinegar soup. In case of kidney qi pain and rib-side pain, take these with *Xiao Hui Xiang* (Fructus Foeniculi Vulgaris) wine. In case of non-freely flowing stools, take these with powdered *Bin Lan* (Semen Arecae Catechu) brewed in honey. In case of qi choking, take these with *Mu Xiang* (Radix Auklandiae Lappae) soup. In case of food retention without dispersion, take these with tea or wine or boiled water.

Xiong Huang Sheng Bing Zi
(Realgar Divine Cake)

[This formula] treats all kinds of alcohol and food damage with heart and abdominal fullness and lack of happiness.

Xiong Huang (Realgar), 5 *qian*
Ba Dou (Semen Crotonis Tiglii), 100 pieces, deoiled, cored & skinned
Wheat flour, 10 *liang*, sifted twice [before use]

Except for the flour of which 8-9 *liang* should be left [aside], powder finely the above ingredients, mix evenly with the flour, and make into cakes the size of the palm with fresh water. Boil these in cooked millet water till the cakes rise and float on the surface. In other words, cook some millet and put it in cold water. Then let it sit for 5-6 days till the millet has fermented and turned sour. Remove these and get rid of [excess] water by pressing. Pound them, [the number of times varying] in accordance with their hardness and make into pills the size of Chinese parasol tree seeds. Then press these into [the shape of a] cake. Take 5-7 cakes each time, possibly increased to [more than] 5-7, 10, or [even] 15. [For every] one cake chewed, [there will be] one [bowel] movement. Two cakes chewed [will induce] two [bowel] movements. Take these either with tea or wine before meals.

Juan Yin Zhi Shi Wan
(Alleviate Rheum Immature Citrus Aurantium Pills)

[This formula] expels rheum and clears phlegm, abducts stagnation and clears the diaphragm.

Zhi Shi (Fructus Immaturus Citri Aurantii), stir-fried with bran, stripped of pulp
Ban Xia (Rhizoma Pinelliae Ternatae), washed with boiled water
Chen Pi (Pericarpium Citri Reticulatae), stripped of the inner white skin, 2 *liang* for each of the above
black *Qian Niu Zi* (Semen Pharbiditis), 8 *liang*, of which only 3 *liang* of the ground sifted powder is left for use

Powder the above and make into pills the size of Chinese parasol tree seeds with cooked flour paste. Take 50 pills each time with ginger soup after meals.

Gan Ying Wan
([Swift] Reacting Pills)

[This formula] treats vacuity of the middle [burner] with accumulation and chill, weak damaged qi, collection and accumulation in the stomach duct with inability to convey and transform, or qi damaged by chilled [food], surfeit following hunger, or drinking excessive alcohol [resulting in] hardness and fullness below the heart, rib-side distention and pain, severe heart and abdominal pain, sudden turmoil with vomiting and diarrhea, frequent defecation, tenesmus with slow, astringent [evacuation], enduring red and white dysentery with mixed blood and pus [in the stool], untransformed rice and grain [in the stool], and remission and relapse [of the illness]. In addition, [this formula] treats wine stroke with retching, vomiting, phlegm counterflow, nausea, a predilection to spitting, spinning head, chest and diaphragmatic glomus and oppression, fatigue of the four limbs, and no desire for eat or drink. [It] also treats damage due to chill in pregnancy and damage freshly [inflicted in child] delivery as well as enduring accumulation and cold with no effect after [administration of] hot medicinals. [Further,] they also treat enduring languished form from years-long chronic disease gradually resulting in vacuity weakness, a yellow facial complexion, emaciated flesh, eating and drinking sometimes increasing and sometimes decreasing, and sometimes constipation and sometimes diarrhea. In addition, they treat accumulation and cold, whether it be enduring or new.

Gan Jiang (Rhizoma Zingiberis Officinalis), blast-fried, 1 *liang*
southern *Mu Xiang* (Radix Auklandiae Lappae), stemmed
Ding Xiang (Flos Caryophylli), 1.5 *liang* each
Bai Cao Shuang (Pulvis Fumi Carbonisati), 2 liang
Rou Dou Kou (Semen Myristicae Fragrantis), skinned, 30 pieces
Ba Dou (Semen Crotonis Tiglii), skinned, cored, stripped of membrane, deoiled & ground, 70 pieces
Xing Ren (Semen Pruni Armeniacae), 140 pieces, soaked with boiled water, skinned, tipped & smashed

Except for the powdered *Ba Dou, Bai Cao Shuang,* and *Xing Ren,* pound the other four of the above seven flavors [or ingredients] into fine powder. Then mix this with the [other] three, grind fine, and finally mix [all this] with casing wax. Wax is commonly applied as a protective coating for various pills. Therefore, such pills have acquired the name of casing wax. However, in this formula, wax is not used as a coating but is mixed in as an ingredient with the other medicinals. The first step is to melt six *liang* of wax. Filter it through a double layer of silk cloth to rid it of impurities, [re]heat, keep it boiling for a while in one *sheng* of good wine contained in a silver or stone vessel, and finally pour it out. Do not collect the wax till the wine has cooled and the wax has risen to the surface. Weigh it and separate it into nuggets for use. In spring and summer, to prepare these pills, first boil one *liang* of sesame oil in a ladle till the scum has dispersed and it emits a fragrant [odor]. Then put in [this] and melt four *liang* of wine-processed wax. Finally, put in and mix the above medicinals in the ladle while [the mixture of oil and wax] is still hot. To prepare these pills in autumn and winter, 1.5 *liang* of sesame oil is used. This is boiled together with wine- processed wax till [the wax] is melted and then mixed with the powdered medicinals. Prepare this mixture as nuggets which are [then] wrapped with single-layer oil paper. Before taking, roll them into [small] pills.

Shen Ying Wan
(Divinely Responding Pills)

[This formula] treats abdominal pain, borborygmus, and untransformed rice and grain [in the stool] caused by chilled things, iced water, sheep milk, and [various] beverages [including wine or boiled fruit juice or pulp].

Ding Xiang (Flos Caryophylli)
Mu Xiang (Radix Auklandiae Lappae), 2 *qian* each
Ba Dou (Semen Crotonis Tiglii)
Xing Ren (Semen Pruni Armeniacae)
Bai Cao Shuang (Pulvis Fumi Carbonisati)
Gan Jiang (Rhizoma Zingiberis Officinalis), 5 *qian* [for each of] the above
Yellow wax, 2 *liang*

[Among] the above, first remove the impurities from the yellow wax by boiling it in vinegar. *Ba Dou* and *Xing Ren* should be stir-fried together till black smoke is no longer seen and then ground into paste. Heat the yellow wax again and put in five *qian* of oil in spring and summer or eight *qian* in autumn and winter. Pour in and mix the smashed *Xing Ren* and *Ba Dou*, but not till the wax is melted. Then put in the powdered *Ding Xiang, Mu Xiang*, and the others. Grind the mixture evenly, roll it into nuggets which should be wrapped in oil paper, and then roll them into pills. Take 30-50 pills each time with warm, thin rice gruel before meals three times a day. These are divinely [or magically] effective.

Bai Zhu An Wei San
(Atractylodes Quiet the Stomach Powder)

[This formula] treats all kinds of diarrhea and dysentery irrespective of mixed blood and pus in the stool, tenesmus and pain, or [diarrhea] day and night without limit. It also treats men's small intestinal qi pain [or hernia], while in females, [it treats] vacuity chill below the umbilicus and postpartum child's pillow conglomeration pain. Child's pillow conglomeration pain refers to a hard, painful lump in the lower abdomen with tenderness traditionally believed to be caused by pillowing of the fetus in the womb. In addition, it treats postpartum vacuity weakness and incessant cold and heat.

Wu Wei Zi (Fructus Schisandrae Chinensis)
Wu Mei (Fructus Pruni Mume), procure and stir-fry to dry the pulp [for use], 5 qian each
Che Qian Zi (Semen Plantaginis)
Fu Ling (Sclerotium Poriae Cocos)
Bai Zhu (Rhizoma Atractylodis Macrocephalae), 2 liang [for each of] the above
Ying Su Ke (Pericarpium Papaveris Somniferi), 3 liang, stripped of the tip, the base, and the pulp, boiled in vinegar overnight, and dry by stir-frying

Powder the above and take five qian each time boiled in 1 1/2 cups of water down to one cupful and taken while warm on an empty stomach after removing the dregs.

Sheng Bing Zi
(Divine Cake)

[This formula] treats red and white diarrhea and dysentery with [peri]umbilical and abdominal gripping pain which endures and does not heal.

Huang Dan (Minium), 2 qian
Ding Fen (Carbonate of lead)
Liu Huang (Sulphur) from abroad
Mi Tuo Seng (Lithargyum), 3 qian [for each of] the above
Qing Fen (Calomelas), a small amount

Grind the above [medicinals] finely. Put in four coins of wheat flour and drip in water [until one] gets a mixture the size of the fingertip. Roll this into a cake and dry in the shade. [Before taking it,] rub it in warm, cooked millet water and take before meals. Black-colored stools prove [its] efficacy.

Dang Gui He Xue San (Dang Gui Harmonize the Blood Powder)

[This formula] treats intestinal afflux with blood in the stool and damp toxins with blood in the stool.

> *Chuan Xiong* (Radix Ligustici Wallichii), 4 *fen*
> *Qing Pi* (Pericarpium Citri Reticulatae Viride)
> *Huai Hua Mi* (Flos Immaturus Sophorae Japonicae)
> *Jing Jie Sui* (Herba Seu Flos Schizonepetae Tenuifoliae)
> *Shu Di* (cooked Radix Rehmanniae Glutinosae)
> *Bai Zhu* (Rhizoma Atractylodis Macrocephalae), 6 *fen* [for each of] the
>   above
> *Dang Gui* (Radix Angelicae Sinensis)
> *Sheng Ma* (Rhizoma Cimicifugae), 1 *qian* each

Powder the above ingredients and take 2-3 *qian* each time with thin rice gruel before meals.

He Li Le Wan (Terminalia Pills)

[This formula] treats intermittent dysentery for which no [previous] medicinals are effective with incessant [diarrhea] day and night, [stools] so foul and stinking as to deter [people] from coming near, and [peri]umbilical and abdominal gripping pain.

> *He Zi* (Fructus Terminaliae Chebulae), cored & tipped, 5 *qian*
> *Chun Gen Bai Pi* (Cortex Cedrelae), 1 *liang*
> *Ding Xiang* (Flos Caryophylli), 30 pieces

Powder the above [medicinals] and make into pills the size of Chinese parasol tree seeds with vinegar and flour paste. Take 50 pills each time with cooked stale rice water mixed with a small amount of vinegar at the fifth watch [*i.e.*, before dawn]. Three doses for three days bring effect.

Endnotes

[1] This formula is composed of: *Xiong Huang* (Realgar), *Ba Dou* (Semen Crotonis Tiglii), and scorpion tails.

[2] This formula is composed of: *Huang Qin* (Radix Scutellariae Baicalensis), *Huang Lian* (Rhizoma Coptidis Chinensis), and *Da Huang* (Radix Et Rhizoma Rhei) mixed with honey and prepared in the shape of pills.

15

Spleen-stomach Detriment Warrants
Regulated Drinking & Eating
And Suitable Cold & Hot [Foods]

The *Shi Si Nan* (14th Difficulty) states, "[For] detriment to the spleen, regulate the eating and drinking and [take] suitable cold and warm [foods]."[1]

> The spleen, stomach, large intestine, small intestine, triple burner, and urinary bladder are the root of the granaries [and] the abode of the constructive [qi]. They are called organs and are capable of transforming wastes and converting flavors and [are responsible for] exiting and entering.[2]

"If food and drink are never burning hot nor chillingly cold but are moderately and appropriately cold or warm, the qi will be sustained and evils will not result in aggregation."[3] [However, if] eating and drinking are unregulated and cold and warm [foods] are not suitable, this will engender disease, there will be diarrhea without limit, or there will be glomus and oppression below the heart, abdominal and rib-side drum distention, loss of enrichment and flavor in the mouth, and encumbrance and fatigue of the four limbs. All this is due to damage of the spleen and stomach. The stomach and intestines are markets where there is nothing that cannot be received and nothing that cannot enter. If the qi of wind, cold, summerheat, dampness, or dryness tends to be overwhelming, these are also able to damage the spleen and cause detriment to the stomach. [Thus] the identification of patterns and the use of medicinals require deliberate study [of these qi]. Readers should note that Li is saying that any of the six environmental excesses may cause damage to the spleen and/or stomach. This is an important observation that is often overlooked.

[If one] obtains a bowstring pulse at the spleen and stomach (ruling the right bar, their [normal] pulse being moderate [or relaxed]), [this indicates] damage by wind evils. [In that case,] *Gan Cao Shao Yao Tang* (Licorice & Peony Decoction)[4] and *Huang Qi Jian Zhong Tang* (Astragalus Fortify the Center Decoction)[5] or [other such] sweet and sour formulas can be used. A surging pulse [at the right bar indicates] damage by hot evils. [In this case,] *San Huang Wan* (Three Yellows

Pills),[6] *Xie Huang San* (Drain the Yellow Powder),[7]and *Tiao Wei Cheng Qi Tang* (Regulate the Stomach & Order the Qi Decoction),[8] or [other such] sweet, cold formulas can be used. A moderate [or relaxed] pulse [indicates] the channels of the spleen and stomach being excessively damaged by damp evils. [In this case,] *Ping Wei San* (Level the Stomach Powder)[9] with *Bai Zhu* (Rhizoma Atractylodis Macrocephalae) and *Fu Ling* (Sclerotium Poriae Cocos) added and *Wu Ling San* (Five [Ingredients] Poria Powder)[10] or [other such] dampness-eliminating, per-colating, bland formulas can be used. A choppy [or rough] pulse [indicates] damage by dry heat. [In that case,] *Yi Gong San* (Wonder-working Powder)[11] with *Dang Gui* (Radix Angelicae Sinensis) added and *Si Jun Zi Tang* (Four Gentlemen Decoction)[12] with *Shu Di* (cooked Radix Rehmanniae Glutinosae) added or [other such] sweet, warm or sweet, moistening formulas can be used. A deep, fine pulse [indicates] damage by cold evils. [In this case,] *Yi Huang San* (Boost the Yellow Powder),[13] *Yang Wei Wan* (Nourish the Stomach Pills),[14] *Li Zhong Wan* (Rectify the Center Pills),[15] and *Li Zhong Tang* (Rectify the Center Decoction)[16] with *Fu Zi* (Radix Praeparatus Lateralis Aconiti Carmichaeli) added in case of severe cold or [other such] sweet, warm formulas can be used. In each of the above instances, it is my assumption that the noted pulse image mani-fests at the right bar associated with the spleen and stomach.

The formulas stipulated above are standard and can be altered in case of varied [conditions].

Wei Feng Tang (Stomach Wind Decoction)

[This formula] treats adults and children [in whom] wind and chill have taken advantage of vacuity to enter and lodge in the intestines and stomach. [This gives rise to] untransformed water and grains, diarrhea pouring downward, abdom-inal and rib-side vacuity fullness, borborygmus, and [intestinal] gripping pain. It is also [appropriate for] intestinal and stomach damp toxins with unstoppable diarrhea day and night with stools like soy sauce or the precipitation of static blood [in the stools].

Ren Shen (Radix Panacis Ginseng), stemmed
Fu Ling (Sclerotium Poriae Cocos), skinned
Chuan Xiong (Radix Ligustici Wallichii)
Gui Zhi (Ramulus Cinnamomi Cassiae), debarked
Dang Gui (Radix Angelicae Sinensis), with the sprouts sorted out
Bai Shao (Radix Albus Paeoniae Lactiflorae)
Bai Zhu (Rhizoma Atractylodis Macrocephalae), all in equal amounts

Coarsely powder the above and [take] two *qian* each time, boiled with several hundred grains of millet in a large cup of water down to 7/10. Take while moderately hot on an empty stomach before meals after removing the dregs. Reduce [this dosage] for children in accordance with their strength.

San Huang Wan
(Three Yellows Pills)

[This formula] treats males and females alike for triple burner accumulation and heat; upper burner heat harassing and surging [upward to give rise to] red, swollen eyes, swelling and pain in the head and neck, and sores in the mouth and tongue; middle burner heat [giving rise to] heart and diaphragm vexation and agitation and no liking for food or drink; and lower burner heat [giving rise to] red, astringent urination and constipation. [It also treats] heat in all the five viscera which invariably gives rise to welling abscesses, boils, and sores. In addition, it treats the five [types of] hemorrhoids with anal pain and swelling or precipitation of fresh blood [in the stool]. The five types of hemorrhoids are 1) bleeding hemorrhoid, 2) feminine hemorrhoid, *i.e.*, an anal fistula, 3) masculine hemorrhoid, which is characterized by marked swelling around the anus, 4) intestinal hemorrhoid, which is characterized by ulceration and swelling around the anus, and 5) vessel hemorrhoid, *i.e.*, an anal fissure.

Huang Lian (Rhizoma Coptidis Chinensis), stemmed
Huang Qin (Radix Scutellariae Baicalensis), stemmed
Da Huang (Radix Et Rhizoma Rhei), 1 *liang* [for each of] the above

Powder the above and make into pills the size of Chinese parasol tree seeds with heated honey. Take 30 pills each time swallowed with well done water [*i.e.*, water boiled for a long, long time]. In case of viscera and bowel congestion and repletion, increase the number of pills administered. [This formula] is appropriate to administer for accumulation and heat in infants.

Bai Zhu San
(Atractylodes Powder)

[This formula] treats vacuity heat with thirst.

Ren Shen (Radix Panacis Ginseng), stemmed
Bai Zhu (Rhizoma Atractylodis Macrocephalae)
Mu Xiang (Radix Auklandiae Lappae)
Fu Ling (Sclerotium Poriae Cocos), skinned

Huo Xiang (Herba Agastachis Seu Pogostemi), with soil cleared
Gan Cao (Radix Glycyrrhizae Uralensis), 1 *liang* [for each of] the above
dry *Ge Gen* (Radix Puerariae), 2 *liang*

Coarsely powder the above [ingredients] and take 3-5 *qian* each time boiled in
one cup of water down to half and taken while warm. As for those drinking much,
boil [the medicinals] and let them drink [the decoction] any time. For thirst with
inability to eat, my late master [Zhang] Jie-gu doubled the amount of *Ge Gen*.
In case of thirst with ability to eat, administer *Bai Hu Tang* (White Tiger
Decoction)[17] with *Ren Shen* (Radix Panacis Ginseng) added.

Jia Jian Ping Wei San
(Modified Level the Stomach Powder)

[This formula] treats spleen-stomach disharmony [with] no thought for food
or drink, heart, abdominal, and rib-side distention, fullness, and stabbing pain,
a bitter [taste] in the mouth or no flavor [*i.e.*, a bland taste in the mouth], chest
fullness, shortness of breath, retching, vomiting, and nausea, belching and swallowing acid [*i.e.*, acid regurgitation], a sallow, yellow facial complexion, generalized emaciation and weakness, fatigue, somnolence, generalized heaviness, joint
pain, frequent diarrhea, or sudden turmoil attacking, the five chokings, the eight
glomuses, diaphragmatic qi, and stomach reflux. The five chokings are qi choking, worry choking, food choking, taxation choking, and reflection choking. The
translators have failed to identify the eight glomuses. Since the Chinese word *ge*
means both the diaphragm and blockage, diaphragmatic qi refers to qi blockage or obstruction around the diaphragm.

Gan Cao (Radix Glycyrrhizae Uralensis), sliced and stir-fried, 2 *liang*
Hou Po (Cortex Magnoliae Officinalis), debarked, processed with ginger,
    and stir-fried until a good smell is emitted
Chen Pi (Pericarpium Citri Reticulatae), stripped of the inner white skin,
    3.2 *liang* each
Cang Zhu (Rhizoma Atractylodis), debarked, soaked with rice water, 5 *liang*

Powder the above [and] take two *qian* each time boiled in one cup of water
together with three slices of raw ginger and two dates down to 7/10. Take while
warm after removing the dregs or take while hot after removing the ginger and
dates alone. [Take] on an empty stomach before meals. Or put in a pinchful of
salt and then take the boiling [decoction] sip by sip. Constant administration of
this decoction regulates the qi and warms the stomach, transforms retained food
and disperses phlegm rheum, and eliminates the untimely qi of wind, cold, cool,
and damp in the four seasons.

In case of red, astringent urination, add *Fu Ling* (Sclerotium Poriae Cocos) and *Ze Xie* (Rhizoma Alismatis Orientalis). In case of untransformed rice and grains [in the stool due to] damage done by overeating and overdrinking, add *Zhi Shi* (Fructus Immaturus Citri Aurantii). In case of unhappy qi in the chest and glomus qi below the heart, add *Zhi Ke* (Fructus Citri Aurantii) and *Mu Xiang* (Radix Auklandiae Lappae). In case of spleen-stomach encumbrance and weakness [with] no thought for food or drink, add *Huang Qi* (Radix Astragali Membranacei) and *Ren Shen* (Radix Panacis Ginseng). In case of glomus and oppression below the heart and abdominal distention, add *Hou Po* (Cortex Magnoliae Officinalis) but reduce [the amount of] *Gan Cao* by half. In summer, add stir-fried *Huang Qin* (Radix Scutellariae Baicalensis). In rainy, wet weather, add *Fu Ling* and *Ze Xie*. In the presence of phlegm drool, add *Ban Xia* (Rhizoma Pinelliae Ternatae) and *Chen Pi* (Pericarpium Citri Reticulatae). Except for *Cang Zhu* and *Hou Po* in the expanded formula, the other ingredients should each be increased by the same amount, for example to five *qian* for one packet. In case of phlegm, add five *fen* of *Ban Xia*. In case of coughing and reduced food intake with a bowstring, fine pulse, add *Dang Gui* (Radix Angelicae Sinensis) and *Huang Qi*. In case of a large, surging, and moderate [or relaxed] pulse, add *Huang Qin* and *Huang Lian* (Rhizoma Coptidis Chinensis). In case of hard stools, add *Da Huang* (Radix Et Rhizoma Rhei), three *qian*, and *Mang Xiao* (Mirabilitum), two *qian*. First thoroughly chew *Tao Ren* (Semen Pruni Persicae), stir-fry with bran, and swallow with the decoction.

San Zhi Qi Tang
(Dissipate Stagnant Qi Decoction)

[This formula] treats mild pain beneath the abdominal skin, glomus and fullness below the heart, no thought for food or drink, inability to dissipate [or disperse] food despite ability to take it in, and frequent presence of glomus qi [*i.e.*, middle burner distention and fullness] as a result of depressed qi bound in the middle ductal.

Dang Gui (Radix Angelicae Sinensis), 2 *fen*
Chen Pi (Pericarpium Citri Reticulatae), 3 *fen*
Chai Hu (Radix Bupleuri), 4 *fen*
mix-fried Gan Cao (Radix Glycyrrhizae Uralensis), 1 *qian*
Ban Xia (Rhizoma Pinelliae Ternatae), 1.5 *qian*
Sheng Jiang (uncooked Rhizoma Zingiberis Officinalis), 5 slices
Hong Hua (Flos Carthami Tinctorii), a small amount

Slice the above ingredients to the size of cannabis seeds and [take] all as one dose boiled in two cups of water down to one cupful. Take while moderately hot before a meal after removing the dregs. Sodden wheat food and wine are prohibited [when taking this formula].

Tong You Tang
(Free the Flow of the Dark Gate Decoction)

[This formula] treats lack of free flow of the dark gate [*i.e.*, the pylorus] with [qi] surging upward and [thus] failing to open the gate of inhalation [or the epiglottis] along with choking and congestion. [This results in] the qi not obtaining ascension and descension. [In this case, priority should be given to] treating the dark gate blockage and difficult defecation. This condition is commonly seen initially [when] the spleen and stomach suffer from heat stroke. It is [also] called lower duct not freely flowing.

jam of *Tao Ren* (Semen Pruni Persicae)[*i.e.*, smashed peach seeds]
Hong Hua (Flos Carthami Tinctorii), 1 *fen* each
Sheng Di (uncooked Radix Rehmanniae Glutinosae)
Shu Di (cooked Radix Rehmanniae Glutinosae), 5 *fen* each
Dang Gui (Radix Angelicae Sinensis)
mix-fried *Gan Cao* (Radix Glycyrrhizae Uralensis)
Sheng Ma (Rhizoma Cimicifugae), 1 *qian* [for each of] the above

Slice the above and take all as one dose boiled in two large cups of water down to one cupful. Take while moderately hot before a meal after removing the dregs.

Run Chang Wan
(Moisten the Intestines Pills)

[This formula] treats [damage done by] food and drink and taxation fatigue, constipation, possible dry, blocked, obstructed, and non-freely flowing [stools], and absolutely no thought for food. Either wind binding or blood binding is capable of [causing such] blockage and obstruction. [In this case,] moisten dryness, harmonize the blood, and course wind and disinhibition will naturally be affected.

Da Huang (Radix Et Rhizoma Rhei), debarked
Dang Gui Wei (Extremitas Radicis Angelicae Sinensis)
Qiang Huo (Radix Et Rhizoma Notopterygii), 5 *qian* [for each of] the above
Tao Ren (Semen Pruni Persicae), soaked in boiled water, skinned & tipped,
     1 *liang*
Huo Ma Ren (Semen Cannabis Sativae), stripped of their shells, 1.25 *liang*

Except for *Huo Ma Ren* which should be ground into paste, all the above [ingredients] should be pounded and finely sifted [together]. Then make into pills the size of Chinese parasol tree seeds with heated honey. Take 50 pills each time with boiled water on an empty stomach.

Dao Qi Chu Shi Tang
(Abduct the Qi & Eliminate Dampness Decoction)

[This formula] treats urinary blockage and obstruction as a result of [damage by] food and drink and taxation fatigue. This is blood astringency [or stasis] resulting in qi not freely flowing and, thereby, astringes [or inhibits] the orifices.

Hua Shi (Talcum), stir-fried yellow
Fu Ling (Sclerotium Poriae Cocos), skinned, 2 *qian* each
Zhi Mu (Rhizoma Anemarrhenae Aspheloidis), grated fine and washed
    with wine
Ze Xie (Rhizoma Alismatis Orientalis), 3 *qian* each
Huang Bai (Cortex Phellodendri), debarked and washed with wine, 4 *qian*

Slice the above and take 0.5 *liang* each time boiled in two cups of water down to one cupful. Take while moderately hot on an empty stomach after removing the dregs. In case of emergency, no definite time [of administration] is stipulated.

Ding Xiang Zhu Yu Tang
(Clove Dispel Stasis Decoction)

[This formula] treats stomach vacuity retching, hiccough, and counterflow vomiting as well as non-free flow of the diaphragm and throat.

Gan Jiang (dry Rhizoma Zingiberis Orientalis)
Huang Bai (Cortex Phellodendri), 2 *fen* each
Ding Xiang (Flos Caryophylli)
mix-fried *Gan Cao* (Radix Glycyrrhizae Uralensis)
Chai Hu (Radix Bupleuri)
Chen Pi (Pericarpium Citri Reticulatae)
Ban Xia (Rhizoma Pinelliae Ternatae), 5 *fen* [for each of] the above
Sheng Ma (Rhizoma Cimicifugae), 7 *fen*
Wu Zhu Yu (Fructus Evodiae Rutecarpae)
Cao Dou Kou (Semen Alpiniae Katsumadai)
Huang Qi (Radix Astragali Membranacei)

Ren Shen (Radix Panacis Ginseng), 1 *qian* [for each of] the above
Dang Gui (Radix Angelicae Sinensis), 1.5 *qian*
Cang Zhu (Rhizoma Atractylodis), 2 *qian*

Slice the above ingredients the size of cannabis seeds and take 0.5 *liang* each time boiled in two cups of water down to one cupful. Take while moderately hot before meals after removing the dregs. Cold food is prohibited [while taking this prescription].

Cao Dou Kou Wan
(Alpinia Katsumada Pills)

[This formula] treats spleen-stomach vacuity overwhelmed by heart fire and [therefore] unable to enrich and construct the upper burner original qi. During winter, when the cold water of the kidneys and urinary bladder is effulgent, since the child is capable of making the mother replete, lung metal and the large intestine mutually struggle [or conspire] to restrain the heart and overwhelm the spleen and the stomach. This is a violent retaliation. The classic says great victory must [be followed by] great retaliation. Thus the original qi expires in the exterior between the skin, the blood vessels, and the partings of the flesh. In addition, the two qi of great cold and great dryness overwhelm in co-operation. This leads to tormenting aversion to wind and cold, tinnitus, contraction between the lower and upper backs causing pain in the chest, inhibited breathing through the nose, inability to smell fragrance and fetor, a cold forehead and pain in the brain, occasional visual dizziness, and disinclination to open the eyes. An abdomen counter-restrained by cold water gives rise to spitting of phlegm and foaming at the mouth, stomach reflux, constant [abdominal] pain and acute contraction of the rib-sides with intermittent pain, flaccid belly, more [frequently] diarrhea than constipation, and incessant flatulence or borborygmus. Counter-restraint is the restrained phase overwhelming the restraining phase. All this is due to extreme spleen-stomach vacuity. [This formula also treats] chaotic qi in the chest with heart vexation and restlessness which is a sudden turmoil in progress, non-freely flowing diaphragm and throat, choking, and, in the extreme, rales, panting and wheezing, and [qi] obstruction which may be relieved a little in the sun or in a warm room but recurs when wind cold is inhaled with counterflow chilling of the four limbs, generalized heaviness with inability to turn over the body and head, and agitation arising upon urination. This formula governs against cool and cold in autumn and winter and is a formula able to greatly restore the qi.

Ze Xie (Rhizoma Alismatis Orientalis), 1 *fen*, reduce to half [in amount] in
   case of frequent urination
Chai Hu (Radix Bupleuri), 2-4 *fen*, the amount depending on the rib-side pain
Shen Qu (Massa Medica Fermentata)
Jiang Huang (Rhizoma Curcumae Longae), 4 *fen* each
Dang Gui (Radix Angelicae Sinensis)
uncooked *Gan Cao* (Radix Glycyrrhizae Uralensis)
mix-fried *Gan Cao* (Radix Glycyrrhizae Uralensis)
Qing Pi (Pericarpium Citri Reticulatae Viride), 6 *fen* [for each of] the above
Tao Ren (Semen Pruni Persicae), washed with boiled water, skinned
   & tipped, 7 *fen*
Jiang Can (Bombyx Batryticatus)
Wu Zhu Yu (Fructus Evodiae Rutecarpae), with its bitter, pungent flavor
   washed off with boiled water, baked dry
Yi Zhi Ren (Fructus Alpiniae Oxyphyllae)
Huang Qi (Radix Astragali Membranacei)
Chen Pi (Pericarpium Citri Reticulatae)
Ren Shen (Radix Panacis Ginseng), 8 *fen* [for each of] the above
Ban Xia (Rhizoma Pinelliae Ternatae), 1 *qian*, washed with boiled water
   7 times
Cao Dou Kou (Semen Alpiniae Katsumadai), 1.4 *qian*, roasted with flour as
   a wrapping till the flour is well done, skinned, only the pulp to be used
powdered *Mai Ya* (Fructus Germinatus Hordei Vulgaris), stir-fried to
   yellow, 1.5 *qian*

Put the [above] 18 flavors [or ingredients] together. [Except that] *Tao Ren* should
be smashed separately. The rest are powdered, mixed evenly together with *Tao
Ren*, and made into pills the size of Chinese parasol tree seeds with boiled water
soaked steamed cake. Take 30-50 pills each time with well done boiled water.
[The dosage] is discretionary. Although Li obviously was enamored with this formula, its use has not stood the test of time.

Shen Sheng Fu Qi Tang (Magically Divine Retaliating Qi Decoction)

[This formula] treats qi retaliation taking advantage of tai yang cold qi and foot
shao yin kidney water effulgence – the child being capable of making the mother
replete – [to cause] the repleted hand tai yin lungs to rebel against earth and subject fire and wood to evils. For example, if the first half of a year sees an abnor-

mal prevalence of cold, then, as a rule, abnormal warmth or heat will prevail during the second half of the year. This warm or hot weather is known as retaliating qi. [This results in] the five blocks with obstruction in the lower and upper backs, pain [in the chest], frequent sneezing, drooling from the mouth, tearing from the eyes, incessant running of turbid nasal mucus or polyp in the nose with inability to smell fragrance or fetor, cough with phlegm and foam, fire-like heat above with ice cold below, intermittent headache, fire sparkling in the eyes, blurred vision, tinnitus, deafness, the head with the mouth and nose averse to wind cold and having a liking for the sun, troubled sleep, a constant sensation of choking by phlegm, non-free flow of the diaphragm and throat, loss of flavor [or taste with] the mouth, acute bilateral rib-side contraction and pain, stirring [or loose] teeth with inability to chew things, genital sweating and chilling of the anterior yin, moving and stepping awry, difficulty attending to one's daily activities, cold in the palms, wind impediment, numbness and tingling, frequent, profuse urination during the day but frequent, scanty urination at night, shortness of breath, panting and wheezing, diminished qi insufficient to [catch] the breath, and sudden [occurrence of] emission [of stools] without limit. In women, [it also treats] white vaginal discharge, great pain in the private gate radiating a dragging pain to the heart with a soot-black, colorless [facial] complexion. The five blocks refer to either of two systems of classification. One includes worry, indignation, qi, cold, and heat blocks. The other includes worry, reflection, anger, fright, and joy blocks. Note that this kind of blockage usually involves the chest and diaphragm. In men, [it also treats] testicular contraction sending a dull, dragging pain to the heart and abdominal region and a reddish brown [facial] complexion. [Further, it treats] decreased eating, unregulated urination and defecation, heart vexation, sudden turmoil, counterflow qi, tenesmus, white-colored abdominal skin, flatulence, inability to exert the abdomen or borborygmus, hypertonicity of the sinews below the knee, and great pain in the scapula. All this [is due to] cold water which is wreaking vengeance upon fire and earth.

black *Fu Zi* (Radix Lateralis Praeparatus Aconiti Carmichaeli), wrapped
    [with flour], blast-fried & skinned
Gan Jiang (dry Rhizoma Zingiberis Officinalis), powdered by blast-frying,
    3 *fen* each
Fang Feng (Radix Ledebouriellae Divaricatae), sliced to the size of beans
Yu Li Ren (Semen Pruni), soaked in boiled water, skinned, tipped & ground
    into paste
Ren Shen (Radix Panacis Ginseng), 5 *fen* [for each of] the above
Dang Gui (Radix Angelicae Sinensis), washed with wine, 6 *fen*
Ban Xia (Rhizoma Pinelliae Ternatae), soaked in boiled water 7 times
Sheng Ma (Rhizoma Cimicifugae), sliced, 7 *fen* each

Gan Cao (Radix Glycyrrhizae Uralensis), sliced
Gao Ben (Radix Et Rhizoma Ligustici Sinensis), 8 *fen* each
Chai Hu (Radix Bupleuri), sliced to the size of beans
Qiang Huo (Radix Et Rhizoma Notopterygii), sliced to the size of beans,
   1 *qian* each
white *Kui Hua* (Flos Altheae Rosae, sunflower), 3 flowers, cored, cut
   fine for use

Boil the above ingredients all as one dose in five cups of water down to two cupfuls. Then put in:

Chen Pi (Pericarpium Citri Reticulatae), 5 *fen*
Cao Dou Kou (Semen Alpiniae Katsumadai), roasted with flour as a
   wrapping & skinned
Huang Qi (Radix Astragali Membranacei), 1 *qian* each

After that, boil [the mixture] down to one cupful and then put in the following ingredients:

Sheng Di (uncooked Radix Rehmanniae Glutinosae), 2 *fen*, washed with wine
Huang Bai (Cortex Phellodendri), soaked in wine
Huang Lian (Rhizoma Coptidis Chinensis), soaked in wine
Zhi Ke (Fructus Citri Aurantii), 3 *fen* [for each of] the above

These last four [ingredients] should be soaked in fresh water for one day before use. Also add:

Xi Xin (Herba Asari Cum Radice), 2 *fen*
Chuan Xiong (Radix Ligustici Wallichii), powdered
Man Jing Zi (Fructus Viticis), 3 *fen* each

Soak the last three flavors [or ingredients] separately in half a large cupful of fresh water the day before. Then pour this into the boiled main medicinals, including *Huang Bai* and the others, with the dregs preserved. Heat these over the fire again and boil them down to one large cupful. Take [the resulting decoction] while moderately hot on an empty stomach after removing the dregs. [This formula] can also treat cheek, lip, and tongue biting, stiffness and hardness of the root of the tongue, and other conditions like [possession by] spirits. Meat soup is prohibited so as not to assist the fire evils in the channels and network vessels. [However,] one should eat meat. This implies that meat broth contains too much fat and that meat should be lean meat. On the whole, administration [of this formula] is appropriate for either cold in the kidney and bladder channels or original qi insufficiency. An interesting yin fire type formula but not one that has withstood the test of time.

Endnotes

[1] *Nan Jing*, 14th Difficulty

[2] *Su Wen*, Ch. 9

[3] *Ling Shu*, Vol. 6, Ch. 29

[4] This is composed of: *Bai Shao* (Radix Albus Paeoniae Lactiflorae) and mix-fried *Gan Cao* (Radix Glycyrrhizae Uralensis), 4 *liang* each.

[5] This is composed of: *Gui Zhi* (Ramulus Cinnamomi Cassiae), mix-fried *Gan Cao* (Radix Glycyrrhizae Uralensis), *Gan Jiang* (dry Rhizoma Zingiberis Officinalis), *Bai Shao* (Radix Albus Paeoniae Lactiflorae), *Da Zao* (Fructus Zizyphi Jujubae), *Huang Qi* (Radix Astragali Membranacei), and *Yi Tang* (maltose).

[6] See the second formula given in this chapter.

[7] This is composed of: *Huo Xiang* (Herba Agastachis Seu Pogostemi), *Zhi Zi* (Fructus Gardeniae Jasminoidis), *Shi Gao* (Gypsum Fibrosum), *Gan Cao* (Radix Glycyrrhizae Uralensis), and *Fang Feng* (Radix Ledebouriellae Divaricatae).

[8] This is composed of: *Da Huang* (Radix Et Rhizoma Rhei), mix-fried *Gan Cao* (Radix Glycyrrhizae Uralensis), and *Mang Xiao* (Mirabilitum).

[9] This is composed of: *Cang Zhu* (Rhizoma Atractylodis), *Hou Po* (Cortex Magnoliae Officinalis), *Chen Pi* (Pericarpium Citri Reticulatae), *Gan Cao* (Radix Glycyr rhizae Uralensis), *Gan Jiang* (dry Rhizoma Zingiberis Officinalis), and *Da Zao* (Fructus Zizyphi Jujubae).

[10] See Ch. 13, present Bk.

[11] See the last formula given in Ch. 12, present Bk.

[12] This is composed of: *Ren Shen* (Radix Panacis Ginseng), mix-fried *Gan Cao* (Radix Glycyrrhizae Uralensis), *Fu Ling* (Sclerotium Poriae Cocos), and *Bai Zhu* (Rhizoma Atractylodis Macrocephalae).

[13] This is composed of: *Chen Pi* (Pericarpium Citri Reticulatae), *Ding Xiang* (Flos Caryophylli), *He Zi* (Fructus Terminaliae Chebulae), *Qing Pi* (Pericarpium Citri Reticulatae Viride), and mix-fried *Gan Cao* (Radix Glycyrrhizae Uralensis).

[14] The translators have failed to find the ingredients of this pill. There is a *Yang Wei Tang* (Nourish the Stomach Decoction) indicated for the same pattern. It is given below for reference only: *Hou Po* (Cortex Magnoliae Officinalis), *Cang Zhu* (Rhizoma Atractylodis), *Ban Xia* (Rhizoma Pinelliae Ternatae), *Huo Xiang* (Herba Agastachis Seu Pogostemi), *Cao Guo* (Fructus Amomi Tsao-ko), *Fu Ling* (Sclerotium Poriae Cocos), *Ren Shen* (Radix Panacis Ginseng), mix-fried *Gan Cao* (Radix Glycyrrhizae Uralensis), *Ju Hong* (Pericarpium Citri Erythrocarpae), *Gan Jiang* (dry Rhizoma Zingiberis Officinalis), and *Wu Mei* (Fructus Pruni Mume).

[15] This is composed of: *Ren Shen* (Radix Panacis Ginseng), *Gan Jiang* (dry Rhizoma Zingiberis Officinalis), mix- fried *Gan Cao* (Radix Glycyrrhizae Uralensis), and *Bai Zhu* (Rhizoma Atractylodis Macrocephalae) made into pills with honey.

[16] This is composed of the same ingredients as the pills above only prepared as a decoction.

[17] This is composed of: *Zhi Mu* (Rhizoma Anemarrhenae Aspheloidis), *Shi Gao* (Gypsum Fibrosum), mix-fried *Gan Cao* (Radix Glycyrrhizae Uralensis), and rice.

16

Methods for Supporting & Rectifying the Spleen & Stomach

This chapter discusses the role of dietary therapy as an adjunct to internally administered medicinals. In a nutshell, it is an explanation of what has come to be known as the clear, bland diet of Chinese medicine. These teachings are also the basis for the Japanese macrobiotic diet.

Rice porridge [or congee, steamed] rice, mung beans, small [red] beans [*i.e.*, aduki beans], and salted fermented beans are all bland percolators and urine-disinhibitors. [In case of] frequent urination, it is not ok to disinhibit urination. In addition, [such disinhibition] greatly drains the yang qi and contrarily [or erroneously] causes movement of the yin tract. Sodden wheat food is absolutely prohibited [in this case. However,] this prohibition can be lifted if [the patient feels] better after eating it.

Medicinals which it is not ok to administer [in this case] include *Ze Xie* (Rhizoma Alismatis Orientalis), *Zhu Ling* (Sclerotium Polypori Umbellati), *Fu Ling* (Sclerotium Poriae Cocos), *Deng Xin Cao* (Medulla Junci Effusi), *Hu Po* (Succinum), *Tong Cao* (Medulla Tetrapanacis Papyriferi), *Mu Tong* (Caulis Akebiae), *Hua Shi* (Talcum), and the like. All these [cause] movement of the yin tract and drain the yang tract [*i.e.*, drain righteous yang and/or clear heat]. In case of thirst, inhibited urination, [or urinary] block, obstruction, and non-free flow, [they can] be administered. [But, as soon as] disinhibition has been obtained [or achieved], they should not be administered any longer.

Great saltiness is prohibited [for] it assists fire evils and drains the true yin of kidney water. In addition, refrain from greatly acrid flavors, [including] garlic, leek, the five peppers, vinegar, aniseed[-type] things [*i.e.*, spices], cinnamon, dry ginger, and the like, for they can all damage the original qi.

If upbearing or sinking medicinals are administered, the first day support and rectify [the stomach by giving it a rest]. Then the next day [the medicinals] should be taken on an empty stomach. After that, [the stomach] should be supported and rectified [or given a rest] for the next 10 days. It is even better to give [the stomach a rest] for 3 days in advance. Otherwise [the medication] will do harm [instead of good].

The methods of the use of medicinals [require that,] for the various diseases in the four seasons, whatever the diseases are, whether they be warm or cool, hot or cold, clear, cool, windy medicinals should be used in spring. Greatly cold medinals should be used in summer. Qi-warming medicinals should be used in autumn, [and] greatly hot medicinals should be used in winter. Thus the source of engendering and transforming will not expire. Qian Zhong-yang [a.k.a. Qian Yi, the great Song dynasty pediatrician] had a deep understanding of this principle in treating children. The *Nei Jing (Inner Classic)* [states that treatment] must anticipate the yearly qi [*i.e.*, weather changes peculiar to a certain year] and avoid infringing on the heavenly harmony [or the natural laws of weather in the four seasons] to be a consummate treatment. It also says that one should not act against the seasons nor should transformation be infringed upon. In addition, it says [that one should] not infringe upon the qi which engenders the living [or vital] qi. The qi which engenders the living qi is the spleen and stomach qi. All this is a common *dao* [or well established approach], a general principle for the use of medicinals. If [one acts] contrary to such a common *dao*, unusual conditions will also be engendered. These then require a special treatment to remedy. If the patient drinks wine, eats too much cold food, or too much hot food, this can increase [the severity of] the disease. In that case, specific medicinals should be considered as a expedient [or stop-gap] measure. [However,] these cannot be used constantly.

17

Nursing

This chapter discusses various lifestyle adjustments Li thinks are important to prevent and adjunctively remedy disease. Most are simple common sense.

It is prohibited to bathing [when exposed to] the wind or [when] sweating. [If one] must, it is necessary to close the sweat pores by rubbing first with the hand. Thus no disease of wind stroke or cold stroke will be contracted. In case of sudden [breaking out of] wind and cold which [one's] clothing is unable to resist, one should exert oneself to activate the qi around the body to ward it off. [Those with] weak qi unable to resist will become diseased.

If [one is wearing] thin clothes and is short of breath, one should put on more clothes and live in a place protected from the wind. [In case] qi remains short, [*i.e.*, the breath remains short, if one inhales] through their nose and mouth the steam [arising from] a bowl of boiling water, they will no longer be short [of breath]. If [a person who is] short of breath and wears thick clothes lives in a place where the wind is not freely flowing [*i.e.*, is poorly ventilated, they] should reduce their clothes, close their sweat pores by rubbing, and live in a well ventilated place. If shortness of breath is the result of having lived for a long [time] in high chambers or in confinement by yin dampness in cold weather, the above steaming method is also applicable. If shortness of breath results from living in a small, tightly shut hut or staying in cool and cold places in intensely hot weather, one should go out to expose oneself to the sun and wind. For any kind of shortness of breath, one should eat enriching, flavorful soups and drinks to regulate and harmonize the stomach. While *qi duan* commonly means shortness of breath, in this paragraph Li seems to be using this term more to convey a general sense of qi vacuity and weakness. At least that is how I read this paragraph.

In case of thirst and a predilection for cold drinks with ability to eat in intensely hot [weather, cold] drinks can be administered as a stop-gap measure, but it is not ok to overindulgence in them. In case of a predilection for hot things in cold winter, these can also be eaten temporarily to accord with the season.

Restless sleep may be a result of heat congestion caused by thick quilts. They should be removed promptly and sweat should be wiped off. In case of restless [sleep] with thin [covers], add more [covers] and sleep will automatically become firm [or steady]. In case of restless sleep due to hunger, one should eat a little. In case of restless sleep due to satiation [or overeating], walk and sit a little.

During changeable cold and windy heavenly qi [or weather] or during persistent wet days, one should take precautionary measures in advance. Generally speaking, one should [stay] comfortably warm, avoid wind and cold, economize speech, and lessen taxation.

18

Distancing Desires [*i.e.,* Keeping Desires at a Distance]

Which is dearer, fame or one's body? Which is worth more, one's body or belongings? [One] would be laughed at by all people if one shot at a bird at a distance of a thousand *ren* with the pearl of Duke Sui. One *ren* equals 2 2/3 meters. Duke Sui was a hero in an ancient fable who is so silly as to throw his priceless Moonlit Pearl at a bird in the hope of catching it. What can justify a trifle acquisition at a prodigious sacrifice? This stub of my body is 60 plus five [years old]. My ears and the eyes have lost half of their vision and hearing. The hundreds of vessels are boiling, [thus giving rise to] heart vexation. [My] body [feels] as if drifting and flowing in a multitude of vessels. Yang Shou-zhong interpreted this as floating in whirls. When [I] close [my] eyes, the ethereal soul departs like the breaking of a wave. This means Li falls asleep immediately whenever he closes his eyes. The spirit qi is [more] debilitated [today than] the day before. [The amount of] food [I] eat is reduced [compared with] former times. When I respond [or attend] to human affairs, [all my symptoms of] disease get worse. [Nevertheless,] the pearl of Duke Sui is no comparison to my possession, [my body. Therefore,] relish oblivion and obscurity, think less, [have] little desire, and [practice] economy of speech in order to nourish the qi. [Refrain from] unnecessary taxation in order to nourish the form, and empty the heart to protect the spirit. [Take] longevity or death, obtaining or losing [without attachment,] being quiet [or at peace] with their number [or amount], and take bereavement lightly. Then blood and qi will naturally be in accord and harmonious, evils will find no place to lodge, and disease will quiet and not increase. If one is able to keep to all this, one follows the *dao,* and one can obtain the true purpose [and/or delight of life].

Great advice! What more can one say?

19

Admonition on Economy of Speech

Qi is the forefather of spirit and essence is the child of qi. In other words, spirit is nothing other than the accumulation of qi in the heart, and essence is made from the surplus of qi and blood sequestered in the five viscera. [Thus] qi is the root of essence and spirit. Qi produces both spirit and latter heaven essence. Great is qi! [When] qi accumulates, it produces essence. [When] essence accumulates, it completes the spirit. This means the blood and essence are necessary to enrich and nourish the spirit in order to keep it healthy. These lines clearly and succinctly elucidate the relationship between spirit, qi, and essence. In terms of this, Li's vision of this relationship is entirely a natural (as opposed to a spiritual/spiritist) one. Keep clear [or serene by all means], keep still [or quiet by all means], and abide by the *dao*. A heavenly man [*i.e.*, an immortal] can do all of these. He has the *dao* and is able [to follow it]. But what am I? It will be ok for me just to practice economy of speech. This final bit of advice is hugely important in my experience. As a professional teacher, I know how debilitating speaking excessively is. One should not underestimate the deleterious effects of speaking unnecessarily.

Appendix:
Representative Dong-yuan Yin Fire Formulas

Formulas from the *Pi Wei Lun*
(Treatise on the Spleen & Stomach)

Bu Pi Wei Xie Yin Huo Sheng Yang Tang
(Supplement the Spleen & Stomach, Drain Yin Fire & Upbear Yang Decoction)

Huang Qi (Radix Astragali Membranacei)
Ren Shen (Radix Panacis Ginseng)
mix-fried *Gan Cao* (Radix Glycyrrhizae Uralensis)
Cang Zhu (Rhizoma Atractylodis)
Chai Hu (Radix Bupleuri)
Qiang Huo (Radix Et Rhizoma Notopterygii)
Sheng Ma (Rhizoma Cimicifugae)
Huang Qin (Radix Scutellariae Baicalensis)
Huang Lian (Rhizoma Coptidis Chinensis)
Shi Gao (Gypsum Fibrosum)

Functions: Fortifies the spleen and boosts the qi, rectifies the qi and upbears the clear, and drains yin fire

Indications: Spleen vacuity with liver depression and depressive or damp heat

Sheng Yang Yi Wei Tang
(Upbear Yang & Boost the Stomach)

Huang Qi (Radix Astragali Membranacei)
Ren Shen (Radix Panacis Ginseng)
mix-fried *Gan Cao* (Radix Glycyrrhizae Uralensis)
Fu Ling (Sclerotium Poriae Cocos)

Ban Xia (Rhizoma Pinelliae Ternatae)
Bai Shao (Radix Albus Paeoniae Lactiflorae)
Fang Feng (Radix Ledebouriellae Divaricatae)
Qiang Huo (Radix Et Rhizoma Notopterygii)
Du Huo (Radix Angelicae Pubescentis)
Chen Pi (Pericarpium Citri Reticulatae)
Ze Xie (Rhizoma Alismatis Orientalis)
Chai Hu (Radix Bupleuri)
Huang Lian (Rhizoma Coptidis Chinensis)

Functions: Supplements the spleen and boosts the qi, harmonizes the liver and relaxes tension, dispels wind and eliminates dampness, clears heat

Indications: Spleen vacuity with a combination of malnourishment of the sinews and vessels and wind damp impediment pain complicated with heat in the liver, stomach, and/or heart. Originally this formula was for the treatment of spleen vacuity resulting in lung disease or, more specifically, the lungs' easy contraction of disease in the fall.

Tong Qi Fang Feng Tang
(Free the Flow of the Qi Ledebouriella Decoction)

Huang Qi (Radix Astragali Membranacei)
Ren Shen (Radix Panacis Ginseng)
Gan Cao (Radix Glycyrrhizae Uralensis)
Chai Hu (Radix Bupleuri)
Sheng Ma (Rhizoma Cimicifugae)
Qiang Huo (Radix Et Rhizoma Notopterygii)
Fang Feng (Radix Ledebouriellae Divaricatae)
Chen Pi (Pericarpium Citri Reticulatae)
Qing Pi (Pericarpium Citri Reticulatae Viride)
Bai Dou Kou (Fructus Cardamomi)
Gao Ben (Radix Et Rhizoma Ligustici Chinensis)
Huang Bai (Cortex Phellodendri)

Functions: Fortifies the spleen and boosts the qi, dispels wind and eliminates dampness, harmonizes the stomach and clears heat

Indications: Spleen qi vacuity with damp encumbrance and qi stagnation complicated by wind damp impediment and some damp heat

Bu Zhong Yi Qi Tang
(Supplement the Center & Boost the Qi Decoction)

Huang Qi (Radix Astragali Membranacei)
Ren Shen (Radix Panacis Ginseng)
Bai Zhu (Rhizoma Atractylodis Macrocephalae)
mix-fried *Gan Cao* (Radix Glycyrrhizae Uralensis)
Dang Gui (Radix Angelicae Sinensis)
Chai Hu (Radix Bupleuri)
Sheng Ma (Rhizoma Cimicifugae)
Chen Pi (Pericarpium Citri Reticulatae)

Functions: Fortifies the spleen and boosts the qi, warmly and sweetly eliminates heat, upbears yang and lifts the fallen

Indications: 1) Spleen qi vacuity with marked fatigue and liver depression, 2) downward fall of central qi with various types of dizziness and prolapse, 3) qi vacuity emission of heat or fever

Huang Qi Ren Shen Tang
(Astragalus & Ginseng Decoction)

Huang Qi (Radix Astragali Membranacei)
Ren Shen (Radix Panacis Ginseng)
Bai Zhu (Rhizoma Atractylodis Macrocephalae)
Cang Zhu (Rhizoma Atractylodis)
mix-fried *Gan Cao* (Radix Glycyrrhizae Uralensis)
Sheng Ma (Rhizoma Cimicifugae)
Chen Pi (Pericarpium Citri Reticulatae)
Shen Qu (Massa Medica Fermentata)
Radix Angelicae Sinensis (*Dang Gui*)
Mai Men Dong (Tuber Ophiopogonis Japonici)
Wu Wei Zi (Fructus Schisandrae Chinensis)
Huang Bai (Cortex Phellodendri)

Functions: Fortifies the spleen and boosts the qi, dries dampness, upbears the clear, and abducts stagnation, nourishes the blood and enriches heart, lung, and stomach yin, and clears heat

Indications: Spleen vacuity with dampness plus food stagnation, yin vacuity, and some vacuity and/or damp heat.[1] Originally, this formula was for summer-heat damaging the latter heaven source qi. It can also be used to prevent fall season allergic rhinitis when taken prophylactically in the late summer.

Chu Feng Shi Qiang Huo Tang
(Eliminate Wind Dampness Notopterygium Decoction)

Huang Qi (Radix Astragali Membranacei)
mix-fried *Gan Cao* (Radix Glycyrrhizae Uralensis)
Fu Ling (Sclerotium Poriae Cocos)
Cang Zhu (Rhizoma Atractylodis)
Qiang Huo (Radix Et Rhizoma Notopterygii)
Fang Feng (Radix Ledebouriellae Divaricatae)
Gao Ben (Radix Et Rhizoma Ligustici Chinensis)
Du Huo (Radix Angelicae Pubescentis)
Chuan Xiong (Radix Ligustici Wallichii)
Chai Hu (Radix Bupleuri)
Sheng Ma (Rhizoma Cimicifugae)
Chen Pi (Pericarpium Citri Reticulatae)
Zhu Ling (Sclerotium Polypori Umbellati)
Ze Xie (Rhizoma Alismatis Orientalis)
Huang Bai (Cortex Phellodendri)
Huang Lian (Rhizoma Coptidis Chinensis)

Functions: Dispels wind and eliminates dampness, fortifies the spleen and rectifies the qi, clears heat and seeps dampness

Indications: Damp heat impediment pain complicated by possible lower burner damp heat vaginitis or cystitis, spleen vacuity and liver depression

Tiao Zhong Yi Qi Tang
(Regulate the Center & Boost the Qi Decoction)

Huang Qi (Radix Astragali Membranacei)
Ren Shen (Radix Panacis Ginseng)
Cang Zhu (Rhizoma Atractylodis)
Gan Cao (Radix Glycyrrhizae Uralensis)
Chai Hu (Radix Bupleuri)
Sheng Ma (Rhizoma Cimicifugae)

Chen Pi (Pericarpium Citri Reticulatae)
Mu Xiang (Radix Auklandiae Lappae)

Functions: Fortifies the spleen and boosts the qi, dries dampness and rectifies the qi

Indications: Spleen vacuity with damp exuberance and either liver depression qi stagnation or stomach and intestine qi stagnation resulting in inhibition of the throat and diaphragm, burping and belching, nausea and vomiting, chest fullness and bodily heaviness, somnolence and lack of strength

Qing Shu Yi Qi Tang
(Clear Summerheat & Boost the Qi Decoction)

Huang Qi (Radix Astragali Membranacei)
Ren Shen (Radix Panacis Ginseng)
Cang Zhu (Rhizoma Atractylodis)
Bai Zhu (Rhizoma Atractylodis Macrocephalae)
mix-fried *Gan Cao* (Radix Glycyrrhizae Uralensis)
Sheng Ma (Rhizoma Cimicifugae)
Chen Pi (Pericarpium Citri Reticulatae)
Qing Pi (Pericarpium Citri Reticulatae Viride)
Shen Qu (Massa Medica Fermentata)
Huang Bai (Cortex Phellodendri)
Ge Gen (Radix Puerariae)
Mai Men Dong (Tuber Ophiopogonis Japonici)
Wu Wei Zi (Fructus Schisandrae Chinensis)
Dang Gui (Radix Angelicae Sinensis)

Functions: Fortifies the spleen and boosts the qi, dries dampness and rectifies the qi, enriches yin, clears heat, and disperses accumulation

Indications: Spleen vacuity due to enduring damp heat with damaged fluids and an element of qi and food stagnation[2]

Sheng Yang San Huo Tang
(Upbear Yang & Scatter Fire Decoction)

Ren Shen (Radix Panacis Ginseng)
uncooked *Gan Cao* (Radix Glycyrrhizae Uralensis)

mix-fried *Gan Cao* (Radix Glycyrrhizae Uralesis)
Chai Hu (Radix Bupleuri)
Sheng Ma (Rhizoma Cimicifugae)
Fang Feng (Radix Ledebouriellae Divaricatae)
Qiang Huo (Radix Et Rhizoma Notopterygii)
Du Huo (Radix Angelicae Pubescentis)
Ge Gen (Radix Puerariae)
Bai Shao (Radix Albus Paeoniae Lactiflorae)

Functions: Fortifies the spleen and boosts the qi, harmonizes the liver and nourishes the sinews, dispels wind and eliminates dampness, clears heat

Indications: Spleen vacuity resulting in qi and blood vacuity with malnourishment of the liver and sinews with simultaneous wind, dampness, and heat due to blood and fluid vacuity dryness. Originally, this formula was meant to resolve, scatter, and clear interior heat and emit fire depression when yang qi was depressed and blocking the spleen and stomach.

Qing Yang Tang
(Clear Yang Decoction)

Huang Qi (Radix Astragali Membranacei)
mix-fried *Gan Cao* (Radix Glycyrrhizae Uralensis)
Hong Hua (Flos Carthami Tinctorii)
Su Mu (Lignum Sappan)
Dang Gui (Radix Angelicae Sinensis)
Huang Bai (Cortex Phellodendri)
Gui Zhi (Ramulus Cinnamomi Cassiae)
uncooked *Gan Cao* (Radix Glycyrrhizae Uralensis)
Sheng Ma (Rhizoma Cimicifugae)
Ge Gen (Radix Puerariae)

Functions: Quickens the blood and dispels stasis, fortifies the spleen and supplements the qi, moistens the sinews and clears heat

Indications: Blood stasis complicated by spleen vacuity resulting in qi and blood vacuity with malnourishment of the sinews and vacuity heat

Wei Feng Tang
(Stomach Wind Decoction)

mix-fried *Gan Cao* (Radix Glycyrrhizae Uralensis)
Gan Jiang (dry Rhizoma Zingiberis Officinalis)
Cang Zhu (Rhizoma Atractylodis)
Da Zao (Fructus Zizyphi Jujubae)
Man Jing Zi (Fructus Viticis)
Cao Dou Kou (Semen Alpiniae Katsumadai)
Huang Bai (Cortex Phellodendri)
Qiang Huo (Radix Et Rhizoma Notopterygii)
Gao Ben (Radix Et Rhizoma Ligustici Chinensis)
Ma Huang (Herba Ephedrae)
Dang Gui (Radix Angelicae Sinensis)
Ge Gen (Radix Puerariae)
Bai Zhi (Radix Angelicae Dahuricae)
Chai Hu (Radix Bupleuri)
Sheng Ma (Rhizoma Cimicifugae)

Functions: Dispels wind and eliminates dampness, frees the flow of the channels and supplements the center, clears heat

Indications: Internal stirring of wind due to vacuity resulting in one-sided paralysis or wind damp impediment complicated by an element of heat

Qing Zao Tang
(Clear Dryness Decoction)

Huang Qi (Radix Astragali Membranacei)
Ren Shen (Radix Panacis Ginseng)
mix-fried *Gan Cao* (Radix Glycyrrhizae Uralensis)
Bai Zhu (Rhizoma Atractylodis Macrocephalae)
Cang Zhu (Rhizoma Atractylodis)
Fu Ling (Sclerotium Poriae Cocos)
Huang Lian (Rhizoma Coptidis Chinensis)
Huang Bai (Cortex Phellodendri)
Chai Hu (Radix Bupleuri)
Mai Men Dong (Tuber Ophiopogonis Japonici)
Wu Wei Zi (Fructus Schisandrae Chinensis)

Dang Gui (Radix Angelicae Sinensis)
Sheng Di (uncooked Radix Rehmanniae Glutionosae)
Zhu Ling (Sclerotium Polypori Umbellati)
Ze Xie (Rhizoma Alismatis Orientalis)
Shen Qu (Massa Medica Fermentata)
Sheng Ma (Rhizoma Cimicifugae)
Chen Pi (Pericarpium Citri Reticulatae)

Functions: Fortifies the spleen and boosts the qi, both dries and seeps dampness, clears heat, nourishes yin, rectifies the qi, and disperses food

Indications: Spleen vacuity with enduring damp heat damaging yin fluids complicated by qi and food stagnation

Sheng Yang Chu Shi Tang (Upbear Yang & Eliminate Dampness Decoction)

Yi Zhi Ren (Fructus Alpiniae Oxyphyllae)
Cang Zhu (Rhizoma Atractylodis)
Gan Cao (Radix Glycyrrhizae Uralensis)
Ban Xia (Rhizoma Pinelliae Ternatae)
Chen Pi (Pericarpium Citri Reticulatae)
Zhu Ling (Sclerotium Polypori Umbellati)
Ze Xie (Rhizoma Alismatis Orientalis)
Mai Ya (Fructus Germinatus Hordei Vulgaris)
Shen Qu (Massa Medica Fermentata)
Qiang Huo (Radix Et Rhizoma Notopterygii)
Chai Hu (Radix Bupleuri)
Sheng Ma (Rhizoma Cimicifugae)

Functions: Fortifies the spleen and supplements the qi, transforms and seeps dampness, abducts stagnation and moves the qi

Indications: Spleen qi vacuity and dampness enduring diarrhea complicated by qi and food stagnation

Yi Wei Tang (Boost the Stomach Decoction)

Huang Qi (Radix Astragali Membranacei)

Ren Shen (Radix Panacis Ginseng)
Bai Zhu (Rhizoma Atractylodis Macrocephalae)
Cang Zhu (Rhizoma Atractylodis)
Yi Zhi Ren (Fructus Alpiniae Oxyphyllae)
Ban Xia (Rhizoma Pinelliae Ternatae)
Chen Pi (Pericarpium Citri Reticulatae)
Dang Gui (Radix Angelicae Sinensis)
Huang Qin (Radix Scutellariae Baicalensis)
Chai Hu (Radix Bupleuri)
Sheng Ma (Rhizoma Cimicifugae)

Functions: Fortifies the spleen and boosts the qi, clears the lungs, liver, stomach, and intestines, transforms dampness and rectifies the qi

Indications: Spleen qi vacuity with damp heat in the stomach and intestines diarrhea with dampness heavier than heat

Qiang Wei Tang
(Strengthen the Stomach Decoction)

Huang Qi (Radix Astragali Membranacei)
Ren Shen (Radix Panacis Ginseng)
Gan Cao (Radix Glycyrrhizae Uralensis)
Ban Xia (Rhizoma Pinelliae Ternatae)
Chen Pi (Pericarpium Citri Reticulatae)
Shen Qu (Massa Medica Fermentata)
Cao Dou Kou (Fructus Alpiniae Katsumadai)
Sheng Jiang (uncooked Rhizoma Zingiberis Officinalis)
Dang Gui (Radix Angelicae Sinensis)
Huang Bai (Cortex Phellodendri)
Chai Hu (Radix Bupleuri)
Sheng Ma (Rhizoma Cimicifugae)

Functions: Fortifies the spleen and boosts the qi, dries dampness, abducts stagnation, and clears vacuity heat

Indications: Taxation malaria-like disease due to spleen vacuity and dampness with vacuity heat

Formulas from the *Lan Shi Mi Cang* (Secret Treasury of the Orchid Chamber)

Liang Xue Di Huang Tang (Cool the Blood Rehmannia Decoction)

Huang Qin (Radix Scutellariae Baicalensis)
Jing Jie Sui (Herba Seu Flos Schizonepetae Tenufoliae)
Huang Bai (Cortex Phellodendri)
Zhi Mu (Rhizoma Anemarrhenae Asphodeloidis)
Huang Lian (Rhizoma Coptidis Chinensis)
Xi Xin (Herba Asari Cum Radice)
Chuan Xiong (Radix Ligustici Wallichii)
Hong Hua (Flos Carthami Tinctorii)
Sheng Di (uncooked Radix Rehmanniae Glutinosae)
Dang Gui (Radix Angelicae Sinensis)
Fang Feng (Radix Ledebouriellae Divaricatae)
Qiang Huo (Radix Et Rhizoma Notopterygii)
Chai Hu (Radix Bupleuri)
Sheng Ma (Rhizoma Cimicifugae)
Gan Cao (Radix Glycyrrhizae Uralensis)

Functions: 1) Dispels wind, eliminates dampness, and clears heat, quickens the blood and frees the flow of the network vessels; 2) Upbears the clear and resolves depression, clears heat and quickens the blood

Indications: 1) Wind damp heat impediment complicated by blood stasis in the network vessels; 2) Uterine bleeding due to heat in the blood in turn due to liver depression/depressive heat

Huang Qi Dang Gui Ren Shen Tang (Astragalus, Dang Gui & Ginseng Decoction)

Huang Qi (Radix Astragali Membranacei)
Ren Shen (Radix Panacis Ginseng)
Sheng Di (uncooked Radix Rehmanniae Glutinosae)
Huang Lian (Rhizoma Coptidis Chinensis)
stir-fried *Shen Qu* (Massa Medica Fermentata)
Ju Hong (Pericartium Citri Erythrocarpae)
Gui Zhi (Ramulus Cinnamomi Cassiae)

Cao Dou Kou (Semen Alpiniae Katsumadae)
Ma Huang (Herba Ephedrae)
Dang Gui (Radix Angelicae Sinensis)
Xing Ren (Semen Pruni Armeniacae)

Functions: Clears heat and transforms dampness, moves the qi and quickens the blood, fortifies the spleen and disperses accumulation

Indications: Spleen qi vacuity with damp heat stasis and stagnation complicated by an element of food damage

Chai Hu Tiao Jing Tang
(Bupleurum Regulate the Menses Decoction)

mix-fried *Gan Cao* (Radix Glycyrrhizae Uralensis)
Cang Zhu (Rhizoma Atractylodis)
Ge Gen (Radix Peurariae)
Du Huo (Radix Angelicae Pubescentis)
Gao Ben (Radix Et Rhizoma Ligustici Chinensis)
Dang Gui (Radix Angelicae Sinensis)
Hong Hua (Flos Carthami Tinctorii)
Chai Hu (Radix Bupleuri)
Sheng Ma (Rhizoma Cimicifugae)

Functions: Supplements and moves the qi, nourishes and quickens the blood, dispels wind and eliminates dampness

Indications: Qi and blood vacuity, stasis, and stagnation complicated by wind damp impediment

Sheng Yang Ju Jing Tang
(Upbear the Yang & Lift The Menses Decoction)

Huang Qi (Radix Astragali Membranacei)
Ren Shen (Radix Panacis Ginseng)
Bai Zhu (Rhizoma Atractylodis Macrocephelae)
mix-fried *Gan Cao* (Radix Glycyrrhizae Uralensis)
Rou Gui (Cortex Cinnamomi Cassiae)
Fu Zi (Radix Lateralis Praeparatus Aconiti Carmichaeli)
Dang Gui (Radix Angelicae Sinensis)

Bai Shao (Radix Albus Paeoniae Lactiflorae)
Hong Hua (Flos Carthami Tinctori)
Tao Ren (Semen Pruni Persicae)
Shu Di (cooked Radix Rehmanniae Glutinosae)
Chuan Xiong (Radix Ligustici Wallichii)
Xi Xin (Herba Asari Cum Radice)
Du Huo (Radix Angelicae Pubescentis)
Qiang Huo (Radix Et Rhizoma Notopterygii)
Gao Ben (Radix Et Rhizoma Ligustici Chinensis)
Fang Feng (Radix Ledebouriellae Divaricatae)
Chai Hu (Radix Bupleuri)

Functions: Fortifies the spleen and supplements the kidneys, boosts the qi and warms yang, moves the qi and quickens the blood

Indications: Spleen-kidney yang vacuity with liver depression qi stagnation and blood stasis possibly complicated by wind damp impediment

Dang Gui Nian Tong Tang
(Dang Gui Assuage Pain Decoction)

Ren Shen (Radix Panacis Ginseng)
Bai Zhu (Rhizoma Atractylodis Macrocephalae)
Cang Zhu (Rhizoma Atractylodis)
Dang Gui (Radix Angelicae Sinensis)
Zhu Ling (Sclerotium Polypori Umbellati)
Ze Xie (Rhizoma Alismatis Orientalis)
Zhi Mu (Rhizoma Anemarrhenae Aspheloidis)
Huang Qin (Radix Scutellariae Baicalensis)
Yin Chen Cao (Herba Artemisiae Capillaris)
Ku Shen (Radix Sophorae Flavescentis)
Sheng Ma (Radix Cimicifugae)
Ge Gen (Radix Puerariae)
Qiang Huo (Radix Et Rhizoma Notopterygii)
Fang Feng (Radix Ledebouriellae Divaricatae)
Gan Cao (Radix Glycyrrhizae Uralensis)

Functions: Supplements the spleen and nourishes the blood, dispels wind, eliminates dampness, and clears heat

Indications: Wind damp heat impediment complicated by spleen vacuity, liver depression,[3] blood vacuity and/or blood stasis

Zhong Man Fen Xiao Wan
(Central Fullness Dividing & Dispersing Pills)

Ren Shen (Radix Panacis Ginseng)
mix-fried *Gan Cao* (Radix Glycyrrhizae Uralensis)
Fu Ling (Sclerotium Poriae Cocos)
Bai Zhu (Rhizoma Atractylodis Macrocephalae)
Gan Jiang (dry Rhizoma Zingiberis Officinalis)
Ban Xia (Rhizoma Pinelliae Ternatae)
Hou Po (Cortex Magnoliae Officinalis)
Zhi Shi (Fructus Immaturus Citri Aurantii)
Jiang Huang (Rhizoma Curcumae Longae)
Huang Qin (Radix Scutellariae Baicalensis)
Huang Lian (Rhizoma Coptidis Chinensis)
Zhi Mu (Rhizoma Anemarrhenae Aspheloidis)
Ze Xie (Rhizoma Alismatis Orientalis)
Zhu Ling (Sclerotium Polypori Umbellati)
Chen Pi (Pericarpium Citri Reticulatae)
Sha Ren (Fructus Amomi)

Functions: Fortifies the spleen and rectifies the qi, drains heat and eliminates dampness

Indications: Spleen vacuity with dampness, liver depression qi stagnation, and replete, depressive, or damp heat resulting in abdominal distention or even possible drum distention

Zhi Shi Xiao Pi Wan
(Immature Aurantium Disperse Glomus Pills)

Ren Shen (Radix Panacis Ginseng)
Bai Zhu (Rhizoma Atractylodis Macrocephalae)
Fu Ling (Sclerotium Poriae Cocos)
Gan Jiang (dry Rhizoma Zingiberis Officinalis)
mix-fried *Gan Cao* (Radix Glycyrrhizae Uralensis)
Ban Xia (Rhizoma Pinelliae Ternatae)
Zhi Shi (Fructus Immaturus Citri Aurantii)
Hou Po (Cortex Magnoliae Officinalis)
Huang Lian (Rhizoma Coptidis Chinensis)
Mai Ya (Fructus Germinatus Hordei Vulgaris)

Functions: Disperses glomus and eliminates fullness, fortifies the spleen and harmonizes the stomach

Indications: Spleen vacuity with stomach duct glomus and fullness

Conclusion

Although some people only remember that Li supplemented earth and cleared heat by the method of using sweet, warm medicinals, this is a gross over-simplification of Li's real methodology and importance to modern practitioners. Of the 330 formulas found in Li's four books,[4] fully 221 or 58.2% include bitter, cold, fire-draining medicinals. Not only did Li eliminate heat with sweet and warm, he also 1) drained fire and upbore yang, 2) drained fire and resolved toxins, 3) cleared and drained dampness and heat, 4) drained fire and cooled the blood, 5) drained heat and cleared glomus, 6) drained fire and boosted yin, 7) cleared and resolved summerheat heat, 8) drained fire and quieted the spirit, and 9) cleared and abated vacuity heat. Likewise, 80 of Li's 330 formulas or 24.2% quicken the blood and transform stasis by either 1) nourishing the blood and transforming stasis, 2) boosting the qi, upbearing yang, and transforming stasis, 3) enriching yin and transforming stasis, 4) warming the channels and/or yang and transforming stasis, 5) moving the qi and transforming stasis, 6) dispersing food and transforming stasis, 7) dispersing phlegm and transforming stasis, 8) transforming stasis and dispersing wind, 9) transforming stasis and stopping bleeding, 10) transforming stasis and freeing the flow of the network vessels, 11) cooling the blood and transforming stasis, and 12) breaking the blood and scattering stasis. Therefore, anyone who says Li only supplemented the spleen and used sweet, warm medicinals clearly has not taken a very good look at Li's actual formulas other than *Bu Zhong Yi Qi Tang*.

Endnotes

[1] Originally this formula was designed to treat the spleen vacuity and fluid damage of summerheat dampness. However, summerheat is really only a species of damp heat. Therefore, this formula can be used in a wider range of situations than originally intended.

[2] This formula differs from *Huang Qi Ren Shen Tang* above in that it addresses more serious qi stagnation.

[3] Because acrid and windy exterior-resolving medicinals upbear and out-thrust the yang qi, they also rectify the qi. Therefore, even though there are no qi-rectifying medicinals in this formula, given its combination of blood-nourishers and exterior-resolvers, it can course the liver and rectify the qi.

[4] I.e., the *Pi Wei Lun, Lan Shi Mi Cang, Nei Wai Shang Bian Hou Lun (Treatise on Discriminating [i.e., Clarifying] Doubts of Internal & External Damages)*, and *Yi Xue Fa Ming (Shining Light on The Study of Medicine)*

Formula Index

General Index

M

Mai Jing, 14, 35, 53, 57
malign and inharmonious facial
  complexion, 37, 57
malign sores, 24, 63
managing qi, 100
mansion of the blood, 212
massive discharge of perspiration,
  158
measles in children, 63
medicinal prohibitions, 59, 62
melancholy, 29, 37, 57, 67
Meniere's syndrome, 152
menometrorrhagia, 152
menopausal syndrome, 152
menorrhagia, adolescent, 152
middle burner, 6, 20, 62, 82, 98, 205,
  211, 217, 220, 257, 274, 281, 283
ministerial fire, 82
minute vessels, 4, 26, 72
mounting disorders, 93
mouth, bitter taste in the, 23, 28, 37,
  60, 122, 282
mouth, bland taste in the, 62, 118-
  119, 176, 282
mucous, sticky nasal, 24
multiple sclerosis, 161
muscles, hot, 50
myasthenia gravis, 91-92, 136, 152
myocardial ischemia, 114

N

Nan Jing, 14, 22, 72, 214, 216, 229,
  231, 264, 290
nasal congestion, 57, 104, 113, 115,
  120, 141-142
nasopharyngeal cancer, 148
Nei Ting, 199
Neoconfucianism, 48
nephritis, chronic, 91, 99
no aversion to cold, 21
no desire to eat, 37, 155
no liking for food, 258, 281
nonhealing sores, 103

O

obstructed diaphragm, 96
oligospermia, 129
On Balancing the Channels, 7
oncology, 10
oppression, 20, 23, 50, 91, 134, 144,
  156, 161-163, 180-182, 186, 191,
  205, 216, 241-242, 247, 258, 260,
  271-272, 274, 279, 283
opthalmological bleeding, 152
oral apthae, 97, 109, 119, 152
oral apthae, recurrent, 97, 152
original qi, 5-8, 11, 17, 22, 33, 57, 60-
  62, 81-82, 87, 89, 155, 158-160,
  162, 173, 179, 185-186, 193-194,
  202-203, 205, 211, 214-215, 219,
  228, 233, 235, 240, 243-244, 265-
  267, 286, 290
original qi of the six bowels, 203
original qi of the triple burner, 62,
  244
otitis media, chronic, 141, 152
Outer Classic, 81, 90
outlet obstruction constipation, 149
overtaxation, 23, 54-55, 101, 202-203

P

pain all along the low back, spine,
  upper back, and scapula, 30
pain below the umbilicus, 21, 88
pain beneath the abdominal skin,
  mild, 283
pain, chest and rib-side 28, 60, 68
pain, fullness and stabbing, 282
pain, migratory, 23
pain in the eye, 21
pain in the shoulders and back, 53
pain in the top of the head, 88
pain in walking, 182
pain, upper abdominal, 110
painful joints, 37, 55
palms, cold in the, 288
parapharyngeal cysts, 123

pediatric enuresis, 152
pediatric hyperactivity, 152
pediatric polyuria, 152
pelvic inflammatory disease, chronic, 152
penetrating vessel, 49, 95-96, 166, 180, 221, 250
penicillin, 111, 123
periodic numbness, 127
perspiration, spontaneous, 19-20, 41-44, 78, 91, 107, 124, 126, 132-133, 147, 155, 170, 172, 211, 219, 253-254
pessimism, 160
PID, 152
Ping Ren Qi Xiang Lun, 4
postpartum urinary incontinence, 99
postpartum urinary retention, 131, 133-134
postpartum vacuity, 276
post-surgical gastrointestinal dysfunction, 130
post-surgical nonhealing of wound, 105
precipitation, 18, 59-61, 63, 89, 130, 190, 242, 263, 265, 280-281
Prednisone, 45, 99, 111-112
pricking pain all over the body, 21
profuse menstruation, 94
profuse urination, 27, 30, 62, 109, 247, 288
Pulse Classic, 15, 35, 53, 57
purpuric nephritis, 45

Q
qi and *wei*, 34, 47
qi and yin vacuity, 22, 101
Qi Bo, 65-66, 197-198, 200, 203-204
qi bordering on expiration, 179
qi choking and food retention, 272
Qi Chong, 5
qi counterflow, 49, 161, 179
qi dryness, 49
Qi Jiao Bian Lun, 67

Qi Jie, 161, 166
qi of heaven, 3, 8, 10, 211, 216, 234
qi weakness, 19, 124, 160

R
raised qi with dyspnea, 85
rales, 286
red and white dysentery, 274
red facial complexion, 56-57
regular hours in living, 65
renal vein compression syndrome, 115
respiratory tract infections, recurrent, 152
restless fetus, 93
retching, 28, 155, 180, 242, 266, 274, 282, 285
retching, frequent, 155
rhinitis, chronic, 94, 141
ringing in the ears, 4, 57, 67, 92
rocking hands and feet, 266

S
sadness, 160
San Jian, 199
San Li, 5, 97, 161-162, 198-199, 201, 203, 209
scapula, great pain in the, 288
sea of water and grain, 5, 169
seasonal disease, 166
seasonal prohibitions, 59-60
seminal emission, 152
sensation of choking by phlegm, constant, 288
serum albumin, 151
seven spirits, 158, 166, 193-194, 233
Shang Ju Xu, 162, 209
shao yang, 9, 55, 60, 87, 166, 172, 199, 202, 213, 223, 233
shao yin, 21, 71, 198, 223-224, 233, 287
Sheng Qi Tong Tian Lun, 8
Shi Si Nan, 279
shortness of breath, 17, 19-21, 24, 29,

46, 49-50, 56, 89, 91, 95, 99, 104-
106, 119-122, 124, 127, 131-132,
138, 146-147, 157-158, 160, 162-
163, 173, 237, 239, 242, 247, 259-
260, 282, 288, 293
Shu Gu, 199
Si Shi Jiu Nan, 263
sinusitis, 54, 142, 152
sinusitis, chronic, 142
sleep fraught with fright, 55
sleep, troubled, 288
sleeplessness, 191
small intestinal qi pain, 276
sneezing, 24, 57, 113, 116, 288
sneezing, frequent, 57, 288
sodden wheat foods, 33-34, 61-62
soft stools, 51, 62, 176
soles of the feet, dull pain in the, 25
solid stools, 63
somnolence, 7, 18-20, 30, 37, 97, 116,
120-121, 132, 136, 155, 163, 239,
270, 282, 303
Song dynasty, 25, 48
sore throat, 56, 62, 94, 111, 113, 115,
123
sore throat, chronic, 94
sores, 24, 63, 69, 97, 103, 109-110,
114, 119, 281
sorrow, 67, 193, 203, 205
spasm, acute, 20, 90, 155
spasms and sudden abdominal pain,
28
spices, 33, 61, 83, 156, 248
spinning head, 242-243, 274
spirit brightness, 4, 8, 72
spleen qi vacuity, 11, 17, 22, 25, 27,
37, 62, 82-83, 85, 88, 125, 201, 205,
215-216, 251, 256-257, 267-268,
300-301, 306-307, 309
spleen-kidney yang vacuity, 22, 30,
310
stiff neck, 54
Still's disease, 111
stomach cancer, 120

stomach heat, 17, 27, 245, 249
stomach qi, 4-5, 7, 9, 26, 34, 39-40,
49, 62, 67, 70, 81-82, 85, 87, 90,
165, 167, 179, 190, 197-198, 202-
203, 209, 211-213, 218, 221-222,
242-243, 262, 267, 269
stones, biliary duct, 152
strangury, 21, 38, 55, 93, 101, 268
Su Wen, 5, 11-12, 22, 46, 52, 63, 68,
73, 152, 167-168, 177, 187, 191,
194, 204, 210, 214, 222, 225, 228,
231, 235, 251, 254, 290
sun, liking for the, 288
superimposition disagreement, 67,
212-214
sweating, lack of, 170
swelling and pain in the head and
neck, 281
swelling, cheek and submandibular,
57
swelling, submandibular, 56-57
swill diarrhea, 9, 65, 69, 71, 163, 179,
185, 187, 195, 238, 263
systolic hypertension, 145

T
tai yang, 54-55, 57, 60-61, 95-96, 199,
201-202, 209, 213, 233, 244, 287
tai yin, 61, 65, 70-71, 165, 172, 181,
185, 190, 198-199, 224, 233, 243,
287
Tai Yin Yang Ming Lun, 65, 185
taxation strangury, 93
testicular contraction, 288
testicles, cold in the, 30
*The Great Treatise on What is
Consummately True,* 47
The Spiritual Pivot Classic, 5
*The Treatise on Qi Images [of the
Pulse] in Healthy People,* 4
The Treatment of Chaos, 200
The Yellow Emperor's Inner Classic, 65
thickened vocal cords, 137
thirst, 19-21, 23, 38-39, 49, 51, 62, 85,

OTHER BOOKS ON CHINESE MEDICINE AVAILABLE FROM:
BLUE POPPY PRESS

5441 Western, Suite 2, Boulder, CO 80301
For ordering 1-800-487-9296 PH. 303\447-8372 FAX 303\245-8362
Email: info@bluepoppy.com Website: www.bluepoppy.com

ACUPOINT POCKET REFERENCE
by Bob Flaws
ISBN 0-936185-93-7

ACUPUNCTURE & IVF
by Lifang Liang
ISBN 0-891845-24-1

ACUPUNCTURE AND MOXIBUSTION
FORMULAS & TREATMENTS
by Cheng Dan-an, trans. by Wu Ming
ISBN 0-936185-68-6

ACUPUNCTURE PHYSICAL MEDICINE:
An Acupuncture Touchpoint Approach to the
Treatment of Chronic Pain, Fatigue, and
Stress Disorders
by Mark Seem
ISBN 1-891845-13-6

AGING & BLOOD STASIS:
A New Approach to TCM Geriatrics
by Yan De-xin
ISBN 0-936185-63-5

BETTER BREAST HEALTH NATURALLY
with CHINESE MEDICINE
by Honora Lee Wolfe & Bob Flaws
ISBN 0-936185-90-2

THE BOOK OF JOOK:
Chinese Medicinal Porridges
by B. Flaws
ISBN 0-936185-60-0

CHANNEL DIVERGENCES
Deeper Pathways of the Web
by Miki Shima and Charles Chase
ISBN 1-891845-15-2

CHINESE MEDICAL PALMISTRY:
Your Health in Your Hand
by Zong Xiao-fan & Gary Liscum
ISBN 0-936185-64-3

CHINESE MEDICAL PSYCHIATRY
A Textbook and Clinical Manual
by Bob Flaws and James Lake, MD
ISBN 1-845891-17-9

CHINESE MEDICINAL TEAS:
Simple, Proven, Folk Formulas for
Common Diseases & Promoting Health
by Zong Xiao-fan & Gary Liscum
ISBN 0-936185-76-7

CHINESE MEDICINAL WINES & ELIXIRS
by Bob Flaws
ISBN 0-936185-58-9

CHINESE PEDIATRIC MASSAGE THERAPY:
A Parent's & Practitioner's Guide to the
Prevention & Treatment of Childhood Illness
by Fan Ya-li
ISBN 0-936185-54-6

CHINESE SELF-MASSAGE THERAPY:
The Easy Way to Health
by Fan Ya-li
ISBN 0-936185-74-0

CLINICAL NEPHROLOGY
IN CHINESE MEDICINE
by Wei Li & David Frierman,
with Ben Luna & Bob Flaws
ISBN 1-891845-23-3

CONTROLLING DIABETES NATURALLY
WITH CHINESE MEDICINE
by Lynn Kuchinski
ISBN 0-936185-06-3

CURING ARTHRITIS NATURALLY WITH
CHINESE MEDICINE
by Douglas Frank & Bob Flaws
ISBN 0-936185-87-2

CURING DEPRESSION NATURALLY WITH
CHINESE MEDICINE
by Rosa Schnyer & Bob Flaws
ISBN 0-936185-94-5

CURING FIBROMYALGIA NATURALLY
WITH CHINESE MEDICINE
by Bob Flaws
ISBN 1-891845-09-8

CURING HAY FEVER NATURALLY WITH
CHINESE MEDICINE
by Bob Flaws
ISBN 0-936185-91-0

THE TREATMENT OF DISEASE IN TCM,
Vol. II: Diseases of the Eyes, Ears, Nose, & Throat

by Sionneau & Lü

ISBN 0-936185-69-4

THE TREATMENT OF DISEASE, Vol. III:
Diseases of the Mouth, Lips, Tongue,
Teeth & Gums

by Sionneau & Lü

ISBN 0-936185-79-1

THE TREATMENT OF DISEASE, Vol IV:
Diseases of the Neck, Shoulders,
Back, & Limbs

by Philippe Sionneau & Lü Gang

ISBN 0-936185-89-9

THE TREATMENT OF DISEASE, Vol V:
Diseases of the Chest & Abdomen
by Philippe Sionneau & Lü Gang

ISBN 1-891845-02-0

THE TREATMENT OF DISEASE, Vol VI:
Diseases of the Urogential System
& Proctology

by Philippe Sionneau & Lü Gang

ISBN 1-891845-05-5

THE TREATMENT OF DISEASE, Vol VII:
General Symptoms

by Philippe Sionneau & Lü Gang

ISBN 1-891845-14-4

THE TREATMENT OF EXTERNAL
DISEASES WITH ACUPUNCTURE
& MOXIBUSTION

by Yan Cui-lan and Zhu Yun-long, trans. by Yang
Shou-zhong

ISBN 0-936185-80-5

THE TREATMENT OF MODERN
WESTERN MEDICAL DISEASES
WITH CHINESE MEDICINE

by Bob Flaws & Philippe Sionneau

ISBN 1-891845-20-9

THE TREATMENT OF DIABETES
MELLITUS WITH CHINESE MEDICINE

by Bob Flaws, Lynn Kuchinski
& Robert Casañas, MD

ISBN 1-891845-21-7

160 ESSENTIAL CHINESE HERBAL
PATENT MEDICINES

by Bob Flaws

ISBN 1-891945-12-8

630 QUESTIONS & ANSWERS ABOUT
CHINESE HERBAL MEDICINE:
A Workbook & Study Guide

by Bob Flaws

ISBN 1-891845-04-7

230 ESSENTIAL CHINESE MEDICINALS

by Bob Flaws

ISBN 1-891845-03-9

750 QUESTIONS & ANSWERS ABOUT
ACUPUNCTURE
Exam Preparation & Study Guide

by Fred Jennes

ISBN 1-891845-22